Sexual Euphoria

A Complete Guide for Men and Women

George Moufarrej

Moufarrej Publishing

Sexual Euphoria—A Complete Guide for Men and Women

By George Moufarrej

Copyright 2011 by George Moufarrej

Published in the United States by
Moufarrej Publishing
305 S. San Gabriel Blvd.
Pasadena, CA 91107

Edition ISBNs:

Paperback: 978-0-578-10194-1
Kindle e-Book: 978-0-578-10195-8
Nook e-Book: 978-0-578-10196-5

Book design by Christopher Fisher
Illustrations by Carol Ruzicka
Cover design by Pete Garceau

All rights reserved. All content contained within *Sexual Euphoria—A Complete Guide for Men and Women* is the sole property of Moufarrej Publishing. It can only be reproduced by Moufarrej Publishing. Any form of copying or reproduction of the information contained within *Sexual Euphoria—A Complete Guide for Men and Women* is strictly forbidden without express permission from Moufarrej Publishing. If the information is copied or reproduced without permission from the author or the publisher, the offender(s) will be prosecuted to the full extent of the law.

Disclaimer and Legal Notice:

The information provided in *Sexual Euphoria—A Complete Guide for Men and Women* does not represent any kind of medical advice. It is only the author's opinion based on the research work of Shere Hite, Alfred Kinsey, Masters and Johnson, and other sources. This book is not a medical manual. It is a reference volume only to help a person make informed decisions about his or her sex life.

The author is not a medical professional nor a licensed sex therapist. If a person needs any medical advice he or she should consult a medical professional. Furthermore, a person should consult a physician or a certified sex therapist before attempting any sexual technique mentioned in the book, or do so at his or her own risk.

Neither the author nor the publisher nor any of their associates will be liable or responsible to any person or entity for any loss, damage, injury, or ailment caused, or alleged to be caused directly or indirectly by the information or lack of information contained in this book.

The author and publisher are committed to offering responsible and practical advice about sexual matters that is supported by legitimate scientific research. While all attempts have been made to verify the information provided in *Sexual Euphoria—A Complete Guide for Men and Women* the author and the publisher do not assume any responsibility for errors, omissions, or contradictory interpretation of the subject matter herein.

In no event shall the author, nor the publisher, be liable for damages of any kind or character.

Contents

Introduction	1
Benefits of Sex	5
The Male and Female Anatomy	9
The Male Sexual Response	23
The Female Sexual Response	29
Pubococcygeus Muscle	37
The G-Spot	43
The Male P-Spot	49
Masturbation	55
Manual Stimulation by the Opposite Sex	69
Oral Sex	81
Anal Sex	103
Pre-foreplay	113
Dressing for Sex	119
Kissing	127
Foreplay	135
Sex Positions	161
After Sex Play	209

SEX TECHNIQUES	215
VARIETY DURING SEX	267
THE CLIMAX DILEMMA	303
NON-PHYSICAL ASPECTS OF SEX	325
DOES SIZE MATTER?	341
FAKING AN ORGASM	347
SAFER SEX	351
SEXUALLY TRANSMITTED DISEASES	361
PREMATURE EJACULATION	373
SEX DURING MENSTRUATION, PMS, AND MENOPAUSE	387
SEX AND PREGNANCY	393
NATURALLY ENLARGING THE PENIS	403
MULTIPLE ORGASMS FOR MEN	409
CONCLUSION	417
BIBLIOGRAPHY	419
INDEX	423

Sexual Euphoria

A Complete Guide for Men and Women

Chapter 1

Introduction

A few centuries ago neither the man nor the woman was supposed to enjoy the sex act. Sex was for the purpose of making children only. It was believed that nature designated the ejaculation of semen only for the purpose of having children. It was believed that the ejaculation of semen for any other purpose including masturbation was wrong and unnatural. Sex for the purpose of pleasure was wrong and unnatural. The woman was supposed to be passive in bed. The fact that the woman was entitled to an orgasm was unthinkable. Female masturbation was believed not to exist.

It was not until the sexual revolution in the 1960s that the pursuit of sexual pleasure during sex was legitimized in western societies. Society's attitudes towards sex changed in the late 1960s, and was partly aided by the widespread use of the birth control pill. The birth control pill made it easier for society to accept the fact that a woman has the right to enjoy sex without making childbearing a requirement. This was because men and women were able to enjoy sex purely for recreation and forget about unwanted pregnancies. Also, it was not until 1972, when the American Medical Association declared masturbation to be normal, that society accepted masturbation as normal.

Despite the fact that society has improved its attitudes towards sex, many people are still not well informed about sex. This is because from the time most people are young they are taught to keep a silence about sex. They are taught not to talk about sex, not to read any sexual material, nor listen to nor watch any sexual material. The fact that many people are not well informed about sex causes them to not be able to take control and gain confidence in their sex life. If a person's sexual functioning was treated the same as other functions like eating and sleeping, most people would be better informed about sex and more accepting of their sexuality. A person would be better informed about sex because he or she would read, watch, and listen to sexual material freely, without being embarrassed or feeling guilty. Also, a person would be better informed about sex because he or she would talk about sex freely, without any hesitation.

Many people keep in silence about sex believing that a person will know how to perform sexually naturally. They believe that sex is based on a person's instincts, and that it does not have to be learned. Unfortunately, the incorrect belief that sexual performance comes naturally causes many couples to not seek out knowledge about sexual matters. It makes them embarrassed to do so. Sex, like other human activities, has to be learned. Just as a person learns how to cook, how to change the tires on the car, or how to clean the house, likewise a person has to learn how to have sex and make the sexual encounter pleasurable to both people. The fact that many people are not well informed about sex causes many to have an unsatisfied sex life.

This book is written to make people more informed about sex and how to have more pleasurable sexual encounters. This book is written for the average person to understand. It is written in a way that makes all the concepts easy to understand. This book explains the male and female sexual response and the male and female anatomy, making it easier for the couple to enjoy the sexual encounter. It describes different sexual techniques, positions, kissing techniques, foreplay techniques, and other ways to add variety to sex. This gives the couple various ways to make the sexual encounters more pleasurable. This book talks about manual stimulation, anal sex, oral sex, the G-spot, and the male prostate giving the man and the woman added ways to spice up their sex life. It dispels myths about sexually transmitted diseases, safer sex, and masturbation. This book talks about how a couple could keep their sex life exciting and alive even after many years of being in a relationship. This is discussed in the Variety chapter. This book also talks about how the man can make the penis larger naturally if he chooses.

This book explains that every healthy man usually orgasms during sex, but two-thirds of the women in our society do not regularly orgasm during sex. This book makes it clear that every woman can orgasm during sex and shows how it can be done in the Climax Dilemma chapter. It makes it clear that most women can experience multiple orgasms during a sexual encounter and shows how it could be done also in the Climax Dilemma chapter. Multiple orgasms is when a woman experiences more than one orgasm in a row without a refractory period. The book shows that some women can only experience one orgasm during an encounter, and that is perfectly fine. This book explains that a small number of men experience multiple orgasms. It shows that the majority of men can experience multiple orgasms during sex if they train themselves to. This is shown in the Multiple Orgasms for Men chapter. It makes it clear that if a man can only experience one orgasm during an encounter that is perfectly fine. The

Introduction

book has a wide range of information in it about sexual matters to make the sexual experience more pleasurable for the man and the woman.

Making the sexual experience more pleasurable for the couple will result in a happier relationship. Making the sexual experience more pleasurable reduces the likelihood that a relationship or marriage will end. Many relationships and marriages end because the sex life becomes boring and the couple's sex life becomes non-existent. When a person knows how to be a great lover, his or her confidence and high self-esteem will show up, making him or her more attractive to the opposite sex. When a person knows how to have more pleasurable sexual encounters, his or her joy will spill into other aspects of his or her life, making his or her life more pleasurable as a whole. This book is designed for heterosexual couples to give both the man and the woman the information that they need to make their sex life more pleasurable and exciting.

Chapter 2

Benefits of Sex

Sex is not just for procreation. Sex has numerous benefits. The most popular benefit of sex is that it is one of the greatest sources of pleasure and happiness to human beings. It can boost a person's personal sense of wellbeing. It is also a manner of human expression. Sex is meant to give two people a way to express their love and commitment to each other with deep pleasure. Sex is important for a couple that cares about each other. Sex is important for a person's health and physical wellbeing. The more sex a person has, the more pleasurable the sex becomes. A person's sexuality affects other aspects of his or her life. Sex can enhance a person's outlook in life, making the person more optimistic. It can also enhance the person's self-esteem. This results in a person having a happier life.

Sex and Relationships

Sex is very important to a relationship between a man and a woman. Lack of sex in a relationship creates emotional discord between the man and the woman. This could lead to the end of the relationship. Sex that is not fulfilling to either partner can also lead to emotional discord between both the man and the woman. This could also lead to the end of the relationship. Therefore, it is important that the sex in the relationship be fulfilling to both partners and be sufficient to both partners. Thus, sex is not enough for a relationship. It has to be good sex.

Good sex is important for people who care about their relationships. It is important because it brings a couple closer. It strengthens the intimacy between the couple. In a monogamous relationship, it acts as glue cementing the bond between both the man and the woman. It makes emotional attachments between partners stronger and encourages a stable happy relationship. If the couple is married it encourages a stable, happy family unit. It can even save a marriage or a relationship.

Good sex makes both people feel closer physically and emotionally. It lets both people feel so close that it seems as if they are one physically and emotionally. The intimacy that both lovers have between each other as a result of good sex tends to be the greatest intimacy that two human beings can have between each other. Intimacy is an essential aspect of a relationship. Even though a person no longer feels the same intense sexual excitement in a long-term relationship that he or she once felt early on in the relationship, the intimate feelings continue to bond a couple. Intimacy is important to a healthy long-term relationship because it reinforces feelings of love, attachment, and sexual interest.

Good sex also helps a person in the relationship with himself. It helps a person feel good about himself and about his sexuality. It makes a person feel sexually confident. Sexual confidence creates greater confidence in many other areas of a person's life. This in turn makes the person more desirable to the opposite sex, and more desirable to his or her partner. Therefore, the person is more likely to experience a healthy and pleasurable relationship with his or her partner as a result of the sexual confidence that good sex causes. Also, sexual confidence makes a person more secure and confident when he or she deals with the opposite sex.

Sex and Health

Sex is very important for a person's health, just as nutrition and exercise are important for a person's overall health. Sex can help boost the immune system of human beings. Levels of immunoglobulin, a microbe-fighting antibody, are higher in people who engage in sex regularly than those that are abstinent. Sex can make a person actually heal faster when he or she is injured. Oxytocin, one of the hormones released during sexual arousal, healed sores on lab rats twice as fast when its quantity was increased by a percentage equal to the percentage of the increase of oxytocin in the human body during sexual arousal. During orgasm, oxytocin surges up to five times its normal blood level. Its concentration in the human blood peaks at orgasm. It regulates body temperature and blood pressure and speeds the healing of wounds and injuries. Sex can reduce depression and physical pain. Just being sexually excited causes various hormones that reduce depression and physical pain to surge in the blood. Oxytocin, which surges in the blood during sexual excitement, is a "feel good" hormone that is an amphetamine-like upper. It also relieves pain, from headaches to cramps and overall body aches. It can lower levels of arthritic pain and whiplash pain. The release of oxytocin triggers the release of endorphins. Endorphins are also natural painkillers and fight depression. Testosterone is another hormone that surges in the human blood during sexual excitement that acts as an antidepressant. It also improves the thinking of a person. Orgasms increase the level of the female sex hormone estrogen in the woman's bloodstream, which also adds to mood improvement and helps ease the discomfort of premenstrual symptoms.

Sex can prolong a person's life. It can strengthen the heart, and reduce the risk of a heart attack. Exercise, even brief physical exercise, can generate major aerobic benefits for the body and the immune system. Therefore, even regular non-marathon sex can have substantial physical benefits for the whole body, especially the heart. It can increase bloodflow to the brain and to all other organs of the body. All that deep breathing and increased heart rate during sex saturate the body's organs and muscles with fresh oxygen and hormones. It causes the used blood to be removed, taking with it the cells' wastes that cause fatigue and even illness. The DHEA (dehydroepiandrosterone) hormone surges in the person's blood during sexual activity. As a matter of fact, during orgasm DHEA levels increase three to five times higher than usual. DHEA is a hormone that reduces the risk of heart disease. DHEA has been found to actually strengthen the heart muscle after a heart attack, and that is why doctors recommend sex as soon as a heart attack victim is strong enough. Sex can increase a woman's estrogen level during an orgasm, and estrogen has been known to strengthen a woman's heart. Sex can also prolong a person's life, by making the risk of cancer less likely. This is because the oxytocin hormone, and the sex hormones estrogen and testosterone, have some role in cell signaling and cell division. These hormones surge in the human body during sexual activity. Estrogen surges in the woman's body, while testosterone surges in both the woman's body and the man's body. But testosterone's concentration in the man's body is more than in the woman's body.

Sex can also increase a person's desire for sex. This is because during sexual activity the DHEA hormone surges in the person's blood, causing an increase in the amount of the DHEA hormone in the human body. The DHEA hormone increases the frequency of sexual thoughts, and increases the sexual desire of a person. Another way that sex is important for health is in the case of postmenopausal women. Postmenopausal women run the risk of having vaginal atrophy from lack of sex. Vaginal atrophy is when the opening of the woman's vagina narrows from disuse. It is a condition that can lead to dyspareunia, or pain associated with intercourse. The estrogen released during orgasm in the woman's body can keep her vaginal tissues more supple. In conclusion, sex is a key to good health that should not be overlooked.

Sex and Sleep

Sex releases the pressures of day-to-day life and reduces a person's blood pressure. Many people use sex to relieve stress and get rid of tension so that they can sleep. Sex allows a person to fall asleep more easily and allows a person to sleep better.

Many people sleep more deeply and restfully after satisfying sex or masturbation. At the point of sexual orgasm human brainwave patterns change radically, thus putting a person into an altered state of consciousness. This causes a person after sex to feel better and more energized. The profound relaxation that typically follows lovemaking with orgasm allows a person to completely let go, surrender, and relax. This profound relaxation causes a person to let go of distracting thoughts. This allows a person to fall asleep more easily and more deeply. People that have sex frequently often report that they can handle stress better.

Summary of Benefits of Sex

Finally, sex is very important to a person's life. It can benefit a person in many ways. It allows a person to express his or her affection to his or her partner in a pleasurable way. It brings both people closer together and helps create a stable relationship between them. It improves a person's relationship with himself, causing him to have a higher sense of self-esteem. It causes a person to have a more optimistic viewpoint about life and causes a person's life to be more pleasurable. It causes a person to have a longer life and a healthier life. It strengthens the heart, relieves pain, clears the sinuses, and even reduces blood pressure. It relieves muscle tension and stress. It allows a person to fall asleep more easily and more deeply. All these benefits can lead to a positive cycle. When a person has sex, his or her body is flooded with healthful natural chemicals like DHEA, endorphins, oxytocin, and so forth. This leads to a person being healthier. If a person has better health, he or she will feel more energetic and happy. If a person feels more energetic and happy, he or she will have a higher sex drive and will be more desirable to the opposite sex. If a person is more desirable to the opposite sex, has a higher sex drive, and is single, he or she will have more dates. More dates will result in more sex. If a person is more desirable to the opposite sex, has a higher sex drive, and is married, he or she will have more sex with his or her spouse.

Chapter 3

The Male and Female Anatomy

A man or woman should learn about the male and female anatomy, for several reasons. The first reason is that the man or woman will appreciate the beauty of his or her partner's anatomy and will feel more comfortable and less inhibited during sex. The second reason is that the man or woman will know how to please his or her partner more during sex, which will help the couple achieve the most pleasure in their sexual encounters. Thus, the man and woman will have their sexual satisfaction enhanced during sex and their sex life will be more exciting.

The Male Anatomy

The male reproductive system is made up of a pair of testes, a scrotum, a penis, a urethra, two Cowper's glands, a prostate gland, a pair of seminal vesicles, and a duct system. The duct system is located on each side of the male body, and consists of a pair of epididymis and a pair of vas deferens. As a result of the male reproductive system, sperm and semen are produced.

Scrotum

The scrotum is a wrinkled sac of skin and muscle beneath the penis. It holds two small, ball-like glands, called the testes. It protects the testes from injury. It also acts as an incubator, and protects the testes from extreme temperatures. It makes sure that the temperature is just right for the testes, since for the sperm to be produced the testes should be about five degrees below body temperature. The scrotum changes size to maintain the right temperature. When the body is cold, the scrotum shrinks and becomes tighter to hold in body heat. When the body is warm, the scrotum becomes larger and more floppy to get rid of extra heat. When a man is cold, physically active, frightened, sexually excited, or about to ejaculate, the muscles in his scrotum contract, pulling the testicles protectively closer to his body. Usually, in the scrotum one testicle hangs lower than the other. Usually, it is the left testicle that hangs lower than the right one. In addition to containing the testes, the scrotum contains the epididymis and the vas deferens. The scrotum is darker in color than the rest of a man's skin. It is covered with fine hair, as well as sweat- and oil-secreting glands.

The Testicles

The testicles are two oval glands that can vary in size. However, on average each testicle weighs about 22 grams and measures about two inches long by one inch wide. It is normal for each testicle to be a slightly different size than the other. One testicle is located on the right side of the man's body and the other testicle is located on the left side. The testicles have two main functions. One function is to produce sperm. The second function is to produce testosterone, the male sex hormone. The testicles hang outside the man's body because sperm production requires a temperature slightly lower than body temperature. Inside each testicle, there are hundreds of tiny coiled tubes that produce sperm. These tubes are called the seminiferous tubules. The testicles produce millions of sperm daily, which are stored in a small area on the back of each testicle, called the epididymis.

Epididymis

The epididymis and the vas deferens, make up the duct system of the male reproductive system. The epididymis is a set of two narrow, tightly coiled tubes. One tube is for each testicle. One tube is located on the back of each testicle, and connects the testicle to the vas deferens. The epididymis operates as a little incubator for sperm to grow in until they are mature enough to leave. Sperm usually spend 4 to 6 weeks in the epididymis before they are mature enough to leave. Once the sperm leave the epididymis, they enter the vas deferens.

Vas Deferens

The vas deferens is the dilated continuation of the epididymis. The vas deferens is composed of two sperm carrying tubes, one for each epididymis. They are long, thin, muscular tubes that carry sperm from the epididymis to the urethra via the ejaculatory duct. As the vas deferens tubes extend from the epididymis, they pass behind the urinary bladder. Then each tube joins with one seminal vesicle to form an ejaculatory duct. Then each tube, as an ejaculatory duct, runs through the prostate gland and opens into the urethra. As the sperm is transferred through the vas deferens into the urethra, it collects secretions from the seminal vesicles and prostate gland. These secretions form a large part of the semen. The main function of the vas deferens and the ejaculatory duct is to transport mature sperm and seminal fluid to the urethra.

Seminal Vesicles

The seminal vesicles are two small glands located above the prostate gland. They are attached to the vas deferens near the base of the bladder. They are located behind the bladder. Each seminal vesicle joins with a vas deferens tube, to produce an ejaculatory duct. It is at the ejaculatory duct that the seminal vesicles add secretions to the sperms.

The secretions account for about 65% of the fluid volume of the semen. The secretions are rich in fructose, which is an important source of energy for the sperm.

Prostate

The prostate is a small gland that is found only in the male reproductive system. It is important because its main purpose is to make fluid that protects and feeds sperm. The fluid produced by the prostate becomes part of the semen. The fluid produced by the prostate accounts for about 30% of the fluid volume of the semen. The prostate sits underneath the bladder and surrounds the top part of the urethra.

Cowper's Glands

The Cowper's glands are two pea-sized glands that are alongside the base of the urethra. They sit near the prostate gland. They produce a clear thick fluid that lubricates the penis when it is erect, so that sperm can pass through. The fluid also neutralizes any urine that may be left in the urethra. This fluid actually appears at the tip of the penis prior to ejaculation. It is sometimes called pre-ejaculatory fluid, and it may contain some sperm. The fluid of the Cowper's glands accounts for about 5% of the fluid volume of the semen.

Urethra

The urethra is a narrow tube that runs from the bladder to the end of the penis. It is made up of two parts: the prostatic urethra and the penile urethra. The prostatic urethra is the part of the urethra that runs from the bladder through the prostate. The penile urethra is the part of the urethra that runs through the penis. The purpose of the urethra is for the passage of urine and semen. It carries urine from the bladder, the storage organ for urine, to the tip of the penis. It carries semen to the tip of the penis, out of the body. Semen and urine do not mix in the urethra, because urine is automatically cut off when semen is being released. A ring of muscle called the internal sphincter is located at the base of the bladder. This muscle closes tightly during ejaculation, and stops urine from flowing through the urethra, when semen is flowing through the urethra. Also, when the internal sphincter tightens, it stops the sperm from passing backwards into the bladder.

Penis

The penis is the external male sex organ that has several functions. One function is to give men and women amazing pleasure during sexual intercourse. The second function is to introduce sperm into the woman's vagina. The third function is to carry urine out of the man's body. The penis is well innervated with nerves and is very sensitive. The entire length of the penis is sensitive to touch, pressure, and temperature. The penis is an extremely sensitive part of the body that when stimulated provides fabulous sensations. The skin covering the penis is hairless, loose, and elastic. The skin stretches, becoming taut and thin, as the penis enlarges during an erection.

The penis is made up of two parts: the shaft and the glans. The shaft is the whole cylinder structure, and it is the main part of the penis. The glans is the tip or head of the penis. The head or tip of the penis is very sensitive. It is more sensitive than the penis shaft. The glans contains numerous nerve endings and plays a great part in the male sexual satisfaction and orgasm. The rim of the head of the penis is called the corona, and it is extremely sensitive since it is full of nerve endings. It is more sensitive than the glans. The frenulum is the skin just below the head of the penis on the underside of the penis. It is above the shaft of the penis. It is where the head and shaft meet. Stimulating the frenulum drives the man wild with pleasure and sexual arousal because the frenulum is the most sensitive area on the penis. At the end of the glans there is a small slit or opening, which is where semen and urine exit the body. The glans is exposed all the time if the penis has been circumcised. On uncircumcised men, the foreskin covers most of the glans until an erection occurs. When an erection occurs, the foreskin automatically retracts, causing the full glans to be exposed. All penises work and feel the same, regardless whether the foreskin has been removed or not.

The foreskin is a loose, hairless skin that covers the glans and is usually several shades darker than the man's regular skin color. A circumcision is performed to remove the foreskin in some males. A circumcision is the surgical removal of the foreskin of the penis. If the penis is not circumcised, the foreskin produces an oily substance to lubricate the head of the penis. When this oil mixes with dead skin cells, it becomes a cheesy white substance called smegma. Smegma is not dirty and there is no truth to the myth that sex with an uncircumcised man increases the risks of cervical cancer or sexually transmitted disease for the woman. Smegma is a waxy substance that may accumulate under the foreskin, so the foreskin needs to be pulled back and washed every day. If the smegma is not regularly removed through daily washing, it can accumulate and cause infections, odor, irritations, and pain in the penis.

The penis does not contain any bones, but it is made up of three cylinders of soft spongy tissue that contain many blood vessels and nerves. Two of the cylinders are the corpora cavernosa, and one of the cylinders is the corpus spongiosum. The two corpora cavernosa lie next to each other on the upper side of the penis, and the corpus spongiosum lies between them on the underside of the penis. The two corpora cavernosa attach to the pubic bone by crura or legs. The bottom of the corpus spongiosum forms the bulb of the penis. The bulb of the penis can be felt between the anus and the scrotum, when the penis is erect. The top of the corpus spongiosum forms the mushroom shaped glans. In the glans, there is a small opening leading to the urethra. The urethra is a tube that runs through the middle of the corpora spongiosum to carry urine and semen out of the body. The urethra is surrounded by the corpus spongiosum. The corpus spongiosum becomes an obvious ridge on the underside of the penis when it is erect.

The penis has no erectile bone; instead it relies entirely on engorgement with blood to reach its erect state. An erection is the stiffening and rising of the penis, which occurs in the sexually aroused male. It occurs because of the automatic dilation of the arteries supplying blood to the penis, which allows more blood to fill the three spongy erectile tissue cylinders in the penis. The engorged erectile tissue presses against and constricts the veins that carry blood away from the penis. Therefore, more blood enters the penis than leaves it until an equilibrium is reached. When that equilibrium is reached, an equal volume of blood flows into the dilated arteries and out of the constricted veins, resulting in a constant erect penis.

During an erection, most of the corpus spongiosum remains softer than the rest of the penis. However, the bulb of the penis becomes quite hard and sensitive. The glans increases in size, and becomes much darker in color. However, it remains somewhat soft. The erection enables the man to have sexual intercourse.

Sperm

The sperms are the male reproductive cells. Under a microscope, they look like tadpoles with a head and a tail. They are produced in the testicles and mature in the epididymis. They pass through the vas deferens to the urethra. As they pass through the vas deferens, they are mixed with secretions from the seminal vesicles and the prostate gland.

Semen

The semen is a milky, whitish fluid that contains millions of sperms. It consists not only of sperms, but also of fluids. The fluids are from the seminal vesicles, prostate gland, and Cowper's glands. About 65% of the fluid volume in the semen is fluid from the seminal vesicles. About 5% of the fluid volume in the semen is fluid from the Cowper's glands. About 30% of the fluid volume in the semen is fluid from the prostate gland. Semen contains vitamins and minerals. It is not dangerous if swallowed, provided the man does not have a sexually transmitted disease.

The Female Anatomy

The female reproductive anatomy is made up of both internal and external structures. The function of the external structures is to allow the sperm to enter the body and to protect the internal organs from infectious organisms. The main external structures are the labia majora, labia minora, clitoris, and mons veneris. The internal structures of the female reproductive anatomy are the vagina, cervix, uterus, two ovaries, and two fallopian tubes.

Vulva

The vulva is an anatomical term for the external structures of the female reproductive anatomy. The vulva includes the mons veneris, labia majora, labia minora, clitoris, urethral opening, and vaginal opening. There are a number of different secretions associated with the vulva. These secretions are urine, sweat, skin oils, and vaginal secretions. Smegma is a white substance formed on the vulva. Smegma collects around the clitoris and the labial folds. It results from a combination of dead cells, skin oils, moisture, and naturally occurring bacteria. It is important that the woman wash her vulva daily, especially the clitoris and the labial folds, so that smegma does not build up.

Mons Veneris

The mons veneris, is also known as the mons pubis. It is a cushion of fat on top of the pubic bone that is covered with skin and hair. It is soft and raised above the surrounding area, due to a pad of fat lying just beneath it. Its size varies with the general level of hormones and body fat. It provides protection to the pubic bone during intercourse. It is a sexually sensitive area because it contains many nerve endings. When touched, it produces erotic feelings and erotic pleasure. Many young women intentionally shave away all their pubic hair from the mons veneris because it makes the mons veneris feel more sensitive to touch.

Labia Majora

The mons veneris divides into the labia majora. Labia majora, literally translated, means large lips. The labia majora are two large folds of skin that extend from the mons veneris to the perineum. Each fold is on one side of the body. The labia majora are the outer lips of the vulva. Within the labia majora, there are the labia minora and the clitoris. The labia minora are two folds of skin that are smaller than the labia majora. They are also known as the inner lips.

The outer surface of the labia majora may be smooth or wrinkled. It is darker in color than the surrounding skin. It is covered with pubic hair. The inner surface of the labia majora is smooth, hairless, and moist, because it contains many sweat and oil secreting glands. These sweat and oil secreting glands give off a scent that some feel is sexually arousing. Sometimes one side of the labia is larger or longer than the other.

The labia majora are large and fleshy. They are made of fatty tissue. They contain nerves, muscle, and blood vessels. The labia majora contain many nerves, making them very sensitive to touch. When touched, they produce erotic feelings and great pleasure. The blood vessels within the labia majora cause the erectile tissue within the labia majora to swell with blood when the woman is sexually excited. This causes the labia majora to become swollen, tight, firm, and larger than usual.

The labia majora's main purpose is to protect the openings to the vagina and to the bladder. The labia majora usually meet and cover the urinary and vaginal openings, when the woman is not aroused, or has her legs together. The fact that the labia majora have many nerves makes it clear that they have another purpose, which is to provide erotic pleasure to the woman during erotic play.

Labia Minora

Labia minora, literally translated, means small lips. The labia minora are two folds of skin within the labia majora that are usually smaller than the labia majora. They are the inner lips of the vulva. Each fold is located on one side of the woman's body. They extend from just above the clitoris to below the vaginal opening. The top of the two labia minora come together and cover the head of the clitoris, forming the clitoral hood. The labia minora also surround the opening to the vagina and the urethra. They are thin stretches of tissue that fold and protect the vagina, urethra, and clitoris.

The labia minora are covered with oil secreting glands. They are hairless and do not contain fat. However, they contain numerous nerves. They contain more nerves than the labia majora. This makes them extremely sensitive to touch, producing erotic feelings and pleasure when touched. Also, they are filled with blood vessels and erectile tissue. This allows them to fill with blood and enlarge when the woman is sexually aroused.

The labia minora may be straight, slightly ruffled, or very wrinkled. Sometimes one side of the labia is larger than the other. The labia minora vary in size from woman to woman. In some women, they are not large, so they hide behind the labia majora, and do not extend beyond the labia majora. In other women, they are so large that they protrude beyond the labia majora. Contrary to a myth, the wrinkling and size of the woman's labia is not increased by masturbation.

Clitoris

The clitoris is located where the labia minora or inner lips meet. It is located between the top of the two labia minora. The tissue of the labia minora normally covers the clitoris, which makes a clitoral hood or prepuce to protect it. The clitoris is located above the opening of the urethra and the vagina. It is about three inches above the opening of the vagina.

The main parts of the clitoris are the head, shaft, and crura. The head of the clitoris, also known as the glans, is tiny. It looks like a tiny, oval button. It is highly sensitive, containing 8,000 nerve endings. The shaft of the clitoris is larger than the glans. The average shaft measures 1 to 2 inches in length and a little over half an inch in width. However, the only visible part of the clitoris is usually the glans and part of the shaft. The shaft of the clitoris is mostly hidden beneath the skin of the vulva. The average length of the external clitoris is a quarter of an inch, but the range of the size of the external clitoris runs from a few millimeters to an inch or more. The shaft of the clitoris extends into the body. The base of the shaft attaches to the pubic bone, and then divides into two crura, or legs, each measuring between 2 and 4 inches long. Each crus of the clitoris extends on one side of the woman's body, and attaches to the arch of the pubic bone located on that side of the woman's body. From the roots of the clitoris to the tip of the clitoris, the average clitoris measures roughly four to six inches long, close to the same size as the average penis. The crura are near the vestibular bulbs, which are now thought by some to be part of the structure of the clitoris. The crura are to the left and right of the urethra, urethral sponge, and vagina.

The shaft, glans, crura, and vestibular bulbs contain spongy tissue called cavernous bodies. This tissue becomes engorged with blood during sexual arousal. When the cavernous bodies become engorged with blood during sexual arousal the glans and the shaft fill with blood and increase in size. In addition to getting bigger, the clitoris becomes harder, redder, and erect. When the clitoris becomes erect it extends from under the clitoral hood, causing the hood to retract and making the clitoral glans more accessible. When the vestibular bulbs swell with blood, they make the opening to the vagina smaller, increasing the gripping and hugging of the penis by the vagina.

It is important to remember that the clitoris is like the penis since it is very sensitive to stimulation and becomes erect when stimulated. As a matter of fact, the clitoris is the most sensitive part of a woman's body, with the sole purpose of bringing sexual pleasure to the woman. The stimulation of the clitoris produces sexual excitement, sexual pleasure, an erection, and an orgasm in the woman.

Urinary Opening and Urethra

Just below the clitoris there is a small opening. This opening is the opening to the urethra. The urethral opening is right above the vaginal opening. The urethral opening and urethra are not part of the sexual anatomy of the woman, but their proximity to other parts of the woman's sexual anatomy makes them important to talk about.

The urethral opening's size is that of a small dimple. The urethral opening is the opening to the urethral tube, which is a short tube measuring about 1.5 inches long, and carries urine from the bladder. The urethra is surrounded by spongy erectile tissue that fills with blood when the woman becomes sexually aroused. The urethra and bladder are so close to the vagina that it is not unusual for the woman to feel as if she needs to urinate at the beginning of intercourse. When there is no infection present, the urethra is free of microorganisms, does not carry germs, and does not transmit diseases.

Vagina

The vagina is a muscular, hollow tube that extends from the vaginal opening to the cervix of the uterus. It is also known as the birth canal. It is situated between the urinary bladder and the rectum. It is about three to five inches long in a grown woman. The vaginal opening is right behind the opening of the urethra. The vagina is made up of three layers of tissue. The vaginal layer on the surface that can be touched is the mucosa. It consists of mucous membranes and contains folds or wrinkles. The folds are called rugae and allow the vagina to stretch and return to its original size. The next vaginal layer of tissue is a layer of muscle concentrated mostly around the outer third of the vagina. The third vaginal layer is the innermost layer, and it consists of fibrous tissue that connects to other anatomical structures in the woman's body.

When the woman is not sexually aroused, the vagina is shaped like a flattened tube, with its sides collapsed on each other. In an unaroused state, the vagina is not a continuously open space or hole, as is thought often by both women and men. Rather, the vagina is a potential space. However, the vagina has the ability to expand and contract because of its muscular tissue. It can adjust to any size so that a finger, a tampon, or any size penis can fit snugly in it. It can adjust its size, so that a baby can pass through during childbirth.

The outer third of the vagina contains nearly 90 percent of the vaginal nerve endings, and therefore is more sensitive to touch than the inner two thirds of the vagina. The number of vaginal nerve endings in the middle third of the vagina, is more than the number of vaginal nerve endings in the deep inner third of the vagina, close to the cervix. There are few nerves at the back of the vagina, so there is little sensation in that area. Around the vagina, there is pubic hair. This hair serves to protect the vagina from infection.

At birth, the vaginal opening may be covered with a thin sheet of tissue called the hymen. The hymen partially covers the opening of the vagina. Whether the hymen is intact or not is incorrectly considered a sign of whether a woman is a virgin or not. This is because of the belief, that the first vaginal penetration would usually tear the hymen and cause bleeding. However, the hymen is a poor indicator of whether a woman has actually engaged in sexual intercourse because non-sexual activities can rupture the hymen. Non-sexual things that may rupture the hymen are an injury, a pelvic examination, and certain activities like horseback riding, bicycling, and gymnastics.

The vagina does have microorganisms present in it. These microorganisms do not cause disease. Rather, they ward off infection and keep the vagina in a healthy state. Therefore, the vagina is considered clean when there is no infection present. The vagina usually is kept clean, moist, and in a healthy state by vaginal secretions. These vaginal secretions are normal. They are a result of secretions produced from small glands in the lining of the vagina. Without these vaginal secretions, the vagina would become dry, uncomfortable, and itchy. Without these vaginal secretions, the vagina would get infections more often and would have an unpleasant smell. These vaginal secretions cause a vaginal discharge in all women from time to time. The vaginal discharge is just vaginal secretions that come out of the woman's vagina. The vaginal discharge appears clear, cloudy white, or yellowish when dry on clothing. It is not unusual for a woman to notice a thick white secretion that coats her panty at the end of the day from time to time. This thick white secretion is a vaginal discharge that results from vaginal secretions.

The vaginal tissue is loaded with blood vessels. These blood vessels, when engorged with blood as a result of the woman becoming sexually aroused, press against the vaginal tissue, forcing the natural tissue fluids through the walls of the vagina. This causes droplets of fluid to appear along the vaginal walls, and eventually to cover the sides of the vagina completely. This fluid serves as a vaginal lubricant. Without this lubricant, a woman would most likely find penile penetration uncomfortable or painful. This fluid, in addition to serving as a natural vaginal lubricant, also aids the sperm into the cervix. The vagina starts lubricating within thirty seconds after the woman becomes sexually aroused.

The vagina has four important purposes. The first purpose is for it to receive a male's erect penis and provide sexual pleasure for both the male and the female. The second purpose of the vagina is for it to receive the male's semen and provide a path for the semen to enter the uterus. The third purpose of the vagina is for it to provide a path for the menstrual fluid to leave the uterus and the female body. The fourth purpose of the vagina is for it to provide a path for the baby to take during childbirth in order to leave the woman's body.

Cervix

The cervix is the lower, narrow portion of the uterus, where it joins with the top end of the vagina. The cervix forms the neck of the uterus. It is cylindrical or conical in shape. Approximately half of it is visible, while the other half lies above the vagina, beyond view. If a person inserts one or two fingers into the vagina, all the way to the back, he or she will touch something that feels firm and rounded, like the tip of the nose. This is the cervix.

The narrow opening of the cervix is called the os. The os is a hole the size of a pencil point. The os is the gateway for sperm to enter the uterus. The os allows menstrual blood to flow out from the uterus during menstruation. During orgasm the cervix contracts and the os dilates, drawing semen in the vagina into the uterus, thereby increasing the likelihood of conception. During pregnancy the os closes to help keep the fetus in the uterus until birth. During childbirth the tiny os dilates so that the baby can come out.

Cells inside the cervix secrete mucus that is thin, clear, and slimy. This mucus is abundant just prior to ovulation. This mucus makes it easier for the sperm to swim up the cervix and into the uterus during the most fertile days. After ovulation, the mucus decreases and becomes thicker.

A small bump, or small bumps, may appear on the cervix. These are nabothian cysts that occur when mucous secreting cells on the cervix become blocked. Most of these cysts are the size of a small green pea, but they may be larger or smaller. These cysts are common and benign. They do not cause problems and do not need any treatment.

Stimulation of certain parts of the cervix during intercourse can be very painful to the woman, and result in a sensation similar to being kicked in the stomach. However, stimulation of certain parts of the cervix produces intense orgasms for the woman. It is up to the woman to find out which parts of the cervix are pleasurable for her when stimulated and which parts of the cervix are painful for her when stimulated. The woman should do so because every woman is different when it comes to which parts of the cervix produce pleasure when stimulated. However, one area of the cervix in particular that produces pleasure to every woman is a ring-like structure that encircles the cervix. This ring-like structure is highly erogenous. This area, when stimulated during sexual intercourse or manually, produces intense orgasms for the woman. This area, in a sexual context, is sometimes referred to as the deep spot.

Uterus

The uterus is the womb of the woman. It is a major female reproductive organ. It is a pear-shaped organ where a fetus can develop. The uterus is about three inches long and two inches wide. One end of the uterus opens into the vagina. The lower narrow portion of the uterus, known as the cervix, opens into the vagina. The other end of the uterus is connected on both sides to the fallopian tubes. The uterus is suspended in the abdominal cavity by ligaments. The uterus is behind the vagina and between the bladder and the rectum.

The thin outside covering of the uterus, is the perimetrium. The uterus has a thick lining and muscular walls. The tissue that lines the interior wall of the uterus is the endometrium. The smooth muscle layer of the wall of the uterus is the myometrium. The uterus has some of the strongest muscles in the female body. These muscles can expand and contract to accommodate a growing fetus, and then they help push the baby out during labor. These muscles contract rhythmically during an orgasm. They do so to help push or guide the sperm up the uterus to the fallopian tubes, where fertilization may be possible. The contractions of the uterus during orgasm contribute to the intensity of the orgasm that the woman experiences. Women who have had a hysterectomy (surgical removal of the uterus) have noted a decrease in the intensity of the orgasm.

The major function of the uterus is to accept a fertilized egg from the fallopian tube and have it develop into an embryo. Every month the inside layer of the uterus, the endometrium, becomes thick and plush. If the egg is fertilized, it attaches to the soft tissue of the endometrium. It becomes implanted into the endometrium and derives nourishment from blood vessels, which develop exclusively for this purpose. The fertilized egg develops into an embryo. If the egg from the fallopian tube is not fertilized, then it is not embedded in the wall of the uterus and the woman begins menstruation. The egg is flushed away and some of the lining of the endometrium exits as menstrual fluid. Usually, an egg is released about once a month. If the egg is not fertilized, then menstrual fluid exists about once a month. If the egg is fertilized, then the menstrual fluid and another egg are not released. They are not released until the fertilized egg or embryo is no longer in the woman's body. It is important to note that sometimes instead of one egg, two eggs or even three eggs are released by the ovary at the same time, and if they are fertilized by sperm, twins or triplets result.

Fallopian Tubes

The fallopian tubes are two narrow tubes that are attached to the upper part of the uterus and extend toward the ovaries. Each fallopian tube attaches to a side of the uterus and connects to an ovary. At the end of each tube, there are fringe like projections called fimbriae. When an ovary does ovulate, or releases an egg, these fimbriae draw the egg into the fallopian tube. The fallopian tubes serve as tunnels for the egg to travel from the ovaries to the uterus. Conception, or the fertilization of an egg by a sperm, normally occurs in the fallopian tubes. The fertilized egg then moves into the uterus, where it develops into an embryo. If the egg is not fertilized, it travels from the fallopian tube to the uterus, where it is flushed away along with menstrual fluid.

Ovaries

The ovaries are small, oval-shaped glands. Each ovary is located on one side of the uterus. Each ovary measures about 1½ inches long and is located at the end of a fallopian tube. The primary function of the ovaries is to release eggs and produce hormones. When the woman is born, these little ovaries each contain about 400,000 eggs. The woman's body does not produce any more eggs during the woman's lifetime. Starting at the onset of menstruation during puberty and continuing until menopause, the eggs generally mature and are released at the rate of about one a month. The process by which the egg is released from the ovary is called ovulation.

Usually one egg matures at a time, and that is the reason why a woman usually gets pregnant with only one baby. However, sometimes two or three eggs mature at the same time. If that happens and they are fertilized by sperm, then twins or triplets are produced. Usually each ovary takes a turn in releasing an egg (or eggs) every month. However, if there was a case where one ovary was absent or dysfunctional, then the other ovary would continue to provide, every month, an egg (or eggs) to be released. If puberty starts on average around the age of 13, and menopause starts on average around the age of 47, then the woman releases about 400 eggs in her lifetime. Eggs that are not released are reabsorbed by the ovaries.

The ovaries produce and release two sex hormones: estrogen and progesterone. These two hormones are important to the woman's sexual health. Estrogen is responsible for the appearance of female secondary sex characteristics at puberty. It is also responsible for the development and maintenance of the reproductive organs of the female. Progesterone promotes cyclic changes in the endometrium and prepares the endometrium for pregnancy. Progesterone helps keep the endometrium in a healthy state, during pregnancy.

Chapter 4

The Male Sexual Response

The male can have sex in many different ways. There is no specific pattern for sex that the man has to follow, but the way the male body responds to sexual stimulation follows a certain pattern. The male sexual response cycle is the name given to the pattern of physical changes that the male body goes through during sexual stimulation. Orgasm is only part of the sexual response. There is a lot of pleasure to be enjoyed by the man on the way to orgasm and returning from orgasm. It is important for the man to understand the physiological factors leading to orgasm and the ones that follow it. If the man understands why his body responds the way it does to sexual stimulation, he will enjoy the sexual experience even more. If the woman understands how the man's body responds to sexual stimulation, she will enjoy the sexual experience even more. The male sexual response cycle was first researched by sexologists William Masters and Virginia Johnson in the 1960's. They discovered that the male sexual response cycle had four stages, similar to the female sexual response cycle. The four stages are excitement, plateau, orgasm, and resolution.

Excitement

The excitement stage is the first stage of the male sexual response cycle. It starts when the idea of sex first comes into the man's mind. The idea comes as urges, fantasies, or lust. It is a result of either physical or emotional stimulation. Once the brain has registered sexual interest, it sends a message to the penis. The unstimulated or flaccid penis becomes erect. It becomes erect as a result of increased blood flow into the penis, and as a result of the blood being held there in the veins by valves. The valves keep the blood from flowing back out as long as there is arousal. In most cases, the man has an erection within seconds. An erection causes the penis to become large and stiff, so that it stands out from the body. The intensity of the erection will tend to fluctuate, and may be lost but regained as a result of continuous physical and emotional stimulation during foreplay. The only two reasons why an erection might not be regained is if the man has anxiety about the loss of the erection or if an external event interrupts the sexual experience. An erection can be stopped easily when a nonsexual event interrupts the sexual experience. Examples of nonsexual events that stop an erection are the doorbell ringing, the telephone ringing, and loud screaming. A critical comment, expressed by the woman when the man has an erection can diminish the man's erection. Erections can be kept for extended periods of time without ejaculation if the man is not anxious and if the stimulation is varied in its type and intensity. When the erect penis is stimulated, it sends more sensual feelings back to the brain and to other areas of the body, causing further excitement.

During the excitement phase the heart rate, the breathing rate, and the muscle tension start to increase. The blood pressure also starts to rise. The glans, or head of the penis, swells with blood and starts to change color. The scrotum starts to thicken in order to slightly increase the temperature of the seminal fluid as it is prepared for expulsion and fertilization of the egg. The testicles start to draw closer to the body and start to swell. Some men also experience nipple erection. Since a man's breasts are less prominent than a woman's breasts, the nipple erection is usually not as noticeable in the man as it is in the woman. Some men may experience a sex flush. A sex flush is a blushing or reddening that occurs over the upper third of the man's body. It covers the man's forehead, face, neck, and chest. It is more likely to occur in a room where the temperature is a little high. It is more likely to occur in situations where the man is in great anticipation of sex. It is not important whether a man experiences a sex flush or not. It is just an additional sign for some men that sexual arousal is taking place. The physical changes that happen during the excitement phase make the man's body extra sensitive to touch and stimulation. This causes the man's pleasure to increase.

Plateau

The second stage of the male sexual response cycle is the plateau phase. During the plateau phase the arousal, pleasure, and excitement deepen and intensify. This is usually a result of sustained physical stimulation. Ideally, the plateau phase is the longest phase of the sexual response cycle. Foreplay usually gets this stage going, but this stage continues as the couple has sex. The man usually has a tendency to rush the foreplay at this stage. The man should not rush the foreplay at this stage, but should go at a comfortable pace. The man should do so because the woman cannot have an orgasm without sufficient foreplay, and she needs more foreplay than a man in order to get aroused. The plateau phase is the period of time during which arousal intensifies in preparation for the sexual release.

During the plateau phase, the rigidity of the erection increases slightly. The glans, or head of the penis, continues to enlarge because of more excess blood coming in. The glans also continues to change color. It deepens in color so that it becomes dark red or a purplish color. The skin of the scrotum continues to thicken. The testes continue to draw closer to the body and continue to swell. At this point, the size of the testicles has increased greatly. During this stage, the heart rate and breathing rate continue to increase. The blood pressure also continues to rise. The muscle tension keeps on intensifying. If a sex flush was present in the excitement phase, it continues to exist at this phase.

During the plateau phase, a small amount of pre-ejaculatory fluid seeps from the penis. This fluid contains live sperm that can get a woman pregnant. This is why withdrawing the penis from the vagina before ejaculation is not a safe method of birth control. The seminal fluid begins to collect in the area around the prostate gland. As the man moves through the plateau phase toward the orgasm phase, he begins to feel that he is reaching ejaculatory inevitability, or the point of no return.

Orgasm

The third stage of the male sexual response cycle is the orgasmic phase. The orgasmic phase is the briefest, most intense, and most internal phase. During the orgasmic phase the sexual excitement continues to increase. The heart rate continues to increase, up to 180 beats a minute. The breathing rate continues to intensify and becomes quicker. The man starts to breathe more loudly. The male orgasmic phase can be described in two parts. In the first part, as the man nears the end of the plateau phase and moves into the orgasmic phase, he feels that his body is getting ready to ejaculate. He is approaching ejaculatory inevitability, or the point of no return. Contractions in the prostate gland occur at intervals of eight tenths of a second. The opening (sphincter) of the bladder closes off. This happens so that no seminal fluid is pushed back into the bladder. This also happens so that no urine escapes during ejaculation. As a matter of fact, most men feel immediately before or after an ejaculation that it is almost impossible to urinate. Near the base of the penis, the seminal fluid gathers. It gathers there to be ready for expulsion. The expulsion occurs during the contractions that occur in the second stage of the orgasmic phase.

During the second part of the orgasmic phase, the sensations become increasingly intense. Both partners experience a peak of pleasure, called orgasm. Orgasm consists of contractions along the seminal duct system and the penis. The contractions of the penis and seminal duct system are eight tenths of a second apart. On average, men usually experience five or six such contractions. The second and third contractions are usually the most intense. However, a man can experience anywhere from three to fifteen contractions. An orgasm lasts approximately anywhere from three to ten seconds. A man experiences an orgasm in the genital area. The orgasms can be long or short, and mild or intense. They vary each time, and they vary from individual to individual. During orgasm, other parts of the body might go through involuntary muscle contractions as well. Other parts of the body are the hands, feet, and face. Involuntary muscular contractions throughout the pelvic region also occur. They release accumulated muscular tension, and start to pump excess blood from the genital area back to the rest of the body. Most men are aware of three different sensations during orgasm in the genital area. The first sensation is a deep internal wave of warmth or throbbing pressure. This quickly leads to the second sensation. The second sensation is the feeling of rhythmic contractions. This leads to the third sensation. The third sensation is the sensation of semen rushing through the urethra. This sensation is experienced as a warm spurting sensation. Orgasm is a release of the built up stimulation. It is a discharge of sexual tension. With men, orgasm is almost always accompanied by the ejaculation of the seminal fluid.

A man can sense when he is about to orgasm because he feels an inevitable need to ejaculate. When he feels the inevitable need to ejaculate, the man has reached the point of no return. When the man reaches the point of no return, or ejaculatory inevitability, the ejaculation will take place. Even if the man tries to stop the ejaculation, he will be unable to. Even if nonsexual events interrupt at this point, the man will still ejaculate. Examples of nonsexual events are the phone ringing, the doorbell ringing, and loud noises. When the ejaculation takes place, orgasm or intense sexual pleasure is experienced by the man. The orgasmic contractions along the seminal duct system and the penis force the seminal fluid up the urethral tube and out the penis tip. In younger men, the force of the expulsion of the seminal fluid is more intense than in older men. The force of the ejaculation decreases with age.

Resolution

The fourth stage in the male sexual response cycle is the resolution phase. During this phase, the body returns to its original unstimulated state. All physical signs of sexual arousal go away from the body. The penis loses its erection and becomes limp because the excess blood leaves the genital area. The excess blood returns to the rest of the body. The heart rate and breathing rate decrease to their normal rate. The blood pressure goes down to its normal level. If a sex flush existed earlier, it disappears at this stage. The muscle tension throughout the body is resolved. The muscles throughout the body become relaxed again. The testicles decrease in size and return to their normal size.

This process is usually a lot quicker for men than women. This is because women can often remain aroused for a while after orgasm, and most women with continued physical stimulation can experience climax for a second or a third time or more, whereas most men after experiencing an orgasm go into a refractory period, where they have to rest before they can experience another orgasm. The refractory period varies from man to man. It depends on the man's age and physical health. A few men can experience multiple orgasms without a refractory period, but they are rare. Unlike women, few men can have sexual intercourse immediately after orgasm without a resting period. However, most men have the ability to experience multiple orgasms without a refractory period if they train themselves to do so.

Some men, if they have been aroused but did not have an orgasm, sometimes will feel agitated. If a man gets aroused but does not have an orgasm several things can happen. The process of his body returning to its original, unstimulated state will take longer than if he had orgasmed and ejaculated. It will take longer for the excess blood in the genital area to return to the rest of the body. It will take longer for the man to completely lose his erection. It will take longer for the muscles throughout the body to relax. Some men sometimes may experience testicular aching, because they were aroused and did not orgasm. "Blue balls" is the term that applies to testicular aching that occurs in men who did not orgasm. A man can get relief from feeling uncomfortable for not experiencing an orgasm by sleeping it off or masturbating to orgasm.

Chapter

5

The Female Sexual Response

To some women, orgasm is the entire goal of sex. This should not be the case, since orgasm is only one aspect of the woman's sexual response. There is a large amount of pleasure that can be experienced by a woman during her sexual response on the way toward orgasm or returning from orgasm. Although there is no specific pattern for sex, the woman's sexual response does, in general, follow a cyclic pattern. The woman's sexual response is the way her body responds to sexual stimulation. If the woman understands the orgasm stage, the physiological factors leading up to it and following it, then she could understand why her body responds the way it does during sex. This understanding will make her sexual experience more pleasurable. The sexual response cycle was researched in 1966, by Doctors William Masters and Virginia Johnson. They did the first detailed study of the woman's sexual response cycle. The research examined muscle contractions, and the flow of blood toward and away from the genitals. They divided the woman's sexual response cycle into four distinct phases. The four phases are the excitement phase, plateau phase, orgasm phase, and the resolution phase.

Excitement Phase

The first stage in the woman's sexual response cycle is the excitement phase. The excitement phase starts when the idea of sex first comes into the woman's head. It can come in a form of an urge, blur of fantasies, or lust. It can result from either physical or emotional stimulation. When this stimulation is received and enjoyed, it results in sexual arousal. This sexual arousal produces external and internal changes on the woman's body. The breasts begin to swell. The blood pressure and the muscle tension start to increase. The breathing rate and the heart rate start to increase. Several hormones and natural chemicals are released into the bloodstream. Blood flow rushes to the vulva and causes erectile tissue to swell. The clitoris becomes larger and erect. It pokes out from under its hood. Its roots stiffen and elongate. The clitoris increases two to three times in length and size. As a result of these changes to the clitoris, the woman might hunger for clitoral stimulation. However, at this stage most women prefer the caressing of the general area around the clitoris, rather than having the head or glans of the clitoris directly caressed.

Other changes that occur during the excitement phase are in the labia majora and the labia minora. The labia majora, or the outer lips, spread out as if opening in preparation for receiving the penis. The labia minora, or the inner lips, become slightly engorged with blood. This causes them to increase in size, extend outward, and form a funnel shape. The opening of the outer lips and the inner lips extending outward and forming a funnel shape are indications that the woman is physically becoming aroused. The cervix, which is located at the back of the vagina, is the opening to the uterus. During the excitement phase, the uterus elevates because of increased arousal. Also, the cervix begins to pull away from the vagina so it will not be in the way of the penis during thrusting.

Usually within ten to twenty seconds after stimulation is received, the vagina starts lubricating itself. The lubrication that occurs at the vagina is moisture from the pores of the skin. They form as little drops along the walls of the vagina. Their function is to lessen friction and improve the pleasure of the penis in the vagina. Although some people think that lubrication of the vagina is a sign of readiness for the penis to enter, entry is most likely not desired by the woman until much later. One other bodily change that might occur in some women during the excitement phase is called a sex flush. The sex flush is a blushing or reddening that occurs over the upper third of the body. It occurs usually over the chest, neck, face, and forehead. It is a result of blood moving to the surface of the skin in those areas. It is more likely to occur in a room where the temperature is a little high. It is more likely to occur in situations where the woman is in extreme anticipation of sex. It should not be important whether the woman experiences a sex flush. A sex flush is just an additional sign for some women that sexual arousal is taking place. It is important to note that not all women experience a sex flush, and that only some of them experience it.

Plateau

The second phase in the woman's sexual response cycle is the plateau phase. It is a continuation of the excitement stage. During the plateau phase, the excitement, sexual pleasure, and sexual desire that were started in the excitement stage deepen and intensify. The plateau phase is a result of sustained physical stimulation. It is foreplay that usually gets this stage going, but this stage continues when the couple has sex. Without sufficient foreplay a woman would not be stimulated enough for the plateau phase to occur. Some women prefer a longer time than others of love play and pleasuring, but all women usually like a longer time than men. This is one of those needs or desires that vary from one person to another and in the same person from one time to another.

During the plateau phase, the nipples stiffen and the breasts continue swelling. For women who have not had children, the breasts may increase in size by up to 25% of their normal size. For women who have had children, the breasts show a little increase in size, if any at all. If the sexual flush was present during the excitement phase, it continues during the plateau phase. During the plateau phase, the heart rate and the breathing rate continue to increase. The muscle tension and blood pressure continue to increase. The uterus becomes fully elevated and swells. The cervix becomes fully pulled away from the vagina. The blood keeps on rushing to the genitals. The fact that blood keeps rushing to the vagina during the plateau phase causes the outer third of the vagina to become extremely congested with blood. As a result of this, the outer third of the vagina swells, becomes tighter, and decreases in size, forming what is called the orgasmic platform. The vaginal opening also tightens. The tightening of the external third of the vagina functions as an extra stimulation to the penis and the vagina. The tightening of the vagina produces a grasping effect, holding the penis firmly in the vagina during intercourse. It is important to note that the orgasmic platform is only the first third of the vagina, or about one and a half to two inches in length. It can tighten or expand. It is the most important part of the vagina for penis contact during intercourse.

The vagina elongates and the deepest two thirds of the vaginal alley balloons to nearly twice its normal width. When the inner two thirds of the vagina balloons out, it forms a pool to keep the seminal fluid that contains the sperm inside the vagina. The labia majora become thicker and spread apart more. Their color changes from pink to dark red. The labia minora become bright red and continue to increase in size. The labia minora become bright red about one minute before an orgasm. Masters and Johnson noticed that if the inner lips' color does not change, then a woman won't have an orgasm.

It is important to know that most women during the sexual response cycle, especially the plateau phase, experience their buildup of sexual arousal in a way that can be described as waves. That means that there is a peak in arousal and then an ebb, or diminishing of the intensity of the feelings of arousal. Then a new wave of sexual arousal happens. If a woman lets herself experience the waves in their peaks and in their ebbs without interruption, then the peaks will tend to intensify and the arousal will increase. However, when the woman feels the sexual arousal is diminishing because of the wave's ebb, if she interrupts the wave by becoming anxious, this will stop her response from occurring in its natural, wavelike pattern. Her anxiety fulfills her fear and ends her arousal. So if the woman knows that her arousal comes in waves that peak and then diminish, then when her arousal diminishes she would not worry. Rather, she would continue to be relaxed and enjoy the stimulation. This will cause her to experience a new wave of sexual arousal, with a new intense peak. During the plateau phase, the body undergoes a series of changes as arousal and excitement build. These changes make the body extra sensitive to touch and stimulation, increasing the woman's pleasure further. During this phase, most women feel so good that they want the sex and this phase to last forever.

Orgasm

The third stage of the woman's sexual response cycle is called the orgasm stage. When sensations become very strong, the woman experiences a climax of pleasure called an orgasm. An orgasm is just a release of sexual tension. Involuntary muscular contractions in the outer third of the vagina, the uterus, and in muscles throughout the pelvic area rapidly release accumulated muscular tension and pump blood from the genital tissue back to where it came from in the rest of the body. During this stage the clitoris, the labia majora, and the labia minora remain basically the same as they were at the end of the plateau phase. However, at this stage the heart rate continues to increase, sometimes reaching up to 180 beats per minute. The blood pressure also continues to increase. The breathing intensifies, becoming deeper, faster and noisier. There may be a large amount of involuntary muscular contractions in the face, arms, legs, back, or lower abdomen of the woman. An involuntary contraction in the foot that many times happens is when the foot straightens out and the toes curl downward and away from the body. The involuntary contractions of the face sometimes look like a frown or grimace. The mouth might open involuntarily, as if gasping for air. Also, some involuntary sounds or words might be uttered.

The feelings of orgasm in the genital area are mainly due to strong vaginal contractions in the orgasmic platform. The orgasm is experienced not only in the vagina, but also in the uterus. The uterus undergoes contractions during an orgasm. Some women experience intense contractions in the uterus that are felt in the lower abdomen. Some women misinterpret these contractions as painful rather than pleasurable because they do not understand what they are. However, once a woman understands that the intense contractions in the uterus are causing those sensations in the lower abdomen, she begins to enjoy the intensity of those contractions, rather than experience them as painful. The sensations that occur during an orgasm tend to originate from the vagina and the uterus and expand to other parts of the body. Sometimes they expand to cover the whole body.

An orgasm is an intense feeling of pleasure that blocks out all other feelings and thoughts for a brief amount of time. The orgasm lasts approximately three to ten seconds. The orgasmic contractions occur at intervals of about eight tenths of a second. That means that a woman will have between three and fifteen contractions during an orgasm. Masters and Johnson measured three to five contractions for a mild orgasm and eight to twelve contractions for an intense orgasm. Just as the clitoris size and vaginal shape vary from woman to woman, also the length and intensity of an orgasm vary from woman to woman. Also, the same woman might have orgasms that vary in length and intensity. For example, one day an orgasm with a woman will be four seconds, and another day it will be eight seconds. Also, one day an orgasm with a woman would be mild and another day it would be very intense. All orgasms are good, regardless how long they last, and how intense they are. On average, a woman needs four to five minutes of direct clitoral stimulation to reach orgasm. This is only an average. If it takes a woman longer than four to five minutes of direct clitoral stimulation to reach an orgasm, a woman should not feel inadequate. Some women do not need direct clitoral stimulation. Indirect clitoral stimulation for four to five minutes will bring some women to orgasm.

Women tend to do what men do after an orgasm. Women build up to a single, giant orgasm and then they rest. Most women do not know that they can experience multiple orgasms. Most women are physically capable of having multiple orgasms. Multiple orgasms are one orgasm spilling into another, without a refractory period between them. Some women can experience two orgasms consecutively, others can experience three, and others can experience even more. Women can have multiple orgasms because the excess blood in their genital area does not rush away quickly after an orgasm. The excess blood stays in the woman's genital area for a while, before going to the rest of the body. Therefore, most women do not have to wait in order to have another orgasm. The key for a woman to have multiple orgasms is for her to keep breathing through an orgasm and not hold her breath, which is typically what most women do. Sometimes women during an orgasm breathe in shallow and unpredictable breaths. But if a woman breathes in shallow breaths during an orgasm, or holds her breath during an orgasm, it is difficult for her to keep going from one orgasm to another. If the woman holds her breath or breathes in shallow breaths during an orgasm, the brain will need oxygen and the excess blood will flow from the genital area back to the brain. If the excess blood flows from the genital area to the brain, then the woman won't have excess blood in her genital area. Therefore, she will not be able to experience another orgasm. However, if the woman keeps her breathing normal during an orgasm, then the excess blood in the genital area will remain because the brain is getting sufficient oxygen. If there is excess blood in the genital area, a woman can have another orgasm.

In order for a woman to experience multiple orgasms, she should keep breathing through an orgasm, even if she feels like she is losing orgasm momentum. She should keep in mind that this is only the first wave of pleasure, and not expect it to feel like one big event. She should concentrate on what feels good. She should mentally focus only on what she is feeling at the moment. She should let go of the goal of having an orgasm. Once the woman experiences her first orgasm, going onto the next orgasm is easier. A woman should not pressure herself to experience multiple orgasms, because that is a definite way to fail. If a woman pressures herself to experience multiple orgasms, it will take away from the pleasure of sex, and from the pleasure of the first orgasm.

Some women cannot experience multiple orgasms. If a woman cannot experience multiple orgasms, she should know that one strong explosive orgasm is wonderful also. A woman should not feel inadequate if she never has multiple orgasms. Some sexually experienced women do not have multiple orgasms because sometimes the clitoris is just too sensitive after an orgasm to be touched until a short period of time has passed. The amount of pleasure that a woman experiences during sex, is not tied to the number of orgasms that she has. One good orgasm that a woman experiences might be more pleasurable than multiple orgasms.

Resolution

The final stage of the woman's sexual response cycle is called the resolution phase. During the resolution phase, if a woman is multi-orgasmic, she can have another orgasm at any point if sexual stimulation is present. If the woman desires and she is capable she can have a number of orgasms at any point in the resolution phase. The woman's body does not need to return to its pre-stimulated state before it can experience another orgasm if the woman is multi-orgasmic. Also, there is no waiting period necessary before the woman can experience a second orgasm if the woman is multi-orgasmic.

During the resolution phase, the whole genital area is relieved of tension and of excess blood. Excess blood located in the woman's genital area moves to the rest of the body. The vulva goes back to its normal size and color, but may remain sensitive for a little while. The uterus returns to its normal position. The breathing rate and the heart rate slow down to their normal rates. The blood pressure goes down, returning to its normal level. The breasts return to their normal size and color, but might remain sensitive for a little while. The sex flush, if it existed, fades away. Muscles throughout the body relax, releasing tension that was built up during the first three phases of the woman's sexual response. The body returns to its normal relaxed state.

If the woman experienced at least one orgasm, then the resolution phase will happen quickly, without the woman feeling any discomfort. However, if the woman did not experience at least one orgasm, then the resolution phase will take a longer time to happen. Sometimes some women will experience discomfort if they did not experience at least one orgasm. This is because the whole body is in a heightened state of excitement and waiting for release. If the woman experiences discomfort, there will be a feeling of heaviness and discomfort in the pelvic area. This is because of pelvic blood congestion experienced by the woman, since she did not have an orgasmic release. Blood is trapped in the pelvic area and needs to be dissipated by orgasm muscle contractions. Eventually, without an orgasm, the body will return to its normal relaxed state and the excess blood in the genital and pelvic area will return to the rest of the body. However, it takes several hours for the excess blood in the pelvic and genital areas to return to the rest of the body. Also, if the woman experiences discomfort she will experience it for several hours. The discomfort that the woman experiences is both physical and emotional. Emotionally, the woman may feel frustrated that she did not experience an orgasm. A woman during that uncomfortable time period can sleep, so that she does not experience discomfort. The woman can also masturbate herself to orgasm, so that she does not experience that uncomfortable time, and so that the resolution phase ends quickly.

Chapter 6

Pubococcygeus Muscle

The pubococcygeus muscle, or PC muscle, is an important anatomical structure for intercourse for both men and women. It is known to some people as the love muscle, for both men and women. It is known to other people as the sex muscle, for both men and women. It is known as the sex muscle or the love muscle because it is the one muscle that is essential for the man and the woman's sexual pleasure and fulfillment during intercourse. It stretches from the front to the back of the pelvic girdle in both sexes. It is a hammock-like muscle that stretches from the pubic bone to the coccyx (tail bone). It forms the floor of the pelvic cavity and supports the pelvic organs. Men have two holes through the PC muscle. The holes are at the anus and the urethra. Women have three holes through the PC muscle. The holes are at the anus, vagina, and urethra. The PC muscle in the man wraps around the base of the penis and the anus. The PC muscle in the woman surrounds the anus, vagina, and urethra. In both men and women the PC muscle reflexively contracts during orgasm, providing much of an orgasm's pleasurable sensations.

A person, whether male or female, can identify the PC muscle by sitting on the toilet with his or her legs spread apart and urinating. While urinating, the person can stop the urination for about three seconds and then continue urinating. The muscle that the person uses to control the flow of urine is the PC muscle. The man or woman tightens the PC muscle to stop the flow of urine. A person can make sure that he or she found the right muscle by checking that his or her control of the urine does not depend on his or her legs being close together. If a person's control of the urine depends on his or her legs being close together, then the person is using his or her thigh muscles and not the PC muscle to control the flow of urine.

Advantages of a Strong PC Muscle

A strong PC muscle can be used by the man to control his arousal level during sex. The higher his arousal, the harder he has to squeeze his PC muscle to stop his arousal from going any higher. Therefore, a strong PC muscle would be more efficient in stopping the man's sexual arousal than a weak PC muscle. The PC muscle is also used by the man to delay or prevent his ejaculation. A man can delay or prevent his ejaculation by squeezing the PC muscle when he feels he is coming close to the point of ejaculation. It is important to note that when the man squeezes the PC muscle during sex, it makes the sensations more intense and pleasurable but it delays his sexual arousal by making the ejaculation delayed. However, when the man squeezes the PC muscle right before orgasming he will orgasm, but without ejaculating. A strong PC muscle is more effective than a weak PC muscle when the man tries to delay or prevent his ejaculation. A strong PC muscle is effective in delaying or preventing ejaculation, allowing the man to experience multiple orgasms. When the woman contracts her PC muscle during sex she makes it easier for her to orgasm. A strong PC muscle makes it easier for the woman to orgasm during sex than a weak PC muscle would. A strong PC muscle also allows the woman to become multi-orgasmic because a strong PC muscle is more responsive and sensitive during sex than a weak PC muscle.

If a man has a strong PC muscle, it will contract harder and create more intense orgasms during sex than a weak PC muscle would. Thus, it will make sex more pleasurable for the man. A strong PC muscle will also make sex more pleasurable for the woman. The nerve endings in the PC muscle are responsible for a lot of the sensations that a woman feels during sexual intercourse. As the penis thrusts in and out of the vagina, the woman's PC muscle stretches and relaxes, stimulating nerve endings and producing pleasurable sensations. A strong PC muscle will contract harder than a weak PC muscle and will create more intense pleasurable feelings for the woman during sex than a weak PC muscle. Men with a strong PC muscle tend to get aroused sexually more easily than men with a weak PC muscle. Women with a strong PC muscle tend to get aroused sexually more easily and lubricate faster than women that have a weak PC muscle.

Kegel Exercise

In 1942 Dr. Arnold Kegel developed a series of exercises for women who needed to improve their urinary control. These exercises strengthened the PC muscle, so that the women would have more urinary control. Today, these exercises are used by many people of both sexes to strengthen their PC muscle and to gain voluntary control over it. They do so, so that their sexual encounters become more pleasurable.

In order to do the Kegel exercise, the person needs to contract and relax the PC muscle twenty times in a row. When the person contracts the PC muscle, he or she should contract it as hard as he or she can and try to keep it contracted for ten seconds. A person should avoid contracting his or her stomach muscle when contracting the PC muscle. A person should do this exercise at least twice in a day, once in the morning and once at night. When doing this exercise, the man does not need to touch his penis. When doing this exercise, the woman does not need to touch her vagina. The wonderful thing about this exercise is that a person can do it at anytime and anywhere. For example, a person could do it in the middle of the supermarket, at his or her work, or in the privacy of his or her own bedroom. A person could do this exercise while standing, sitting, or lying. A person could also do this exercise while doing another daily activity such as ironing, washing dishes, taking notes at the board meeting, working at the computer, or waiting at the grocery store checkout counter.

The Kegel exercise may be difficult or tiring for some people at first. A person should start slowly with the exercise and do as much as he or she can. A person should do what is comfortable and pleasurable for him or her. For example, if a person can do only two PC muscle contractions in a row while holding the contractions for ten seconds, then that is okay. With time, the exercise will become much easier. For example, if a person could only do two contractions in a row, after a while he or she might be able to do four contractions in a row. With time, the person's control over the PC muscle will increase and his or her PC muscle will improve in strength. Like any exercise, the more consistent the person is in doing it, the faster he or she will see results. Like any exercise, the more the person does it, the faster he or she will see results. If a person wants to do it more than twice a day, he or she can do it as many times as he or she wants in the day.

A woman can also do another variation of the Kegel exercise. She can do vaginal squeezes. For vaginal squeezes, the woman lies down or sits down on the edge of a bed, and inserts two lubricated fingers into the vagina. Usually, the two fingers are the index finger and the middle finger. The two fingers should be next to each other, and they should be inside the vagina as much as possible. The woman should squeeze the PC muscle with her fingers inside the vagina. She should feel a slight contraction of the vaginal walls approximately one inch from the entrance of the vagina. When the woman squeezes the PC muscle, she should contract it as hard as she can for ten seconds, then she should let go. The woman should do the PC muscle contractions twenty times in a row. Then after doing twenty contractions in a row, or as much as she can do, the woman should spread both fingers apart as if she is making a peace sign. She should spread both fingers apart while they are still in the vagina. Then she should contract the PC muscle again and see if she can bring both fingers together. If she cannot, that means that she still needs to strengthen her PC muscle using vaginal squeezes or the Kegel exercise. Once she can bring both fingers together by contracting the PC muscle, that means that her PC muscle is strong. A woman can use either the Kegel exercise or the vaginal squeezes exercise to strengthen the PC muscle. She can also use both exercises, to strengthen the PC muscle.

Benefits of the Kegel Exercise

The Kegel exercise is the most common method used by both men and women to strengthen their PC muscle. People who do the Kegel exercise regularly, after several months of regular practice, discover that their enjoyment of sex and orgasms increases. By building up the strength of the PC muscle, they increase the blood flow to it. Since good blood flow plays a very important part in sexual arousal, the increased blood to the PC muscle increases their sexual desire, and increases their sexual arousal during sex. When doing the Kegel exercise, contracting the PC muscle increases the sexual energy in the pelvic area of both the man and the woman and spreads a warm flush of arousal throughout their body. As a matter of fact, some men and women, when they do the Kegel exercise, get so turned on from the way contracting the PC muscle feels that it makes them want to masturbate.

For men, the Kegel exercise makes them have stronger erections, stronger orgasms, and better ejaculatory control, since two or three inches of the man's penis is rooted in the PC muscle. Exercising the PC muscle makes the man sensitive and responsive in his genital area, which makes the sex more pleasurable for him. During sex, during the emission phase of orgasm, the man's PC muscle contracts and pulls the base of the penis up against the prostate. The effect of that is that it increases prostate stimulation, which contributes to the occurrence of the rhythmic muscular contractions in the prostate. The rhythmic muscular contractions in the vas deferens, prostate, and seminal vesicles force the sperm and the seminal fluids to collect at the base of the penis, thus forming semen. Then in the expulsion phase of orgasm, the PC muscle contracts and the man ejaculates. In other words, a stronger PC muscle as a result of the Kegel exercise gives the man a greater sensation during both phases of orgasm, especially during the ejaculation phase. It gives a greater sensation during the ejaculation phase because the ejaculation is produced in part by the PC muscle's rhythmic contractions.

Exercising the PC muscle also allows the man to become multi-orgasmic. The man would become multi-orgasmic because he would have a stronger PC muscle and greater control over his PC muscle. This allows him to control his sexual encounter and orgasm without ejaculating. The man would contract the PC muscle when he is close to ejaculating, before the point of ejaculation. When he contracts the PC muscle before the point of ejaculation, he delays ejaculation and experiences an orgasm with no ejaculation. Experiencing an orgasm with no ejaculation will allow the man to experience a second and maybe even a third orgasm after that. He would experience those orgasms with no refractory period in between, thus making him multi-orgasmic. Also, if a man exercises his PC muscle regularly, he can overcome his premature ejaculation. Exercising the PC muscle makes the man's recovery time between orgasms shorter.

For women, exercising their PC muscle increases blood flow to their pelvis. This makes them more aware of sensations in their pelvis, and increases their sexual arousal.

This increases the vagina's sensitivity, and responsiveness to sexual stimulation. The fact that the woman's vagina is more sensitive and responsive to sexual stimulation causes the woman to have an orgasm more easily during sexual intercourse. Strengthening the PC muscle is the most important thing a woman can do to improve her chances of having multiple orgasms. If the woman exercises the PC muscle it makes her vagina well-toned and tighter, which greatly increases the pleasure of the male during sex. Also, during sex the woman's PC muscle will cause harder vaginal contractions against the man's penis, because it is stronger as a result of PC muscle exercises. This will result in a more pleasurable sexual encounter for both the man and the woman. If the woman exercises the PC muscle, it will improve her vaginal lubrication before sex since there is greater blood flow to the pelvis as a result of the Kegel exercise. The vagina can tighten or expand to receive any size penis during intercourse. It can even expand to deliver a baby. The ability of the vagina to tighten or expand can be enhanced by the Kegel exercise. For women who usually have trouble experiencing an orgasm, or experience an orgasm from time to time, the Kegel exercise makes them more likely to experience an orgasm.

As a woman grows older, the strength of the PC muscle decreases unless it is regularly exercised. If a woman has had several vaginal births, the PC muscle is further weakened. Exercising the PC muscle will increase the woman's muscular support of the vagina and uterus after childbirth and with aging. If the woman exercises the PC muscle, its elasticity will improve which is beneficial during the birth process. The best exercise for the woman to use for the PC muscle is the Kegel exercise.

Flexing the PC Muscle During Sex

Both the man and the woman can tighten and release their PC muscle during sex in order to increase their sexual sensitivity and responsiveness. This will increase the sexual pleasure for both of them during sex. When the woman contracts her PC muscle during sex, it will increase the blood flow to the vagina and perineum, which increases her sexual responsiveness and sexual energy. Contracting the PC muscle during sex several times will allow the woman to have orgasms from clitoral and vaginal stimulation more easily. Flexing the PC muscle during sex several times makes the vagina tighter, which increases the pleasure for the man and the woman.

Flexing the PC muscle during sex several times allows the woman to grip and massage the man's penis while he is inside her, increasing his pleasure and her pleasure. The woman would contract her PC muscle while the shaft of the penis is in the vagina so that the vaginal contractions squeeze around the shaft of the penis. This will energize the man's whole body and allow him to experience very high levels of pleasure during sex. It will also cause the man's ejaculation to delay because the vaginal contractions are squeezing the shaft of the penis while it is erect. By the vaginal contractions delaying the man's ejaculation, the amount of time that the couple makes love together is prolonged, increasing both of their pleasure. The woman can contract her PC muscle, as the man's penis is withdrawn from the vagina. Doing that is extremely stimulating, because it creates suction against the vaginal walls. By the woman contracting the PC muscle during lovemaking, it becomes more probable that she will experience an orgasm and multiple orgasms because her vagina becomes more sensitive and responsive.

The man can tighten his PC muscle during sex to make his penis move up and down while it is erect and inside the woman's vagina. He would do that during intercourse for variation if he wants to make his penis dance inside the woman. During orgasm, pelvic contractions occur in the man's body that involve his prostate gland. By the man contracting his PC muscle during orgasm, he can deepen the orgasmic contractions, making them more intense and more pleasurable. When the man contracts his PC muscle on the prostate during orgasm, he will feel a pleasurable shaking or chill throughout his body.

Conclusion

The PC muscle is the one muscle that is essential for the man and the woman's sexual pleasure and fulfillment. It is known as the love muscle, or the sex muscle. For men and women, strengthening the PC muscle is an important part of maintaining general health and realizing their sexual potential. By carrying out the Kegel exercise, the woman and the man can increase the quality and quantity of their orgasms. Therefore, if a person does not have a well exercised PC muscle, then he or she should start working it out.

Chapter 7

The G-Spot

The G-spot is a small spot that is located about one and a half to two inches from the opening of the vagina. It is located on the front wall of the vagina, between the pubic bone and the cervix. It is a tiny bean-shaped area. Its size varies from woman to woman. When unstimulated, its size could be the size of a dime to a nickel. It is a bumpy region that feels like a small lump. It is bumpy because it is a dense patch of soft ridgy tissue. It is made of erectile tissue, like the penis and the clitoris. This erectile tissue becomes hard, swollen, bigger, and full of blood when it is stimulated. It swells to the size of a quarter or even a half dollar when stimulated. With proper stimulation, it becomes a tiny female erection. It is not responsive to gentle touching. It responds best to firm, deep, continuous pressure. The G-spot is a highly sensitive area inside the vagina.

Stimulation of the G-spot could trigger not only an orgasm, but also female ejaculation. The ejaculation occurs before or during the woman's climax. It usually occurs at the woman's climax. The ejaculation can be anywhere from a few drops to more than a cup. Sometimes the amount of the ejaculation is so small that the woman does not realize that she ejaculated. Rather, the ejaculation is mistaken to be normal vaginal secretions. The quantity of the ejaculation that is ejaculated by the woman varies from woman to woman and from one sexual encounter to another. Sometimes the ejaculation comes out as a series of spurts and at other times it just leaks out quietly and unnoticed. The ejaculation is a thin fluid that is colorless, clear, or milky, but not yellow. It does not smell like urine and it does not stain the sheets. The ejaculation is different from urine and it is very similar to the sugary mix that is produced by the prostate in men (the mix which the sperm join in order to become semen). The female ejaculation comes from the paraurethral glands, located around the lower end of the urethra. The female ejaculation seems to occur more frequently with the second or third orgasm; in other words, after prolonged intense stimulation. It tends to occur more frequently in women with strong PC muscles.

However, the G-spot does not appear to be present in all women. Each woman appears to have a different response when the area where the G-spot is supposed to be located is stimulated. Many women have a G-spot, and when it is stimulated it produces an orgasm. Other women have no G-spot, and when the area where the G-spot is supposed to be is stimulated, it does not produce an orgasm. Rather, it only produces a great deal of pleasure, and that area becomes their favorite place. Also, some women ejaculate regularly and some ejaculate occasionally when they orgasm from G-spot stimulation. Others do not ejaculate at all when they orgasm from G-spot stimulation.

Ejaculation Versus Incontinence of Urine

Some women are embarrassed by what they believe is incontinence of urine when they have sex. Some doctors, gynecologists, and psychiatrists incorrectly assume that a woman has incontinence of urine when she has sex and assume incorrectly the she needs surgery or psychotherapy. The ill-informed doctors need to realize that what they assume is incontinence of urine during sex is female ejaculation. Women that used to be embarrassed that they were urinating during sex should not feel embarrassed. Instead, they should realize that they were ejaculating during sex, which is normal and desirable. As a matter of fact, women that ejaculate during sex and know that it is ejaculation say that it feels great.

The wet spot that the couple finds after sex is a circle of dampness that seems too big to blame solely on the man's ejaculation. Some women marvel at the wet spot, and wonder how it got there. Other women assume that the wet spot is a result of them wetting the bed during sex. This is far from the truth. The wet spot is usually a result of the woman's ejaculation. Once women come to realize that the wet spot is normal and a result of female ejaculation, they will feel more liberated during sex and enjoy their sexual encounters more.

Why it is Difficult for a Large Number of Women to Locate the G-Spot

It is very common that a large number of women have never found their G-spot. One reason is that they do not bother to look for it because they assume that since they never felt it, it must not exist. A second reason the G-spot is hard to find is because it is barely noticeable when the woman is unaroused. A third reason the G-spot is hard to find is because it is made of erectile tissue that does not become hard, swollen, bigger, and full of blood unless the woman is aroused. A fourth reason the G-spot is hard to find is because it has to be stimulated properly to really be felt. It responds best to firm, deep, continuous pressure. It does not respond to gentle touching. A fifth reason the G-spot is hard to find is because when the woman is aroused and the G-spot becomes noticeable because its size increased, the woman is greatly occupied with satisfying herself sexually instead of looking for the G-spot.

A sixth reason the G-spot is hard to find is because its size varies considerably among women. When unstimulated, its size can range from that of a dime to a nickel. When stimulated, its size increases ranging from that of a quarter to a half dollar. A seventh reason why it is hard for the woman to locate the G-spot is because the sensation of the G-spot being stimulated is easily confused with the feeling that the woman needs to urinate. There is a simple anatomical reason for this. When the woman's G-spot is stimulated, it results in stimulation of the urethral wall, which results in the sensation of having to urinate. The sensation that is produced when the G-spot is stimulated is pleasure mixed with the sensation that the woman has to urinate immediately. In reaction to this sensation, a woman tenses up, stops thinking of the pleasurable sensations, and focuses only on not urinating by accident, thus making it hard for her to locate the G-spot. An eighth reason why a woman cannot locate a G-spot is because sometimes she cannot locate it on her own and she needs to have her partner show her where it is. It takes patience and sensitivity between the woman and her male partner to find the G-spot. Finally, some women cannot locate a G-spot because some women do not have a G-spot.

Locating the G-spot

In order to locate the G-spot, the first step is for the woman to get herself sexually aroused. She should do so because when she is not aroused the G-spot is difficult to find, since it is barely noticeable. The G-spot is made of erectile tissue that gets hard, swollen, bigger, and full of blood when the woman is sexually aroused. When the G-spot is swollen and larger in size as a result of the woman being sexually aroused, it is easier for the woman to find. The more aroused the woman becomes, the more noticeable the G-spot becomes. The woman could get herself aroused sexually by stimulating her clitoris with her index finger. She could stimulate the clitoris indirectly by putting her index finger on the clitoral hood and rubbing it in any direction she sees fit until she becomes sexually aroused.

When she becomes sexually aroused, she can sit on the toilet. Then, using her index finger, she can stimulate the upper front wall of her vagina by rubbing it, while at the same time applying firm downward pressure on the outside of her abdomen with her other hand. When she rubs the front wall of the vagina, she should rub it with firm, deep, continuous pressure. She should not rub it gently, since that does not stimulate the G-spot. When she rubs the front wall of her vagina with her index finger, she can also explore the front wall of her vagina and look for the G-spot. When she explores the front wall of her vagina, halfway between her vagina opening and cervix, she should feel a small lump that is the size of a quarter to a half dollar. This is her aroused G-spot. The woman should sit on the toilet because during her search for the G-spot when she unknowingly rubs the G-spot, she might feel the urge to urinate and stop her search for the G-spot without knowing that she has discovered it. If she is on the toilet when she feels that urge to urinate, she can continue to rub the G-spot and discover that she has found it. She can do that because she is on the toilet and is not concerned about urinating.

Sometimes there can be difficulty for the woman in locating the G-spot. She might need the help of her male partner to show her where it is. It takes patience and sensitivity between her and her partner to find the G-spot. One way for the man to search for the woman's G-spot is for the woman to lie on the bed on her back with her legs apart. Then the man can insert two fingers into her vagina with his palm up and begin exploring the front wall of her vagina. The two fingers that the man inserts inside the vagina are the index and the middle finger. The man could explore the front wall of the vagina by rubbing it with firm, continuous, strong pressure, and not with gentle strokes. He should rub it this way so that the G-spot is aroused and becomes noticeable. Halfway between the woman's vagina opening and her cervix, the man should feel a small lump. This is the woman's aroused G-spot.

The search for the G-spot, whether done solely by the woman or jointly with her male partner, is supposed to be a fun exploration, and not a sweaty distressing chore. It is important that in both cases the woman be relaxed, because when she is relaxed the G-spot is more likely to be found. It is more likely to be found when the woman is relaxed, because when the woman is tense it is smaller and very hard to notice, while when the woman is relaxed, it is larger and easier to notice. The woman should not be discouraged if the first several attempts of finding her G-spot, whether done alone or with her male partner, are not successful. It sometimes takes multiple explorations before the G-spot is found, and locating it can be a lot of fun. However, some women do not have a G-spot. Therefore, after a large number of unsuccessful attempts of searching for the G-spot, the woman should accept that she does not have a G-spot.

G-Spot Stimulation and the Urge to Urinate

When the G-spot is stimulated, the woman sometimes experiences an uncomfortable feeling that is confused with sensations of having to urinate. This happens because when the G-spot is stimulated, it results in the stimulation of the urethral wall. The woman's feeling that she has to urinate as a result of the G-spot being stimulated is very normal. However, it is the woman's ignorance of that fact that causes her to tense up, stop thinking of the sexual stimulation and pleasure, and start worrying about urinating by accident. This eventually causes her to stop the sexual stimulation and go to the bathroom believing that she has to urinate, although in reality she does not have to urinate.

However, the proper course of action for the woman to take is to urinate before being stimulated sexually. That way she knows for certain she does not have to urinate when her G-spot is stimulated. When her G-spot is stimulated and she feels the urge to urinate, she should have the sexual stimulation continue unchanged. She should do so because after 2 to 20 seconds of G-spot stimulation the urge to urinate should turn to erotic pleasure and the G-spot area should begin to swell. As the G-spot area swells, the area should feel warm and wonderful. The continued stimulation of the G-spot eventually will lead to an orgasm.

Feelings of Inadequacy

Some women feel inferior and inadequate because they do not seem to have a G-spot. Other women feel inferior and inadequate because they cannot ejaculate during sex. There is a minimal difference in the psychological and physiological sexual satisfaction between the women who have a G-spot and those who do not. Also, there is a minimal difference in the physiological and psychological sexual satisfaction between the women who ejaculate during sex and those who do not. Therefore, a woman should not feel inferior and inadequate if she does not seem to have a G-spot or if she does not ejaculate during sex, because there is a little difference in the physiological and psychological sexual satisfaction between the women who have these things and the ones that do not. In other words, if the woman has a G-spot or ejaculates during sex, that is wonderful. But if she does not seem to have a G-spot or does not ejaculate during sex, that is wonderful also. Female ejaculation should not become something a woman strives for during sex. If the female ejaculation happens, then it happens. If it does not happen, then it does not happen. The G-spot is just one more avenue of pleasure to investigate, nothing more.

The Existence of the G-Spot and Female Ejaculation Debated

Since its discovery, the existence of the G-spot has been hotly debated by doctors and sex therapists. There is no agreement among the experts whether the G-spot actually exists. Controversy over the existence of the G-spot has many medical professionals divided. On one hand, there are medical professionals that believe that the G-spot actually exists. While on the other hand, there are medical professionals that believe the

G-spot does not actually exist. They believe that the concept of the G-spot is nothing more than wishful thinking that has no real scientific backup. Some medical professionals believe that the G-spot has no significance.

Furthermore, medical professionals are divided over whether female ejaculation actually exists. Skeptics from the profession have maintained that women that seem to ejaculate are not ejaculating, but are simply peeing during sex. To them female ejaculation is simply a minor medical problem called stress incontinence. They believe it should be treated with surgery or Kegel exercises to tighten up the pelvic muscles.

However, such controversies in the medical profession should not confuse the average person. The G-spot does exist in a large number of women. But there are some women that do not seem to have a G-spot. Also, a large number of women ejaculate during sex. But there are some women who do not ejaculate during sex.

History of the G-Spot

The G-spot is named after gynecologist Ernst Grafenburg, who first described it in 1950. However, before Grafenburg described it and made it known to the western world, it was well known to the ancient Chinese and Indians. In ancient Chinese and Indian writings, the G-spot is described as a sacred spot. In these writings, this area was thought to hold the key to female sexual pleasure. Today, the G-spot is thought by some to be the equivalent of the prostate gland in men.

Chapter 8

The Male P-Spot

The P-spot is found exclusively in men, and not in women. It is known as the male G-spot. It is the male prostate gland. The prostate gland is a gland the size of a walnut that lies just below the man's bladder, at the base of the penis. It is located behind the pubic bone and just in front of the rectum. It is at the center of the man's internal sexual organs. Its shape is that of a walnut. It is a firm organ. Its main job is to produce the milky fluid that is one of the main components of semen. This fluid helps the sperm survive in the vagina.

Most people, when they think of male sexuality, they simply think of the penis and testicles. They overlook the prostate. This is the case because most people do not know that the prostate is an erogenous zone. The prostate is one of the most erotic parts of the male body because it is surrounded by numerous nerve bundles. These nerve bundles pass by the prostate on their way to the penis. They are essential for the male erection. Pressing on those nerves is extremely pleasurable. The prostate responds to direct stimulation by producing intense pleasurable feelings, leading to intense orgasms. During orgasm, the prostate contracts, helping produce extremely pleasurable sensations. During orgasm, the prostate contracts, helping produce an ejaculation.

Locating and Stimulating the P-Spot

There are two ways to locate and stimulate the prostate gland. One way is internally through the anus, and the other way is externally through the perineum. Both ways produce extreme pleasure to the man, leading to an intense orgasm.

Before using either method to stimulate the P-spot, the woman should make sure to cut her fingernails very short and to smooth out any ragged edges. She should also use either a glove, a condom, or a finger cot to cover her finger and nail during the prostate massage, internally or externally. The woman should cut her fingernails and cover her finger and nail to make the man more comfortable during the internal or external P-spot stimulation. The tip of the nail can cause a lot of damage to the walls of the anus and rectum when the prostate is stimulated internally. However, if the tip of the nail is covered with a glove, condom, or a finger cot, and cut short, then the tip of the nail won't cause any damage.

The rectum, anus, and perineum do not produce their own lubrication, so a woman should lubricate her finger, the man's rectum, and his anus if she is going to stimulate the prostate from inside. However, if she is going to stimulate the prostate externally through the perineum, then the woman should lubricate her finger and the man's perineum. It is important that the woman lubricate her finger and the area that she is going to stimulate because without lubrication friction will be produced during the stimulation of the P-spot. This friction will lead to a decrease in the pleasurable sensations produced, and maybe even to pain.

For more intense P-spot stimulation, the couple should try stimulating the prostate gland internally through the anus. The man should lie on his back with his knees bent and the soles of his feet resting on the floor. His legs should be wide open so that the woman kneels between them. Then the woman should gently stroke the opening of the man's anus. If the man becomes aroused, the woman should start to insert her index finger into the anal opening. She should insert her index finger with the palm of her hand up, so that the finger points towards the stomach as it enters. If she notices that the man's anus is tightening up when she inserts the index finger, she should not force her way inside. Instead, she should maintain the same pressure until she notices the tightening loosen. Then it is safe for the woman to push her finger in further, following the natural course of the anus and rectum.

The woman will most likely notice a definite tightening of the anus several times as she pushes her finger further in before reaching the front wall of the rectum. These are the anal sphincters at work. It is important that if the woman feels that the man's anus is tightening that she does not force her way inside. Rather, she should wait until the anal muscles relax while maintaining the same pressure. While waiting for the muscles to relax, the woman could massage or lick the man's scrotum, penis, or inner thighs, which would help the man's anal muscles relax.

When the woman's finger is in as far as it can reach, at the front wall of the rectum, she will notice a small bulge. This is the prostate gland. It should feel firm, the size of a walnut. Below the prostate the woman may feel a small soft dimple, which some men find as sensitive as the prostate, if not more so. The prostate is not inside the rectum. It is very near the wall of the rectum. Stimulating the front wall of the rectum, where the prostate is close to it, should stimulate the prostate. The prostate gland is reachable with the smallest lady index finger because it can be reached two or three inches inside the anus.

To stimulate the prostate, the woman should slowly massage the front wall of the rectum. She should massage the front wall of the rectum by moving her index finger gently, as if she was beckoning another person to come to her. She should move her index finger from the bottom of the front wall of the rectum to the top of it when she moves it as if she is beckoning another person to come to her. It is important that the front wall of the rectum is stroked and not poked. It is important that the stroking of the front wall of the rectum is done gently and slowly, so that the man gets the most pleasure from the experience. Also, the stimulation should be a sustained, regular rhythm, so that it gives the maximum pleasure.

When the woman strokes the front wall of the rectum properly as described, she will stimulate the prostate gland, the area surrounding it, and the dimple below it, producing extreme pleasure. Although stimulating the prostate gland produces extreme pleasure to the man, also stimulating the area around the prostate produces extreme pleasure to the man, and should not be overlooked. The dimple below the prostate should be as sensitive as the prostate when stimulated, and in some cases it might be more sensitive than the prostate. Under no circumstance should it be overlooked by the woman when she stimulates the front wall of the rectum. Continued proper stimulation of the prostate should cause the man eventually to experience an intense orgasm. The woman can consistently bring the man to orgasm when she manually stimulates the prostate gland. As a variation, the woman could try stimulating the prostate and the area around it by moving her index finger along the front wall of the rectum gently in a circular fashion. As an alternative, when the woman is stimulating the man's prostate through the anus, she can keep her other hand or mouth busy, too, by pleasuring his scrotum, perineum, or penis. If this is done, then the combination of the sensations produced can be delightful. Always after the woman stimulates the prostate gland through the anus, she should immediately wash her hands.

Usually there are no feces in the anus and the lower rectum, and the woman usually should not run into any feces when stimulating the man's prostate gland through the anus. However, occasionally there is a small amount of feces that may remain in the anus or the lower rectum, and if the woman is concerned about the possibility of running into them when she is stimulating the man's prostate, then she should wear a glove, a finger cot, or a condom on her index finger. Also, if the woman is having this rare problem with her male partner often, then she should ask her partner to use an enema to clean the lower rectum prior to the prostate gland stimulation.

The second way that the woman could stimulate the man's prostate gland is from the outside of his body without putting her finger inside his anus. She would do that by taking her index finger and the middle finger and stimulating the spot of flesh between the scrotum and the anus, which is known as the perineum. She would stimulate it three quarters of the way down from the scrotum, where a small indentation under the skin is felt. She would stimulate the perineum at that location, because the prostate gland is located above the dent. The prostate gland rests directly on top of the perineum at that location, and stimulating the perineum at that location will stimulate the prostate. This will cause the man a lot of pleasure and will lead to an intense orgasm. Also, the perineum has plenty of nerve endings of its own, so rubbing the perineum to stimulate the prostate stimulates not only the nerves of the prostate indirectly, but it also stimulates the nerves of the perineum directly. This leads to more pleasure than just stimulating the nerves of the prostate. The woman would stimulate the prostate gland by rubbing the perineum at the dent from side to side, top to bottom, or in a circular fashion gently, using the index finger and the middle finger. She would rub gently since this is a delicate little gland.

All of the perineum, from the scrotum to the anus, is a very sensual area. Also, as a variation the woman could stimulate the prostate gland by stimulating all of the perineum, not only the area where the prostate is located. She could stimulate the whole area while emphasizing the area where the prostate is located using the index and the middle finger. Using the index and the middle finger, she would rub from side to side, top to bottom, or in a circular fashion. She would rub gently and not too hard. She should rub gently since this is a delicate area. If the woman stimulates the perineum when the man is aroused, it will squeeze more blood into the man's penis, causing the man to feel more pleasure. If the woman performs the external stimulation of the prostate gland through the perineum and combines it with manual stimulation of the man's penis or oral sex on the man's penis, this will give the man tremendous pleasure and might lead to a full body orgasm.

Most men and women judge a man's arousal by the angle of his erection. This should not be done, since the angle of the man's erection does not give a clue of his arousal, nor the degree of pleasure that he is experiencing. As a matter of fact, when a woman stimulates different parts of the man's body such as his perineum or prostate gland, it is possible that he does not experience an erection or that he loses the one that he has, even though he is experiencing intense pleasure and is greatly aroused. This happens because men sometimes lose their erection or do not experience an erection when they are receptive sexually. Once the man takes the initiative in the sex act, he usually experiences an erection or regains his lost erection.

Reluctance to Stimulate the P-Spot

Many men are reluctant to have their female partner stimulate their P-spot. The main reason why they are reluctant is because they had no experience with their prostate being stimulated. The fact that they had no prior experience where they had their prostate stimulated makes them afraid of the unknown. They are afraid of the experience, not knowing what to expect. They are not sure whether they will like the experience or be repulsed by it. The fear towards the experience also includes the fear that they may experience pain as a result of the experience. A second reason why many men are reluctant to have their female partner stimulate their P-spot is because they incorrectly believe that such an experience is dirty, unnatural, and awkward. The third reason why some men are reluctant to have their female partner stimulate their P-spot is because if they did have an experience involving their prostate, it was with a doctor in an examining room, and that experience was painful and unpleasant.

The man should understand that there is nothing unknown or painful about the experience of having the P-spot stimulated. Rather, the man should understand that the experience will definitely be a pleasurable experience and that it will lead to an intense orgasm. Furthermore, the man should understand that there is nothing unnatural, dirty, or awkward about the experience where the woman stimulates his P-spot. The man should understand that if the experience was unnatural or awkward, it would not be pleasurable and it would not lead to an intense orgasm. In addition, the man should understand that if he ever had an experience involving a doctor examining his prostate, that experience was painful and unpleasant because the doctor did not stimulate his prostate properly. The doctor did not stimulate his prostate properly because he or she was giving him a health exam. However, the man should understand that since his female partner will be stimulating his P-spot properly, he will only experience pleasure and no pain.

Benefits of Stimulating the P-Spot

Stimulating the prostate gland has several benefits. The first benefit is that it maintains a healthy prostate. The second benefit is that it cures an inflamed prostate. It does so by getting rid of built-up pus and dead cells. When it cures an inflamed prostate it makes a man's life more pleasant because it stops the previous blockage of the flow of urine that resulted from the prostate being inflamed. Third, it relieves pelvic congestion that results from a man not having any form of sex for a while. Fourth, it pleasures the man, giving him an intense orgasm. Fifth, it decreases the chance that the man will get prostate cancer.

History of the P-Spot

The prostate, is a well-documented joy button throughout history. In ancient Indian writings, stimulating the prostate is described as being very pleasurable to the man. In the early 1900s, women were urged to buy prostate massagers to service their husband during intercourse. During World War II, American military medics would give prostate massages to servicemen to relieve them of pelvic congestion that resulted from not having any form of sex for a while.

Before antibiotics were widely used, the prostate was stimulated to relieve it of built-up pus and dead cells. This was done in order to shrink it if it was inflamed. Shrinking an inflamed prostate put an end to the blockage of the flow of urine that resulted from an inflamed prostate. Also, the prostate was stimulated before antibiotics were widely used to maintain a healthy prostate.

Similarities Between the P-Spot and the G-Spot

The P-spot and the G-spot are very similar in many ways. The first way they are both similar is they both are the size of a walnut. The second way they both are similar is that both of them are made up of textured erectile tissue that swells with arousal. The third way they both are similar is that they are wrapped around the urethra. The fourth way they are both similar is that they produce ejaculatory fluid. The fifth way they both are similar is that they both produce extreme pleasure and even an orgasm when stimulated. The sixth way they both are similar is that the G-spot is located between the bladder and the clitoris, while the P-spot is located between the bladder and the penis. The seventh way they both are similar is that the G-spot has nerves that connect to the clitoris, while the P-spot has nerves that connect to the penis.

It should not be a surprise that the P-spot and the G-spot are similar since all embryos start out female with the same basic infrastructure, nerves, and tissue types. All embryos, when they start out, look exactly the same. Embryos with a Y chromosome then develop the male sex organs. The clitoris becomes the penis. The ovaries become the testicles. The uterus and vagina remain undeveloped and become the prostatic utricle, or male uterus. The male uterus is about a quarter of an inch long and is located in the center of the prostate. Most important of all, the G-spot becomes the P-spot or prostate gland. The fact that the G-spot becomes the P-spot in the male embryo explains the similarities between the G-spot and the P-spot.

Chapter 9

Masturbation

Masturbation is when a person, male or female, stimulates his or her genital for sexual pleasure, most often to reach orgasm. Masturbation was once thought to have negative effects on the human body. It was believed that masturbation caused insanity, hair loss, acne, heart disease, seizure, idiocy, blindness, warts, memory loss, physical weakness, impotence, and defects in new born babies. It was believed that masturbation was a dangerous waste of male or female fluids. It was also believed that masturbation altered the shape of the male or female genital. Some people believed that if the woman pulled on her labia during masturbation, that it will stretch out of shape. Some people believed that if the man used his right hand to masturbate his penis, his penis will start to curve towards the right. These old myths that prevailed in the past cause some people to this day to be frightened of masturbation and think that it is unhealthy. Some people to this day cannot get rid of these incorrect myths, thus they incorrectly find masturbation as wrong, evil, uncivilized, depressing, lonely, empty, dirty, and cheap. But masturbation should not frighten anyone because the American Medical Association has declared masturbation to be normal. An almost unanimous perspective in the field of sexuality today is that masturbation is healthy, desirable, and an important part of adult sexual behavior.

Masturbation is healthy, natural, normal, and it has no negative side effect. It is a natural and healthy part of sexual behavior for people of all ages. It is not a dangerous waste of male or female fluids since the fluids are always replenished by the body. Most important of all, masturbation does not alter the shape of the man's genital or the woman's genital. Today, most men and women view masturbation as a natural part of life. However, most people still do not admit to masturbation, nor discuss it.

The basic reason for a man or a woman to masturbate is simply he or she wants to have an orgasm. But in fact, masturbation has benefits beyond just feeling good. It keeps a man or woman's organs working in proper order. It keeps the man or the woman's sex muscles in shape and working in proper order. Many people use masturbation to relieve stress and to get rid of tension so that they can sleep. The emotional and physical release as a result of masturbation decreases tension and irritability. Some people masturbate to relieve sexual frustration. Masturbation gives a person a sexual outlet if circumstances prevent him or her from having sex with a partner. Masturbation relieves menstrual cramps in some women. It gives a person something to do if he or she is bored and alone.

Through masturbation, a person can learn to orgasm. By masturbating regularly, a person can make his or her orgasms bigger, quicker, and more reliable. Through masturbation, a person can learn to bring himself or herself to orgasm at will. Books and therapists may give good advice about climaxing, but a person has to feel what actually works for him or her in order to climax. This a person can do through masturbation. A person can determine his or her sexual potential through masturbation. This is so because masturbation indicates a person's natural desires and sexual behavior. Masturbation allows a person to learn about his or her sexuality and come to terms with it. Masturbation is a highly effective way for a person to become fully orgasmic.

Masturbation is important for increasing a person's sexual pleasure during sex. It allows a person to find out where and how he or she likes to be touched to orgasm. The person then can communicate this information to his or her partner so that his or her partner satisfies him or her sexually. This brings greater pleasure to the couple's sexual experience together.

Masturbation is the way a person can learn to make the most of sex. A woman, through masturbating herself, will learn the difference between the clitoris, labia, urethra, and vagina. She can learn the specifics of how to stimulate her clitoris and vagina in order to have an orgasm. Women who have never had an orgasm with a partner can almost always have one during masturbation quite happily and quickly. This means that a woman can learn to orgasm during sex from masturbation. Men can try to hold off orgasm during masturbation to learn how to prolong sex with a partner. The man during masturbation can get in touch with the feelings that come before he reaches the point of ejaculation. Then he can identify those feelings during sex, and therefore hold off on ejaculation until the woman is ready. If a man learns to masturbate for a half hour or more before he ejaculates, then he can probably teach himself to last longer during sex. Masturbation also increases blood flow to the man's genital and the woman's genital and makes orgasms easier for them to achieve during sex. Masturbation will enable the man and the woman to assume responsibility for their share of the sex act and will make them more capable of giving and receiving pleasure.

Proof that Masturbation is Normal

Proof that masturbation is natural and normal is that animals naturally do it. Female mammals may resort to rubbing their sensitive genitalia rhythmically on the ground or on sharp projections, thus creating the stimulus of a penis jerking in and out. Female cats do this kind of stimulated intercourse. Further proof that masturbation is natural and normal is that some children begin masturbating at a young age without even knowing what it is they are doing. Others, when they are teenagers, stumble upon masturbation by accident. They feel an urge between their legs, then begin to rub themselves, and then unexpectedly reach orgasm.

Masturbation and Relationships

People in a relationship, especially married people, are more likely to masturbate than people that are single and not in a relationship. People in a relationship tend to masturbate more than people that are single and not in a relationship because they view masturbation as a valuable complement to the sex that they have with their partner. If people in a relationship masturbate, it does not mean that their partner does not turn them on. It just means that they like experiencing sexual pleasure by themselves in addition to the sex that they enjoy with their partner. Another reason people in a relationship masturbate is that they might have a higher sex drive than their partner and just need some more sexual stimulation to be satisfied sexually. Furthermore, people in a relationship might masturbate because of a physical condition that prevents them from having sex with their partner. For example, the woman might have just had a baby and cannot have sex for the next six weeks, so the man could masturbate to satisfy himself sexually during that time.

It is important that when a person sees his or her partner masturbate, that he or she realizes that it does not mean that he or she is an inadequate lover, and that there is nothing wrong with the love or the sex in the relationship. The person should not view the fact that his or her partner masturbates as a criticism of his or her desirability, nor as a personal rejection. Also, the person that masturbates should let his or her partner know that his or her partner is an adequate lover and that in addition to the wonderful sex that they have together, masturbation is something he or she enjoys doing on his or her own.

When Masturbation Becomes a Problem

Masturbation becomes a problem if a person lets it interfere with his or her normal life. There are several ways it could interfere with a person's normal life. The first way is that a person masturbates a lot that it distracts him or her from his or her work and does not allow him or her to perform his or her work properly. The second way is that it distracts a person from his or her friendships and family relationships. The third way is that a person masturbates to the point that he or she does not want to have sex with his or her partner. If a person masturbates often, even a couple of times a day, that is okay as long as it does not interfere with his or her normal life. In order to make sure that masturbation is not a problem, a person should make sure that it in no way interferes with his or her work, friendships, family relationships, sexual relationship with his or her partner, and any other aspect of his or her life.

If a person is in a relationship or married, sex with his or her partner should take precedence over masturbation. If a person lets masturbation take precedence over sex with his or her partner, then that will sabotage his or her relationship, causing both partners to become distant from each other. In a relationship, a person has a responsibility to create an amazing sex life with his or her partner. Therefore sex with a partner should take precedence over masturbation. If a person chooses masturbation over sex with his or her partner, then the person has a problem, and he or she has to correct it by changing his or her attitude.

Another instance where masturbation becomes a problem is if a person experiences emotional distress or guilt because of it. Masturbation has no negative physical or emotional effect, however if a person has been conditioned to think that masturbation is wrong, dirty, evil, or uncivilized, then when he or she does it, he or she will experience unnecessary emotional distress and guilt. The way for a person to overcome such a problem is for him or her to realize that masturbation is healthy, clean, and normal behavior. Once a person comes to realize that, then when he or she masturbates, he or she will not experience emotional distress or guilt.

Masturbation Techniques for Males

Males masturbate in many different ways because each body has a unique way that stimulates it. Every man has his own masturbation style. Before masturbating, a person should make sure that the atmosphere is completely relaxed and that he will not be disturbed. A person could do that by disconnecting the phone, closing the curtains, and shutting the room door. A person should give himself enough time to masturbate, so that he does it without rushing, and so that he remains relaxed. Some men masturbate while standing up. However, usually a man masturbates by lying on the bed, so that he is completely relaxed. Some men even get totally naked when they lie down on the bed, so that they are fully relaxed when masturbating. Whatever position the man chooses to masturbate, he usually ejaculates into tissues, a towel, or clothing.

In order to start a masturbation session, a man should decide what is the best way for him to start a masturbation session. There are several ways that a person could start a masturbation session. The first way is by a person thinking up a fantasy. The second way is by a person checking out pictures in a pornographic magazine. The third way is by a person watching an X-rated movie. The fourth way is by a person calling a phone sex hotline. The fifth way is by a person doing nothing before masturbating. Before masturbating, the man could place some water-based lubricant on his hands. He would do so to reduce friction during masturbation and to increase the pleasurable sensations during masturbation. The friction produced from masturbating without a lubricant might be painful in some cases.

Before masturbating, the man could fondle his flaccid penis. Then he could shake the penis a little and rub it all over. He would do that until the penis starts to stiffen. When it starts to stiffen, he could begin masturbating.

The first masturbation technique is for the man to grip his penis with one hand and move his hand back and forth from the base to the head, and then from the head to the base. The man could double his pleasure by gently stroking, tugging, massaging, or holding his scrotum and testicles with the second hand at the same time he is masturbating. In addition to touching his testicles, a man can also caress his perineum while masturbating. The second masturbation technique is for the man to place one hand on the base of the penis and then use the other hand to go up and down the shaft and head of the penis while gripping it. The third masturbation technique is for the man to grip his penis with one hand, and move his hand back and forth from the base to the head, and then from the head to the base. The man should gently twist his hand in one direction on the way up, and in the opposite direction on the way down. The fourth masturbation technique is to concentrate stimulation directly on the head of the penis. The person could do that by gripping the head of the penis with one hand, and using that hand to directly stimulate only the head by moving back and forth on the head. The man could grip the shaft of the penis with the second hand and only stimulate the shaft with the second hand by moving the hand back and forth on the shaft. The man would move both hands simultaneously. The head of the penis is one of the most sensitive parts of the penis.

The fifth masturbation technique is for the man to grip the penis with one hand at the head of the penis, and then move his hand from side to side continuously. The sixth masturbation technique is for the man to grasp the penis with both hands, one on top of the other, and then move both hands up the shaft and head of the penis and back down again. The man will have the sensation of thrusting deeply into a long, tight vagina. The man could add variety to this technique by twisting one hand in one direction and the other in the opposite direction as he moves both hands up and down the penis. A seventh masturbation technique is for the man to place one thumb on each side of the frenulum. Then he should move the thumbs up and down, in opposite directions along the frenulum. An eighth masturbation technique is for the man to place one palm of his hand on each side of the penis with his hands open. Then he should move the palms of his hands back and forth, along the length and head of the penis. As an alternative, the man could move the palms of his hands from side to side instead of back and forth.

A ninth masturbation technique is for the man to grasp the penis on the coronal ridge and frenulum with the index finger and thumb and move his fingers up and down on the coronal ridge and frenulum while maintaining them at the coronal ridge and frenulum. The coronal ridge and the frenulum, in addition to the head of the penis, are the most sensitive parts of the man's penis. The sensation produced from this ninth masturbation technique is extremely intense, and some men like climaxing from this kind of movement alone. A tenth masturbation technique is for the man to rub the penis along the bottom of the shaft only, using both of his thumbs. He could rub it by moving both thumbs simultaneously up and down the bottom of the shaft only. An eleventh masturbation technique is for the man to grasp the head of the penis with his right hand and slide his right hand down the shaft of the penis. As he reaches the base of the penis, he should grasp the head of the penis with his left hand. Then he should slide his left hand down the shaft of the penis as his right hand releases and goes back up to the head of the penis. The man should repeat this milking motion, alternating his hands. As an alternative, the man could grasp the penis at the base with his right hand and slide his hand up the shaft and the head. As he reaches the head, he should grasp the penis at the base with his left hand. Then with his left hand he should slide up the shaft as his right hand releases and goes back to the base of the penis.

The man should try all the techniques and choose the ones that he likes. He could use a combination of the techniques in one masturbation session, or he could use just one technique during one masturbation session. Also, the man could use a different technique or a different combination of techniques in each masturbation session, or he could use the same technique or the same combination of techniques in each session. There is no right or wrong way to do it, as long as the man does what brings him the most pleasure and satisfaction.

When masturbating, the man should not put too much pressure on the penis nor too little, since that will decrease the pleasurable sensations. When masturbating, a man could contract and release his PC muscle to increase blood flow to the genital area. This will make the pleasurable feelings during masturbation and during orgasm more intense. While masturbating, a person could breathe slow and deep breaths so that his arousal increases, so that the degree of the pleasurable sensations increases, and so that the intensity of the orgasm increases. When most men masturbate they stroke themselves very quickly, and orgasm as quickly as possible. While masturbating, a man should slow down and enjoy the sensations, since that could lead to more intense pleasurable sensations, and it could lead to a more intense orgasm. When masturbating, the man should find a rhythm that is comfortable to him. Once he finds the rhythm, he should keep it up. It is the continuous rhythm that gives him the stimulation and brings him to orgasm. The man could delay orgasm during masturbation for a short while in order to intensify his orgasm when he climaxes. He could do that by stopping the stimulation of the penis when he feels he is coming close to orgasming. He could stop until the urge to orgasm has subsided. Usually that is around 30 seconds. Then he could resume masturbating and repeating the process as many times as he likes. The more he does this process, the more intense the pleasurable feelings during masturbation and the more intense the pleasurable feelings will be when he orgasms. Then when the man feels he is ready to orgasm he can continue masturbating until he orgasms. No matter how a person masturbates, the outcome of masturbation is usually orgasm and ejaculation.

Masturbation Techniques for Women

Each woman has her individual preference in regards to masturbation. Each woman's body likes to be stimulated differently in order for her to orgasm. In order to start a masturbation session, a woman should make sure that she will not be distracted in any way. She could do that by making sure that the phone is disconnected, the door is closed, the windows are shut, and that the curtains cover the windows. She should give herself ample time to masturbate. That way, she is relaxed and not in a rush. The woman could masturbate either standing up or lying down. Usually, most women masturbate lying down in bed, since that is the most relaxing position to be in. A woman could masturbate with her clothes on, or totally in the nude. Usually, most women masturbate in the nude, since that is extremely relaxing. Therefore, in order to masturbate most women usually lie down in bed, making themselves comfortable by using pillows and blankets and by being totally in the nude.

The woman, in order to get herself aroused sexually for a masturbation session, could either watch an X-rated movie, read a pornographic magazine, or fantasize sexual fantasies. Some women do none of these and just start masturbating. However, before masturbating a woman should put some water-based lubricant on her hands and genital area. A woman should do so because without lubrication the physical stimulation that occurs during a masturbation session might be uncomfortable to her and often painful. With lubrication, the stimulation that occurs during a masturbation session is more pleasurable. It is better for a woman to have too much lubricant than too little.

The woman could start the masturbation session by exploring her body very gently with her hands. She could touch her legs, breasts, stomach, and chest very gently. She should feel the texture and warmth of her skin as she touches her body parts. After that, she should bring her hands down between her legs. She can pull her pubic hair in small tufts, working her way slowly from where her pubic hair starts to where it ends. Pulling her pubic hair causes an exquisite pricking sensation. She can use one, two, or three fingers to trace her labia majora from top to bottom, gently and lightly. Then she can use one, two, or three fingers to trace her labia minora gently and lightly. She can trace her labia minora by going from the bottom of one labium minora to the top of it, over the clitoris hood, and then down the other labium minora. For a variation, the woman could pull the labia minora and the labia majora gently as she touches them with her fingers. The pulling move will intensify the pleasurable sensations that the woman feels as she touches them, because stretched skin tends to have greater feeling. Then she could slide her fingers lightly and gently along the space between her labia majora and the sides of her clitoris. Then she could touch lightly and gently around the clitoris in a circular manner. Then, using her fingers, she could circle the entrance to her vagina lightly and gently, but not enter it yet. The woman should have her fingers linger at the entrance to her vagina and around the clitoris until she is very wet and engorged. The more lubricated and engorged she is, the more pleasurable her masturbation will be. It is important that up to this point, the woman does not rub any part of her genital area. It is important that up to this point, the woman only touches lightly and gently the parts of her genital area.

Once a woman starts to masturbate, she usually goes to the clitoris. One way a woman could masturbate is by removing the clitoral hood, placing her finger on the head of the clitoris, and then rubbing the head of the clitoris directly with her finger in a circular manner. When she rubs the head of the clitoris, she should touch it only lightly, and gradually build up pressure as she becomes more aroused. She should rub the head of the clitoris this way, because it is the most sexually sensitive part of a woman's body. It is so sensitive, that it is painful to the woman if it is stimulated too roughly. A second way for the woman to masturbate is by her stimulating the clitoral ridge and the tip of the clitoris. The clitoral ridge and the tip of the clitoris would be in between the index and the middle finger, and the woman would move the fingers straight up and down or in a circular motion. The woman could also move the fingers in a combination, both straight up and down and in a circular motion. Often, a woman uses this technique to stimulate herself. A woman could also use the palm of her hand, to stimulate the ridge and the tip of the clitoris. A third way a woman could masturbate is by her having the shaft of the clitoris between the index and the middle finger, and rubbing it by going up and down with both fingers. The shaft of the clitoris is less sensitive than the head of the clitoris. Therefore, some women might find this technique not as pleasurable as the technique where the head of the clitoris is stimulated directly. A fourth way for the woman to masturbate is for her to slide a finger up and down the left side of her clitoris shaft several times. Then she could slide her finger up and down the right side of her clitoris shaft several times. She would repeat this process until she climaxes. This technique produces extreme pleasure. The woman can vary the direction of the movement of her fingers along the shaft. Instead of her moving her fingers up and down the shaft, she can move them from side to side.

All the methods of masturbating previously mentioned are direct methods of stimulating the clitoris. However, some women do not like direct stimulation of their clitoris because it is too sensitive. For most women, indirect stimulation of the clitoris is perfectly adequate to reach orgasm. The following ways of masturbating are indirect ways of stimulating the clitoris. A fifth way a woman could masturbate is by rubbing the clitoral hood. The woman could rub the clitoral hood firmly and gently using one finger, two fingers, three fingers, or the whole hand. As a result of the rubbing, the woman should feel the clitoris become erect. The sixth way a woman could masturbate is by rubbing the area surrounding the clitoris, including beneath it, in an up-and-down motion, side-to-side motion, or in a circular fashion. The woman would do so using a finger, two fingers, three fingers, or the palm of her hand. Rubbing around the clitoris will probably be more pleasurable than massaging the clitoris itself because the clitoris may be too tender to massage directly. The seventh way a woman could masturbate is by rubbing the labia minora. By the woman rubbing the labia minora, she indirectly stimulates the clitoris. The labia minora are the delicate pair of inner lips that surround the clitoris. They are highly sensitive. They seem to be very important as sources of erotic arousal. A majority of women who masturbate do so by stroking both the labia minora and the clitoris. The labia majora are the pair of outer lips. They tend to be much less erotically sensitive than the inner ones.

As an alternative, a woman could masturbate by stimulating the clitoris indirectly for a while, and then she could stimulate the clitoris directly for a while. She could keep on repeating this process until she orgasms. As a variation, the woman using her fingers could rub from the clitoris to the vagina and then back again. She could also rub from underneath the clitoris, right over the clitoris head, to above the clitoris using her fingers. She could also rub across the head of the clitoris from one side to the other using her fingers.

When using any masturbation technique to stimulate the clitoris directly or indirectly, the woman should start out very gently touching the skin, and then gradually build up pressure as she becomes more aroused. The woman should start out masturbating extremely slowly. Then she should increase the speed of her hand movement gradually during masturbation until she reaches a speed that she feels is ideal. As a woman approaches orgasm, it is important that she maintains a steady rhythm. It is not proper for her to vary the pace, pressure, or activity as she approaches orgasm.

The other area a woman could stimulate in order to masturbate is the vagina. The more engorged the woman's vagina is, the more sensitive it will be. The more sensitive it is, the more intense the pleasurable feelings produced during masturbation will be. In order for the woman to get her vagina engorged as much as possible, she can massage her labia majora and labia minora and draw them away from her vagina. She can also try rubbing them together. The entrance to the vagina is an erogenous zone for most women. It is only the couple of inches of the vagina at the vaginal entrance that are richly supplied with nerve endings. The deep interior walls of the vagina have few nerve endings and are quite insensitive when stroked or lightly touched. Therefore, when the woman masturbates using the vagina, she should be concerned only with the outer couple of inches of the vagina, at the vagina entrance. She should not be concerned with the deep interior walls of the vagina. In order for the woman to masturbate the vagina, she should slowly insert a clean forefinger into the vagina. When she inserts the finger inside the vagina she should enter it slowly, since by entering it slowly it is more arousing to the vagina. If she enters the vagina slowly, her vagina will be more sensitive and receptive to stimulation. This will make the pleasurable feelings produced during masturbation, more pleasurable.

The woman should use the finger to touch different parts of the vagina, including the top, bottom, and side walls. She should also touch the rough end of the passageway, at the cervix. She should see how each area feels when touched. She will probably find that some areas are more sensitive than others, and that the sensitive areas produce a more pleasurable feeling than the other areas. She should use her finger to stimulate the areas that are more sensitive than the rest. She could stimulate those areas by rubbing them with her finger in an up-and-down motion, a side-to-side motion, or in a circular motion. This will produce a pleasurable sensation that seems to extend vaguely into parts of her body. It is a warm sensation, making a woman breathless and perhaps wanting to tense her legs. The more the woman stimulates those areas with her finger, the more the sensation will increase. This sensation is not an orgasm, but it is the prelude to one. If the woman keeps it up, sooner or later the orgasm will follow. The orgasm will be a sudden intense climax of the pleasurable sensations that occur as a result of the stimulation.

When the woman is masturbating using the vagina, if she has a G-spot she can stimulate the G-spot. The G-spot is located at the upper inner wall of the woman's vagina. Many women get a great deal of pleasure from the stimulation of this sensitive area on the front wall of their vagina. However, some women do not seem to have a G-spot. In order for the woman to locate her G-spot, she should stimulate her labia and clitoris before starting to look for it. She should do so because it is easier for her to find the G-spot if she is fully aroused. The G-spot will be felt more clearly the more aroused she becomes. Then she should slide two fingers into her vagina, keeping her hand palm side up so her fingertips can brush against the front top part of her vaginal wall. She can press her fingers against the front wall of her vagina, as she moves them in and out in search of the G-spot. She can also move her fingers in a side-to-side motion, circular motion, or a zigzag motion in search of the G-spot. If she has a G-spot, she will feel a small knob of firm flesh, about the size of a bean or two. It feels like a small lump. It is located midway between her cervix and pubic bone.

The G-spot will increase in size as the woman stimulates it. The G-spot does not respond well to gentle touching and stroking. It responds best to firm, deep, continuous pressure. The woman could rub the G-spot on the upper inner wall of the vagina, using the fingertips of her index and middle finger. She could have the index and middle finger continuously press firmly with deep pressure against the G-spot as they rub it. Another way for the woman to stimulate the G-spot is to exert a steady pressure with her finger on the spot, pushing for a count of ten, then letting go, then pressing again. It is pressure on the G-spot rather than light stroking that brings on the erotic sensations and can trigger climax. The woman can press on her abdomen with the other hand to heighten the pleasurable sensations felt, while masturbating the G-spot. The woman goes wild and sometimes gushes fluid when she climaxes from stimulation of the G-spot. Many women say orgasms from the G-spot are more powerful than clitoral orgasms.

It is important to note that some women feel discomfort or even the urge to urinate when the G-spot is rubbed. This is normal, and is because of the G-spot's proximity to a woman's urethra and bladder. If the woman patiently continues to stimulate the G-spot, despite the discomfort or the urge to urinate, then the discomfort and the urge to urinate will generally turn to pleasure. If a woman is worried about this seeming need to urinate, she can empty her bladder first, or try finding the spot herself in the privacy of the bathroom.

Many women, whether they have a G-spot or not, find it very pleasurable to have the top of their vagina stimulated during masturbation. A woman could make her index finger into a shape of a hook, pointing upward, and insert it into the vagina. She could use the finger in such a shape to stimulate the top of the vagina by moving it in an up-and-down manner, side-to-side manner, or in a circular manner. The sensations produced are extremely pleasurable. Also, a woman could squeeze the vaginal muscles while her finger is stimulating the vagina, this will intensify the pleasurable feelings produced during masturbation. Also, squeezing the vaginal muscles while the finger is stimulating the vagina produces a sucking feeling. While stimulating the vagina, the woman should use a slow and gentle hand. The cervix is usually deep inside a woman's vagina, and the woman should avoid hitting it during masturbation because that can be painful.

Another masturbation technique is for the woman to stimulate the vagina and the clitoris at the same time. She can use one or two fingers of one hand to stimulate around the clitoris in a circular motion, while she uses a finger or two of the other hand to rub inside the vagina in an in-and-out motion. If the woman stimulates the vagina and the clitoris at the same time, it can lead to extremely intense explosive orgasms. If the woman has a G-spot, she can stimulate the G-spot at the same time she stimulates the clitoris. She can use a finger or two of one hand to stimulate around the clitoris in a circular motion while she uses a finger or two of the other hand to rub the G-spot in an in-and-out motion. This will lead to the most intense full body orgasm that a woman could experience.

In order to make the masturbation session more pleasurable, the woman could do the following. First, if a masturbation technique involves the use of one hand only, she can use the other hand to stimulate her nipples, breasts, inner thighs, buttocks, or anus. Second, a woman could put a vibrator in her vagina when masturbating the clitoris, even though she does not use the vibrator to stimulate the vagina. Women that do this find that having something to contract around during an orgasm is far more satisfying than orgasming with an empty vagina. Third, in order to intensify the pleasurable feelings during masturbation and orgasm, the woman could delay orgasm several times during a masturbation session. The woman could do so by stopping stimulation when she gets close to an orgasm. She would wait until the urge to orgasm subsides then she could resume masturbation. She could repeat this process as many times as she likes. The more she does it the more intense the pleasurable feelings during masturbation become and the more intense the pleasurable feelings during orgasm will be. When the woman feels like it, she can masturbate until she orgasms. Fourth, a woman should not stroke one spot for too long during masturbation, because that will decrease the pleasurable sensations and could even numb the area. Fifth, a woman should contract and release her PC muscle during masturbation to increase blood flow and arousal. This will make the orgasm easier and more intense. Sixth, a woman could breathe slowly and deeply. If a woman breathes slowly and deeply, that will increase her arousal and the intensity of the pleasurable feelings during masturbation and orgasm. Seventh, a woman should keep a steady rhythm during masturbation, since that will increase the pleasurable feelings during masturbation. Eighth, when the woman masturbates, she should rub slowly and gently back and forth or in a circular motion. She should not rub too hard or too fast because that will cause an orgasm not to occur. If she tries to force an orgasm, it will end up causing an unpleasant sensation instead. Ninth, a woman should know that not all orgasms are the same. She should know that sometimes she will experience a very powerful and intense orgasm, while at other times her orgasm is just a gentle wave of release. Finally, every woman is different, and it is best for the woman to find out, what masturbation techniques she likes. The best way for the woman to climax as quickly as possible is to relax and do exactly what pleases her.

Any woman can achieve an orgasm if she masturbates. Most women can even achieve multiple orgasms during masturbation. Most women can achieve an orgasm in three to five minutes when masturbating alone. If a woman is slower than average in climaxing, she can improve with practice. During masturbation, many women can reach orgasm just as fast as males. Many women do not know how to masturbate automatically. They discover through practice the proper ways for them to masturbate. Masturbation can put a woman on the right path to orgasm. She can learn exactly what moves will bring her to a climax through masturbation. Masturbation lets a woman acquire control over her own sexual response.

A Woman Masturbating During Pregnancy

It is safe for a woman to masturbate during pregnancy. The increased blood flow in the genital region of the woman due to pregnancy causes the woman's genital region to become very sensitive. Thus, the sensations produced when the pregnant woman masturbates including orgasms are a lot more pleasurable. The pregnant woman should use a lot of lubricant during masturbation so that she does not experience pain as a result of friction. She should use a lubricant during masturbation to increase the pleasurable sensations.

A woman can use a vibrator during masturbation, even if she is pregnant. However, a woman should not use a vibrator inside the vagina during masturbation after the second trimester. It is safe to use a vibrator during the first and second trimester of the woman's pregnancy. However, the vibrations of a vibrator may feel too intense and uncomfortable because of the increased blood flow to the vulva, clitoris, and vagina, as a result of the pregnancy.

Chapter 10

Manual Stimulation by the Opposite Sex

Manual stimulation by the opposite sex is the same as masturbation, except instead of the person stimulating himself or herself manually, his or her partner stimulates him or her manually. Manual sex serves an important role. It gets a person accustomed gradually to a sexual situation where another person is in physical control. Manual stimulation is very satisfying to the person receiving it, whether the person is male or female. A woman giving manual stimulation to a man is often called giving the man a hand job. It can also be called masturbating the man or jerking the man off. A man giving the woman manual stimulation is called giving the woman a hand job or masturbating the woman.

Manual Stimulation Techniques for Males

Every woman likes to manually stimulate her partner differently, and every male likes to be manually stimulated by his partner differently. Before manual stimulation, the man and the woman should make sure that the atmosphere is completely relaxed and that they will not be disturbed. The couple could do that by disconnecting the phone, closing the curtains, and shutting the room door. The couple should give themselves enough time for manual stimulation, so that they do it without rushing, and so that they remain relaxed. Some couples do the manual stimulation with the man and the woman standing up, facing each other. Other couples do it with the man standing and the woman kneeling, facing him.

However, the most comfortable position for the couple is for the man to lie on his back with his legs straight, and for the woman to be in a kneeling position between his legs, facing his upper body and not his feet. The couple could do it with both partners fully clothed, or with one partner fully clothed. However, the most comfortable, relaxing, and arousing way, is for both partners to be totally in the nude. Whatever position the couple chooses, usually the woman has tissues, a towel, or clothing nearby for the man to ejaculate into.

Before starting the manual stimulation session, the woman could place some water-based lubricant on her hands. She would do so to reduce friction during manual stimulation and to increase the pleasurable sensations to the man. The friction produced from manually stimulating a man without a lubricant might be painful in some cases. To begin the manual stimulation session, the woman should gently place her hand palm down on the man's penis. The woman should then place her other hand palm down on the man's scrotum and cover his scrotum with her hand. She should just let both hands rest there for a while and not move them. The man should feel the natural heat and energy from the woman's hands and start to get aroused, anticipating what is to come. Then the woman could shake the penis a little, and rub it with one hand. With the second hand, the woman could caress the scrotum. She would do that until the penis starts to stiffen. When the penis starts to stiffen, she can start manually stimulating the man.

The first manual stimulation technique is for the woman to grip the man's penis with one hand, and move her hand back and forth from the base to the head, and then from the head to the base. The woman could double the man's pleasure by gently stroking, tugging, massaging, or holding his scrotum and testicles with the second hand at the same time she is manually stimulating him. In addition to touching the man's testicles, a woman can caress his perineum while manually stimulating him. The second manual stimulation technique is for the woman to place one hand on the base of the penis and then use the other hand to go up and down the shaft and head of the penis while gripping it. The third manual stimulation technique is for the woman to grip the man's penis with one hand and move her hand back and forth from the base to the head, and then from the head to the base. The woman should gently twist her hand in one direction on the way up, and in the opposite direction on the way down. The fourth manual stimulation technique is for the woman to concentrate stimulation directly on the head of the penis. The woman could do that by gripping the head of the penis with one hand and using that hand to directly stimulate only the head by moving back and forth on the head. The woman also would grip the shaft of the penis with the second hand and only stimulate the shaft with the second hand by moving the hand back and forth on the shaft. The woman would move both hands simultaneously.

The fifth manual stimulation technique is for the woman to grip the penis with one hand at the head of the penis and then move her hand from side to side continuously. The sixth manual stimulation technique is for the woman to grasp the man's penis with both hands, one on top of the other, and then move both hands up the shaft and the head of the penis and back down again. The man will have the sensation of thrusting deeply into a long tight vagina. The woman could add variety to this technique by twisting one hand in one direction and the other in the opposite direction as she moves both hands up and down the penis. A seventh manual stimulation technique is for the woman to place one thumb on each side of the frenulum. Then she should move the thumbs up and down and in opposite directions along the frenulum. An eighth manual stimulation technique is for the woman to place one palm of her hand on each side of the man's penis with her hands open. Then she should move the palms of her hands back and forth along the length and head of the penis. As an alternative, the woman could move the palms of her hands from side to side instead of back and forth.

A ninth manual stimulation technique is for the woman to grasp the penis on the coronal ridge and frenulum with the index finger and thumb. Then she should move her fingers up and down on the coronal ridge and frenulum while maintaining them at the coronal ridge and frenulum. The sensation produced from this ninth manual stimulation technique is extremely intense, and some men like climaxing from this kind of movement alone. A tenth manual stimulation technique is for the woman to rub the penis along the bottom of the shaft only using both of her thumbs. She could rub it by moving both thumbs simultaneously up and down the bottom of the shaft only. An eleventh manual stimulation technique is for the woman to grasp the head of the penis with her right hand and slide her right hand down the shaft of the penis. As she reaches the base of the penis, she should grasp the head of the penis with her left hand. Then she should slide her left hand down the shaft of the penis as her right hand releases and goes back up to the head of the penis. The woman should repeat this milking motion, alternating her hands. As an alternative, the woman could grasp the penis at the base with her right hand and slide her hand up the shaft and the head. As she reaches the head, she should grasp the penis at the base with her left hand. Then with her left hand she should slide up the shaft as her right hand releases and goes back to the base of the penis.

During manual stimulation, the woman should experiment with the man by varying the techniques that she tries on him. When she experiments with the man, she should see what seems to give him the most pleasure. She should make mental notes of which places give the man the most pleasure when stroked during manual stimulation. She should also make mental notes of the manual stimulation speed and rhythm that gives the man the most pleasure. Then the woman should concentrate on doing the things that the man finds extremely pleasurable during manual stimulation in order to increase the man's pleasurable sensations. This will make the experience extremely pleasurable to the man.

The woman should try all the techniques and choose the ones that both she and her partner like. She could use just one technique during a manual stimulation session, or she could use a combination of techniques. Also, the woman could use a different technique or a different combination of techniques in each manual stimulation session, or she could use the same technique, or the same combination of techniques in each manual stimulation session. There is no right or wrong way to do it, as long as the couple gets the most pleasure and satisfaction from the experience. While manually stimulating the man, if a technique requires the use of one hand only, the woman could use the second hand to stroke the anus, chest, thighs, stomach, butt, or any other area on the body. The woman could do that to add variety to the manual stimulation technique and to increase a man's pleasure. It is pretty easy for a woman to learn to give a good hand job. Once she learns the basic techniques, she can develop her own style practicing what is most erotic and exciting for her partner.

When manually stimulating the man, the woman should not put too much pressure on the penis nor too little, since that will decrease the pleasurable sensations. The woman should apply a steady pressure during manual stimulation. Once the woman finds the amount of pressure that the man likes, she should keep it up until the moment of the man's orgasm. When the man is manually stimulated by the woman, he could contract and release his PC muscle to increase blood flow to the genital area. This will make the pleasurable feelings during manual stimulation and during orgasm more intense. While being manually stimulated by the woman, the man could breathe slowly and deeply so that his arousal increases, so that the degree of the pleasurable sensations increases, and so that the intensity of the orgasm increases. While manually stimulating the man, the woman should slow down since that could lead to more pleasurable sensations, and it could lead to a more intense orgasm. When manually stimulating the man, the woman should find a rhythm that is comfortable to the man. Once she finds the rhythm, she should keep it up because it is the continuous rhythm that gives the man the stimulation and brings him to orgasm. The woman could stop manually stimulating the man when the man lets her know that he is about to climax in order to delay orgasm. Then after the urge to orgasm subsides she could resume stimulating the man's penis. She could do that several times during a manual stimulation session, in order to intensify the pleasurable sensations and to intensify the man's orgasm when the man finally climaxes. During manual stimulation, the woman should put all her attention on pleasuring the man. No matter how a man is manually stimulated by a woman, the final outcome is usually orgasm and ejaculation. Generally, the man's orgasm during manual stimulation comes from penile stimulation, with the right amount of pressure in the places that feel the best, as well as a steady rhythm.

Manual Stimulation Techniques for Women

Each woman has her individual preference in regards to how she likes to be stimulated manually by the man. Each woman's body likes to be stimulated differently during manual stimulation in order for her to orgasm. In order to start a manual stimulation session, both the man and the woman should make sure that there will be no distractions in any way. They could do that by making sure that the phone is disconnected, the door is closed, the windows are shut, and that the curtains cover the windows. The man and the woman should make sure that there is enough time for them to do the manual stimulation session. This is important. That way, the woman is manually stimulated while she is relaxed and not in a rush.

The woman could be manually stimulated while she stands up facing the man, who is standing up also. The woman also could be manually stimulated while she stands up, facing the man, who is in a kneeling position. The woman could be manually stimulated while she lies on her back with her legs straight and the man kneels between her legs facing her. The most common way for the woman to be manually stimulated is for her to lie on her back with her legs straight and the man to kneel between her legs facing her. This is very common because it is the most relaxing position to the woman, and causes the woman to experience the most pleasure during manual stimulation. During the manual stimulation session, both the man and the woman could be wearing their clothes. However, the most relaxing and arousing way is for the man and the woman to be totally in the nude. By both people being totally in the nude during manual stimulation, the experience will be a lot more pleasurable for the woman.

Before touching the woman, the man should put some water-based lubricant on his hands, and on the woman's genital area. A man should do so because without lubrication the physical stimulation that occurs during manual stimulation might be uncomfortable to the woman, and can often be painful. With lubrication, the stimulation that occurs during a manual stimulation session is more pleasurable. It is better for the man and the woman to have too much lubricant than too little.

The man could start the manual stimulation by exploring the woman's body very gently with his hands. He could touch her legs, breasts, stomach, and chest very gently. He could feel the texture and warmth of her skin as he touches her body parts. After that, he should bring his hands down between her legs. He can pull her pubic hair in small tufts, working his way slowly from where her pubic hair starts to where it ends. When the man pulls the woman's pubic hair, it will cause an exquisite pricking sensation. The man can use one, two, or three fingers, to trace the woman's labia majora from the top to the bottom, gently and lightly. Then the man can use one, two, or three fingers, to trace the woman's labia minora gently and lightly. He can trace her labia minora by going from the bottom of one labium minora to the top of it, over the clitoris hood, and then down the other labium minora. For a variation, the man could pull the labia minora and the labia majora gently as he touches them with his fingers. The pulling move will intensify the pleasurable sensations that the woman feels as the man touches them because the stretched skin tends to have greater feeling. Then the man could slide his fingers lightly and gently along the space between the woman's labia majora and the sides of her clitoris. Then he could touch lightly and gently around the clitoris in a circular manner. Then, using his fingers, he could circle the entrance to the woman's vagina lightly and gently, but not enter it as yet. The man should have his fingers linger at the entrance to the woman's vagina and around the clitoris, until the woman is very wet and engorged. The more lubricated and engorged the woman is, the more pleasurable the manual stimulation will be. It is important that up to this point the man does not rub any part of the woman's genital area. It is important that up to this point the man only touches lightly and gently the parts of the woman's genital area.

The man can then start to masturbate the woman. Once a man starts to masturbate the woman, he usually goes to the clitoris. One way a man could masturbate the woman is by removing the clitoral hood, placing his finger on the head of the clitoris, and then rubbing the head of the clitoris directly with his finger, in a circular manner. When the man rubs the head of the clitoris, he should touch it only lightly and gradually build up pressure as the woman becomes more aroused. The man should rub the head of the clitoris this way because it is the most sexually sensitive part of a woman's body. It is so sensitive that it is painful to the woman if it is stimulated too roughly. A second way for the man to masturbate the woman is by him stimulating the clitoral ridge and tip of the clitoris. The clitoral ridge and tip of the clitoris would be in between his index and middle finger, and the man would move the fingers straight up and down, or in a circular motion. The man could also move the fingers in a combination, both straight up and down and in a circular motion. Often, a woman uses this technique to stimulate herself. A man could also use the palm of his hand, to stimulate the clitoral ridge and tip of the clitoris.

A third way a man could masturbate the woman, is by having the shaft of her clitoris between the index and middle finger, and rubbing it by going up and down with both fingers. The shaft of the clitoris, is less sensitive than the head of the clitoris. Therefore, some women might find this technique not as pleasurable, as the technique where the head of the clitoris is stimulated directly. A fourth way for the man to masturbate the woman, is to slide a finger, up and down the left side of her clitoris shaft, several times. Then the man could slide his finger, up and down the right side of the woman's clitoris shaft, several times. He would repeat this process, until the woman climaxes. This technique, produces extreme pleasure to the woman. The man can vary the direction, of the movement of his fingers, along the shaft. Instead of him moving his fingers up and down the shaft, he can move them from side to side.

All the previous methods of masturbating the woman that were mentioned, are direct methods for the man to stimulate the clitoris. However, some women do not like direct stimulation of their clitoris, because it is too sensitive. For most women, indirect stimulation of the clitoris is perfectly adequate to reach orgasm. Therefore, it is important for the man to ask the woman, if she likes direct stimulation of the clitoris or not. If she does not like direct stimulation of the clitoris, then the man should only stimulate the clitoris indirectly. The following ways of the man manually stimulating the woman, are

Manual Stimulation by the Opposite Sex

indirect ways of stimulating the clitoris. A fifth way a man could manually stimulate the woman, is by rubbing the clitoral hood. The man could rub the clitoral hood firmly and gently using one finger, two fingers, three fingers, or the whole hand. As a result of the rubbing, the woman should feel the clitoris become erect. The sixth way a man could manually stimulate the woman, is by rubbing the area surrounding the clitoris including beneath it, in an up-and-down motion, side-to-side motion, or in a circular fashion. The man would do so using a finger, two fingers, three fingers, or the palm of his hand. When the man rubs around the clitoris, it will probably be more pleasurable than if he massages the clitoris itself, because the clitoris may be too tender to massage directly. The seventh way a man could manually stimulate the woman, is by rubbing the labia minora. By the man rubbing the woman's labia minora, he indirectly stimulates the clitoris. The labia minora, are the delicate inner lips that surround the clitoris. They are highly sensitive. They are an important source of erotic pleasure.

As an alternative, a man could manually stimulate the woman by stimulating the clitoris indirectly for a while, and then stimulating it directly for a while. He could keep on repeating this process, until the woman orgasms. As a variation, the man using his fingers could rub from the clitoris to the vagina, and then back again. He could also rub from underneath the clitoris, right over the clitoris head, to above the clitoris, using his fingers. He could also rub across the head of the clitoris, from one side to the other using his fingers.

Another way the man could manually stimulate the woman and bring her a lot of pleasure, is by him making circles and wavy lines on her stomach using his fingers. He would do this very gently and lightly. Then he should slowly move towards the clitoris, while making the wavy lines and circles lightly and gently. Then when he gets very close to the clitoris he should not change his approach, but rather he should continue to make wavy lines and circles with light touches. This should give the woman shivers, and cause a sensation that is enormously pleasurable. The man should continue to make wavy lines and circles with light touches close to the clitoris, so that indirectly he stimulates the clitoris. The man should continue to do so, until the woman orgasms.

Another way for the man to manually stimulate the woman, is for him to lightly stroke from inside of both thighs, and work towards the clitoris. He would do so using both hands, with one hand on each thigh. When he strokes, he should do so slowly using a finger, two fingers, or three fingers of each hand. The reason behind this technique is to relax the woman, so that there is a greater sensation through her entire genital and pelvic area. Once the man gets to the genital area, he should stroke the genital area around the clitoris and vagina, until the woman is greatly aroused. Once she is greatly aroused, the man should stroke the clitoris either directly or indirectly. He should continue to do so, until the woman orgasms.

When the man uses any manual stimulation technique to stimulate the clitoris directly or indirectly, he should start out very gently touching the skin, and then gradually build up pressure as the woman becomes more aroused. The man should start touching the skin very slowly. Then he should increase the speed of his hand movements during manual stimulation gradually, until he reaches a speed that he feels is ideal. As the woman approaches orgasm, it is important that the man maintains a steady rhythm.

The other area a man could manually stimulate for the woman to orgasm is the vagina. The more engorged the woman's vagina is, the more sensitive it will be. The more sensitive it is, the more intense the pleasurable feelings produced during manual stimulation will be. In order for the man to get the woman's vagina engorged as much as possible, he can massage the woman's labia majora and labia minora and draw them away from her vagina. He can also try rubbing them together. When the man manually stimulates the woman's vagina, he should be concerned only with the outer couple of inches of the vagina, at the vagina entrance. He should not be concerned with the deep interior walls of the vagina. This is so because only the couple of inches of the vagina at the vagina entrance are richly supplied with nerve endings. The deep interior walls of the vagina have few nerve endings and are quite insensitive when stroked or lightly touched.

In order for the man to manually stimulate the vagina, he should slowly insert a clean forefinger into the vagina. When he inserts the finger inside the vagina, he should enter it slowly since by entering it slowly it is more arousing to the vagina. If he enters the vagina slowly, it will be more sensitive and receptive to stimulation. This will make the pleasurable feelings produced during manual stimulation, more pleasurable. The man should use the finger to touch different parts of the vagina, including the top, bottom, and side walls. He should also touch the rough end of the passageway, at the cervix. He should see how the woman responds when each area is touched. He will probably find that some areas are more sensitive to the woman than others, and that the sensitive areas produce more pleasurable feelings than the other areas. He should use his finger to stimulate the areas that are more sensitive than the rest. He could stimulate those areas by rubbing them with his finger in an up-and-down motion, a side-to-side motion, or in a circular motion. This will produce a pleasurable sensation that seems to extend vaguely into parts of the woman's body. It is a warm sensation, making a woman breathless and perhaps wanting to tense her legs. The more the man stimulates those areas with his finger, the more the sensation will increase. This sensation is not an orgasm, but it is the prelude to one. If the man keeps it up, sooner or later the orgasm will follow. The orgasm will be a sudden intense climax of the pleasurable sensations that occur as a result of the stimulation.

When the man is manually stimulating the woman using the vagina, he can stimulate the G-spot. The G-spot is located at the upper inner wall of the woman's vagina. Many women get a great deal of pleasure from the stimulation of this sensitive area on the front wall of their vaginas by their male partner during manual stimulation. However, some women do not seem to have a G-spot. In order for the man to locate the woman's

G-spot, he should stimulate her labia and clitoris before starting to look for it. He should do so because it is easier for the man to find the G-spot if the woman is fully aroused. The G-spot will be felt more clearly the more aroused the woman is. The man should slide two fingers into the woman's vagina, keeping his hand palm side up, so his fingertips can brush against the front top part of the woman's vaginal wall. He can press his fingers against the front wall of the vagina as he moves them in and out in search of the G-spot. He can also move his fingers in a side-to-side motion, circular motion, or zigzag motion in search of the G-spot. If the woman has a G-spot, he will feel a small knob of firm flesh, about the size of a bean or two. It feels like a small lump. It is located midway, between her cervix and pubic bone.

The G-spot will increase in size, as the man stimulates it. The G-spot does not respond well to the man's gentle touching and stroking. It responds best to the man's firm, deep, continuous pressure. The man could rub the G-spot on the upper inner wall of the vagina, using the fingertips of his index and middle finger. He could have the index and middle finger continuously press firmly with deep pressure against the G-spot as they rub it. Another way for the man to stimulate the G-spot is to exert a steady pressure with his finger on the spot, pushing for a count of ten, then letting go, and then pressing again. It is pressure rather than light stroking that brings on the erotic sensations and can trigger climax. The man can press on the woman's abdomen with the other hand to heighten the pleasurable sensations she feels during manual stimulation of the G-spot. The woman goes wild and sometimes gushes fluid when she climaxes from manual stimulation of the G-spot. Many women say that orgasms from manual stimulation of the G-spot are more powerful than clitoral orgasms from manual stimulation.

It is important to note that some women feel discomfort or even the urge to urinate when the G-spot is rubbed during manual stimulation by the man. This is normal and is because of the G-spot's proximity to a woman's urethra and bladder. If the man patiently continues to stimulate the G-spot manually, despite the woman's discomfort or urge to urinate, then the discomfort and the urge to urinate will generally turn to pleasure. If the man or the woman is worried about the woman's seeming need to urinate during manual stimulation, the woman can empty her bladder before being manually stimulated by the man.

Many women, whether they have a G-spot or not, find it very pleasurable to have the top of their vagina stimulated by the man during manual stimulation. A man could make his index finger into a shape of a hook, pointing upward, and insert it into the vagina. He could use the finger in such a shape to stimulate the top of the vagina by moving it in an up-and-down manner, side-to-side manner, or in a circular manner. The sensations produced are extremely pleasurable to the woman. Also, a woman could squeeze the vaginal muscles while the man's finger is stimulating the vagina. This will intensify the pleasurable feelings produced during manual stimulation. Also, squeezing the vaginal muscles while the man's finger is stimulating the vagina produces a sucking feeling. While stimulating the vagina, the man should use a slow and gentle hand. The cervix is usually deep inside a woman's vagina, and the man should avoid hitting it during manual stimulation because that can be painful to the woman.

Another manual stimulation technique is for the man to stimulate the vagina and the clitoris at the same time. He can use one or two fingers of one hand to stimulate around the clitoris in a circular motion while he uses a finger or two of the other hand to rub inside the vagina in an in-and-out motion. If the man stimulates the vagina and the clitoris at the same time, it can lead to extremely intense and explosive orgasms. If the woman has a G-spot, the man can stimulate the G-spot at the same time he stimulates the clitoris. He can use a finger or two of one hand to stimulate around the clitoris in a circular motion while he uses a finger or two of the other hand to rub the G-spot in an in-and-out motion. This will lead to the most intense full body orgasm that a woman could experience.

In order to make the manual stimulation session more pleasurable to the woman, the following could be done. First, if a manual stimulation technique involves the use of one hand only by the man, the man can use the other hand to stimulate the woman's nipples, breasts, inner thighs, buttocks, or anus. Second, a man could put a vibrator in the woman's vagina when manually stimulating the clitoris, even though the vibrator is not stimulating the vagina. The man puts the vibrator inside the woman's vagina while manually stimulating her because many women find that having something to contract around during an orgasm is far more satisfying than orgasming with an empty vagina. Third, in order for the man to intensify the pleasurable feelings of the woman during manual stimulation and orgasm, the man could delay a woman's orgasm several times during a manual stimulation session. The man could do so by stopping the stimulation when the woman is close to orgasming. He can wait until the urge to orgasm subsides. Then the man can resume manual stimulation of the woman. The man could do so as many times as he likes. The more he or she does it the more intense the pleasurable sensations during manual stimulation will be, and the more intense the pleasurable sensations during orgasm will be when orgasm occurs. Then, when the man feels like it, he can bring the woman to orgasm. Fourth, a man should not stroke one spot for too long during manual stimulation because the pleasurable sensations will decrease and the area might even become numb. Fifth, a woman should contract and release her PC muscle during manual stimulation to increase blood flow to the genital area. This will make the orgasm easier and more intense.

Sixth, a woman could breathe slowly and deeply when the man is manually stimulating her. The woman would do so because that will increase her arousal and the intensity of the pleasurable feelings during manual stimulation and orgasm. Seventh, a man should keep a steady rhythm during manual stimulation, since that will increase the woman's pleasurable feelings. Eighth, when the man manually stimulates the woman, he can rub slowly and gently back and forth or in a circular motion. If he increases his speed and the hardness of his rubbing to the point that it becomes painful to the woman, he should quickly slow down and lighten the pressure of his rub to a level that he sees is the most pleasurable to the woman. If the man tries to force a woman to have an orgasm by rubbing too fast or too hard, it will never happen. Ninth, a woman should know that during a manual stimulation session, not all orgasms are the same. She should know that sometimes she will experience a very powerful and intense orgasm, while at other times her orgasm is just a gentle wave of release.

Tenth, the man should stop stimulating the woman manually after she orgasms, unless she wants more. The man should do so because some women's clitoris and vagina become very sensitive after orgasm, and they do not want any more stimulation. However, most women, when they have an orgasm, want to have another orgasm right after it. Finally, every woman is different, and it is best for the man to find out what manual stimulation techniques she likes. The best way for the man to have the woman orgasm as quickly as possible is to have her relax and do exactly what pleases her. Once the man learns the basic manual stimulation techniques, he can develop his own style, practicing what is most erotic and exciting for his female partner.

Manually Stimulating the Woman During Pregnancy

It is safe for a man, to manually stimulate the woman during pregnancy. The increased blood flow in the woman's genital region due to pregnancy causes the woman's genital region to become very sensitive. Thus, the sensations produced during manual stimulation of a pregnant woman, including orgasms, are a lot more pleasurable. The man should use a lot of lubricant on his hands and on the woman's genital area when manually stimulating her so that she does not experience pain as a result of the friction produced during manual stimulation.

A man can put a vibrator in the woman's vagina if she is pregnant. However, he should not do so after the second trimester. It is safe for him to do so during the first and second trimester of the woman's pregnancy.

Keeping Manual Stimulation Safe from Sexually Transmitted Disease

Although the possibility of getting a sexually transmitted disease through manual stimulation is low, it is possible for both the man and the woman to get infected. Bacteria and viruses in the woman's vaginal secretions can be transmitted through small cracks of the man's skin on his fingers and hands. Bacteria and viruses in the man's penile secretions can be transmitted through small cracks of the woman's skin on her fingers and hands. So if a person is not sure about the health status of his or her partner, he or she should use latex gloves or a finger cot (a latex sleeve that covers one finger), to protect his or her hands or fingers from vaginal or penile secretions during manual stimulation. The person, after using the gloves or finger cot on his or her partner, should be sure to change them before touching his or her own genital area.

Mutual Masturbation

Many couples find manual stimulation to be more fulfilling if both partners stimulate each other at the same time. Mutual masturbation is when both partners simultaneously stimulate each other's genitals with their hands. It allows both partners to get sexual pleasure at the same time. As for the techniques for the man and the woman to use during mutual masturbation, they are the same techniques as the manual stimulation techniques, except the man and the woman perform them simultaneously on each other. When both partners are mutually masturbating each other, they can also kiss each other to add more pleasure to the experience. Also, when both partners are mutually masturbating each other, they can fondle each other's body parts to make the experience more pleasurable. Both partners can talk erotically to each other when they are mutually masturbating each other to make the experience extremely more delightful.

During mutual masturbation, the man and the woman can stand facing each other. Also, they can both lie down next to each other, on their backs with their legs straight. However, the most relaxing position for both the man and the woman during mutual masturbation is for both of them to be lying on their side facing each other. This position gives both people full access to each other's genital area and allows them to experience the most pleasure because they both are extremely relaxed.

Mutual masturbation brings both partners closer to each other and makes them feel in sync because it allows both people to climax simultaneously. Both people can climax simultaneously because one partner can slow down until the other partner is close to orgasm, then they both can orgasm at the same time. Another plus to mutual masturbation is that both people get familiar with how their partner responds to touch. As a result of mutual masturbation, both people gain knowledge of their partner's body and orgasms, while sharing an amazing sexual experience. Most people think that mutual masturbation is very important because it leads to a mutually satisfying sex life.

Mutual masturbation while the woman is pregnant can be a great substitute for intercourse. However, it should not be done after the second trimester. It is safe to be done during the first and second trimester of the woman's pregnancy.

Chapter 11

Oral Sex

Oral sex is one of the most intimate of sexual delicacies shared between the man and the woman. It can be intensely pleasurable for both the giver and the receiver. When a person is giving oral sex, he or she is up close and personal with the most intimate part of his or her lover's body and all his or her senses (sight, hearing, smell, taste and touch) are stimulated. The mouth can create many more sensations than any other part of the body. Most people (male and female) admit that what makes them have the most intense and pleasurable orgasms is oral sex. Most people love having their partner between their legs. There is not anything that feels better to them. Many people like oral sex because they view their partner's mouth on their genital area as a sign of total acceptance of them. Oral sex makes the couple very intimate and is very satisfying for both the giver and the receiver. Oral sex for the receiver, whether male or female, is so pleasurable that some people prefer it to intercourse. A person, whether male or female, can have a great orgasm as a result of oral sex and he or she does not have to do anything but lie there. It is a way of receiving pure pleasure without having to do any work or effort. For many people, performing oral sex is just as great of a thrill as receiving it. Even though oral sex is widely performed by millions of people, that does not mean that oral sex necessarily comes naturally to everyone. As a matter of fact, to some people it does not come naturally. Oral sex feels great to many because orgasm can happen quickly and intensely because stimulation is concentrated on the genital. The tongue is more flexible and softer than fingers, so it can stimulate the genital area in a way that is totally unique.

Oral sex, like any kind of sex, is a way to express love. Oral sex is an important part of many people's sex lives. It can be part of foreplay, a way to get ready for intercourse. If the woman is not multi-orgasmic and the couple does not want to have a break during sex then oral sex could be performed as part of foreplay to get the partner aroused, but not orgasm. The tight, warm, wet lips wrapped around a man's penis can help a man become aroused during foreplay and help him get a firm erection in preparation for intercourse. A warm wet tongue on the woman's clitoris can help a woman become aroused during foreplay and well lubricated in preparation for intercourse. However, if the couple wants a break during the sexual encounter then oral sex can be performed until orgasm as part of foreplay on the man and the woman even if the woman is not multi-orgasmic. This is because the man or the woman can rest after an orgasm during the sex break and regain their ability to have another orgasm. During the sex break the couple could touch and kiss each other while saying terms of endearment to each other. The sex break makes the two encounters into one long encounter. If a woman is multi-orgasmic oral sex can be performed on the woman until orgasm as part of foreplay, even if there is not going to be a break. Oral sex can be a substitute for sex, when people want to wait to have intercourse, or if one or both partners are not able to have intercourse due to illness or disability. Oral sex can be a sexual variation to be enjoyed simply for the pleasure it brings.

Oral sex is one of the most misunderstood sexual acts. By some, it is not viewed as real sex, because one person's mouth is used to stimulate the sexual organ of the other person. In fact, some young couples have turned to oral sex as a substitute for intercourse. They feel that it lets them explore their sexuality without actually doing it. The fear of pregnancy has also increased the popularity of oral sex. There is no need to worry about pregnancy as a result of oral sex. Some people like oral sex because they feel powerful when they give their partner pleasure through oral sex, since at no other time do they feel such complete control of their partner's pleasure. Some people find it very arousing to watch their partner enjoy receiving pleasure from oral sex. Oral sex is the quickest way to have a person orgasm.

Some people worry if oral sex is natural. Anything that two adults engage in and find mutually pleasurable is natural as long as it does not harm themselves or others. So oral sex is natural because it brings pleasure to both people and it does not cause anyone harm. Some people do not like to give or receive oral sex because they worry that the genital area is unclean. As long as a person (male or female) keeps his or her genital area clean by washing it daily, then it certainly can be as clean as the mouth. It is enlightening to know that the variety and concentration of bacteria in a person's mouth easily rivals the concentration and variety of bacteria on a person's genital area. Some people who like oral sex feel lonely during it. The genital stimulation is terrific, but there is nobody to hug, hold, or kiss. The fact that a person's entire face is directly in front of the partner's genital makes this a highly intimate act and makes most people delighted, while it makes other people uncomfortable.

Some people do not like to receive or give oral sex because they have a lot of hang ups. They may worry that their genital area smells, tastes bad, looks funny, or is out of the ordinary. They might worry that their partner's mouth will get tired after a while or that their partner will get hair in his or her teeth or throat. If a person has kept up with basic good hygiene, he or she should not worry that his or her genital area smells or tastes bad. Each person's genital area has a distinct taste and smell and that is that person's natural aroma. Each person has a genital shape that is distinct. He or she should not worry about how it looks. A person should not worry that his or her partner will get hair in his or her teeth or throat. If a person frees himself or herself of these worries, and does not think of them, then he or she will be able to find pleasure in a whole new way.

Some tips that might help a person get past his hang ups about oral sex are as follows. First, before oral sex both partners are to shower or bathe. They could shower together if they want to. Second, both partners should have oral sex at a time and a place that is comfortable to them. Third, both partners can relax and take deep breaths. Instead of worrying they can think about the good feeling that oral sex can bring. One thing that might help a person overcome his or her hang up about giving oral sex is if his or her partner gives him or her oral sex. This will help the person overcome his or her hang-up because of an unspoken bargain. If a person receives oral sex and he or she likes it, it is only natural that he or she would like to return the favor. Sometimes it takes a little time to help a person overcome his or her hang up of giving oral sex by giving him or her oral sex. At other times, a person overcoming his or her hang up of giving oral sex never happens.

One way to make oral sex more pleasurable is for the woman to have her pubic hair shaved. As a matter of fact, many couples enjoy having the male trim and shave the woman's pubic hair. They enjoy it as a form of erotic foreplay. Another way to make oral sex more pleasurable is for the man to shave his face. The man should rub the inside of his wrist on his face, particularly just below the lower lip. If he feels anything scratch, so will the woman. Some women, if they have sensitive skin, develop a rash on the inside of their thighs because of the man's facial hair. The man should especially make sure that around the mouth and lower lip there is no hair. A third way to make oral sex more pleasurable is for the person about to perform oral sex to move his or her hand through the hair on the genital area of his or her partner. This will seem like a caressing move, but in actuality the person that is about to perform oral sex is removing loose hairs. A fourth way to make oral sex more pleasurable is for the person receiving oral sex to put melted chocolate or whipped cream on his or her genital area.

Some people shy away from oral sex because they worry that they are not good enough at performing oral sex. It is easy to learn the proper techniques to perform oral sex. Just reading this chapter in the book should provide the reader with sufficient information about the proper techniques to perform oral sex. A person should not expect to be perfect the first time he or she tries the techniques. It takes time to learn how to apply the techniques in real life.

Oral sex is called cunnilingus when the man does it to the woman. It involves manipulation of the clitoris or vagina by the man's tongue. It is a great way to pleasure a woman and to experience her sensuality. For a woman, receiving oral sex is the quickest way to have her desire brought to a boil and to become fully lubricated. It is the woman's easiest route to orgasm and very gratifying to her. Her partner can experience her orgasm in a very up close and personal way, which is different from intercourse. Women love the feeling of oral sex simply because of the unique sensations of a warm, wet tongue on their vulva. When a man performs oral sex on a woman he does more than just make her have an orgasm. He gives her pleasure by doing all sorts of things with his tongue and mouth. Satisfying a woman orally is one of life's sweetest tasks, and one that nearly every man would love to master. Oral sex performed on a woman seems to cause every woman to orgasm if performed correctly. A woman may find the man's lips and tongue more arousing than his fingers because they are gentler and can produce a much greater variety of sensations. More subtly, some women find cunnilingus pleasurable because they view the man going down on the woman as an act of honoring, like foot washing or a bow. During cunnilingus, the man puts himself below the woman in a position of seeming inferiority in order to give her a special gift of pleasure. Lots of women like that.

Oral sex is called fellatio when the woman does it to the man. It consists of manipulation of the penis by the mouth. Men derive such great pleasure from fellatio that most of them consider it their favorite sex act. For some men, just thinking about a warm, wet mouth around their penis can drive them wild. Fellatio is also known as giving head, giving a blow job, and going down on the penis. When a woman performs fellatio on the man, she not only gives him an orgasm, but also gives him pleasure by doing all sorts of things with her tongue and mouth. A man may find the woman's mouth and tongue more arousing than her fingers or vagina because they are gentler and can produce a much greater variety of sensations. More elusively, some men find fellatio attractive because the woman is going down on the man as an act of respect and honoring. During fellatio, the woman puts herself below the man in a position of seeming inferiority in order to give him pleasure. Numerous men like that. Some women have the unfounded fear that the man will urinate in their mouth during fellatio. It is very difficult for a man with an erection to urinate, and the man cannot ejaculate and urinate at the same time. Some men are self-conscious on the amount of semen they produce. A man should be aware that it is normal to have less ejaculate when he is older or if he has a lot of sex. A woman's mouth and tongue, allow her to pleasure her partner with pressure and precision that is rare during intercourse. Fellatio remains the quickest way to excite or resuscitate a man's erection when his heart is willing but his body is not quite ready.

Etiquette

As with any kind of sex, no one should be forced to have oral sex if they do not want to. If the man or woman objects to oral sex, the other partner has to accept that it really does not appeal to the man or woman. Instead, the other partner should consider other things to do for foreplay and sex. The partner who objects to oral sex should not feel obligated to do it. If the partner feels obligated to give or receive oral sex, then that person will be resentful if he or she performs it. This will only serve to increase his or her distaste for oral sex. The reluctant partner should remember that he or she is in charge of what he or she does sexually, and that what he or she does sexually should bring him or her pleasure. If what the reluctant partner does sexually does not bring him or her pleasure, then the reluctant partner should not do it at all. Also, if a person is uncomfortable receiving or giving oral sex, then the person should not do it at all. This is because if the person does it, he or she is not likely to receive pleasure nor give his or her partner much pleasure.

Sometimes a partner will feel uncomfortable with the idea of giving or receiving oral sex but will still agree to give it a try. If this is the case the other partner should be very patient and understanding. The other partner should take it slowly and not rush his or her reluctant partner. The other partner should guarantee that he or she will stop the oral sex act as soon as his or her lover asks him or her to. This will reduce the reluctant partner's anxiety. The reluctant partner should give it a try if he or she is unsure about whether to do it or not. That way he or she experiences what it is like. Then the reluctant partner can make the decision of whether he or she should give and receive oral sex or not. If the reluctant partner tries receiving or giving oral sex, he or she might enjoy receiving or giving oral sex more than he or she anticipated. With a little practice, the reluctant partner might find that oral sex is a very erotic, intimate, and intensely personal experience. It is important to remember that some people, after trying receiving or giving oral sex, still dislike it. That is normal and the other partner should accept it and not feel that he or she was inadequate, because everyone is an individual and everyone has a different set of likes and dislikes.

It is important that both partners get their ideas, hopes, and fears about oral sex into perspective. Reading this chapter can help both partners get an accurate picture about oral sex and can help both partners get rid of unrealistic ideas, hopes and fears, about oral sex. A partner can talk with his or her other partner to make sure that the other partner has realistic ideas, hopes, and fears about oral sex. It is important that the reluctant partner talks about his or her anxiety and receives reassurance from his or her partner. It is important that both partners have a clear, accurate, and realistic picture about oral sex, because the issue of oral sex sometimes becomes a huge relationship issue. Many relationships have ended because of disagreement between the couple about oral sex. Many marriages have ended because of disagreement about oral sex.

The woman might want the man to perform oral sex or receive oral sex. Or the man might want the woman to perform or receive oral sex. The solution is for the couple to agree on some sexual activities that they both like and accept.

Fellatio Positions

It is important to find a fellatio position that is comfortable for both partners. The best position for fellatio is with the man lying on his back with his legs stretched out straight and the woman kneeling, lying, or sitting between his legs facing him. If the man's penis angles tightly against his abdominal wall when it is erect, the woman needs to lean forward over his body to get the right angle that pulls the erect penis down towards her without being uncomfortable for him. Another position is with the man lying on his back with legs stretched out straight while the woman kneels, sits, or lies at his side and bends over his genital at an angle. She can place pillows under his buttocks to make it easier on her neck. When the man is lying on his back, the woman has the most control of the situation. A different position is with the man standing and the woman, while facing him, to kneel in front of him. The last position is with the man sitting on the edge of the bed or chair and the woman, while facing him, to kneel in front of him.

Fellatio Techniques

The first step for the woman to give the man pleasure during fellatio is for her not to start caressing, licking, or sucking the penis at the beginning. Rather, the woman should start by licking, kissing, and caressing the inner thighs, since they tend to be extremely sensitive. A man usually finds the licking, kissing, and caressing of his inner thighs extremely pleasurable. The woman then should move to the man's chest and start kissing, licking, nibbling, and caressing his chest. Then she should gently suck on the man's nipples because they are very sensitive. A man usually likes his nipples to be stimulated. The woman should then move to the navel. The woman should kiss, caress, and lick the navel. A man usually finds it erotic that the woman is kissing, licking, or caressing the navel. The woman should then move to the lower abdomen. When the woman moves to the lower abdomen, the man usually becomes very excited that the woman is coming close to his penis. The woman should also kiss, lick, nibble, or caress the lower abdomen.

To make things interesting for the man, the woman at no time should reveal to him when she will stimulate the penis. Rather, she should keep him guessing. She can keep him guessing by moving to the inner thighs right after she has kissed, licked, and caressed his abdomen. At the inner thighs she can kiss, lick, nibble, and caress them. Then she could go back to the lower abdomen to kiss, lick, and caress it. She can do that as many times as she likes. By now, the man should be excited greatly and wondering when his penis is going to be stimulated. This will make the fellatio more pleasurable for him.

The pubic bone is a very sensitive area for many men. Next, the woman should move to the pubic bone and start licking, caressing, and sucking on it. When the woman does that, most men get aroused greatly and begin anticipating when the woman will stimulate the penis. But at that instant the woman should go back to the man's inner thighs and start kissing, licking, nibbling, and caressing them. Then she should go back to the man's pubic bone. She can do that as many times as she likes. She should keep the man guessing as to when she will stimulate his penis. This will make the fellatio exciting and more pleasurable. Then the woman should kiss lightly, with several small kisses, the man's scrotum. This will greatly arouse the man. Then she should lightly kiss the man's penis several times. Next, she should go back to kissing the man's scrotum lightly several times and then she should go back to the man's penis and start kissing the penis lightly several times. She can do that as many times as she likes. This will cause the man to be greatly stimulated and look forward to have her begin sucking his penis. In a sense, the man is teased that his penis is not stimulated as yet, but this will make the fellatio a lot more pleasurable.

But then the woman should move to the area beneath the man's scrotum, but before the anus. This area is called the perineum. It is extremely sensitive to touch, licking, kissing, and nibbling. The woman should caress, lick, and kiss the perineum. The man will find this very pleasurable. Then the woman should move to the scrotum. The woman should kiss, lick, and caress the entire surface of the scrotum. The woman can gently take one testicle into her mouth as she is licking the scrotum. She should take both testicles into her mouth one at a time. A man usually loves it when the woman does that. The woman can then slide her tongue under the man's scrotum and lift it with her tongue. A man usually finds that very erotic and intimate. He finds himself teased that she has not stimulated his penis yet. He finds himself wanting his penis inside of her mouth.

All the kissing, licking, caressing, and nibbling that the woman has done up to this point should have been done slowly and gently. If the woman goes slowly and gently the man will get greater pleasure from the experience. But if the woman goes fast, the man will not enjoy the experience greatly. The woman can rub her breasts against the man's thighs and genital area at this point. Or she can skip this step and move on. She can try doing this step at times and at other times skipping it. This way there is variety in her technique and it keeps the oral sex between her and the man very interesting, exciting, and not boring. The man should be erect by now, but if the man is slow to get aroused and his penis is still soft and not erect as yet, a woman can take his penis inside her mouth. This is an excellent way to raise his sexual energy. It is the quickest way to help the man become erect.

Once the man has an erection, there are several ways that the woman can stimulate the man to orgasm using oral sex. The first method is as follows. The woman should begin to kiss and lick the man's penis. The woman should make her tongue flat and lick the penis like an ice cream cone. She should start at the base of the penis and work her way up to the head of the penis. The woman should spend some time at the corona and the very sensitive frenulum and then lick back down again. She can repeat the process as many times as she likes. The corona is the penis glans outer rim. The frenulum is a strip of skin just below the glans, on the underside of the penis. The saliva the woman generates is a great lubricant and will make the rest of the blow job easier and more pleasurable. The woman should lick up and down the penis shaft. She should make sure that she covered all of the penis shaft with her licking.

The woman then should hold the base of the penis with her hand and take the head of the penis into her mouth, leaving her lips slightly parted. The woman should move her tongue in a circle around the head of the penis. Then she should let the front of her tongue stroke the underside of the penis several times. Next, the soft underside of the tongue should stroke the front of the penis several times. The woman could breathe through her mouth to enhance sensations for the man during fellatio. Now the woman, with the penis still inside her mouth, should flick her tongue rapidly all over the surface of the glans, around the entire corona, and at the frenulum. The woman should linger briefly at the frenulum. As the woman does that, she should observe his reactions. She should be able to tell by his reaction if this is what he likes.

The woman then should start to slide her mouth gradually down the man's penis to its base, and then back again, so that her lips are resting at the glans of the penis. The woman should continue to move her mouth up and down the man's penis until the man orgasms. Men enjoy the fact that their penis is always being touched by the woman during this fellatio technique. Another variation to this technique is for the woman to move the penis in and out of her mouth by moving her mouth up and down on it. Unlike the previous technique, the penis is not being touched by the woman when it is out of her mouth. The fact that the penis is not being touched by the woman when it is out of her mouth on the backstroke offers a different set of sensations to the man than when the penis is still being touched by the woman during fellatio on the back movement. The woman should press slightly around the penis with her lips as she moves. The woman can increase the pressure of her lips on the man's penis as she becomes more excited. Some men will be perfectly happy with this simple in and out movement of the woman's mouth on the penis. The action of the woman moving her mouth up and down the man's penis is often what gives the man the most stimulation during fellatio. But if the woman wants the man to be ecstatic, she needs to learn more advanced moves and variations.

There are three main spots on the man's penis that are extremely sensitive and bring great pleasure to the man when stimulated. The first spot is the skin just below the glans on the underside of the penis, known as the frenulum. It is the most sensitive spot on the penis. The second spot is the rim of the head of the penis. It is called the corona. This spot is very sensitive, but not as sensitive as the frenulum. The third spot is the head of the penis. This spot is very sensitive, but not as sensitive as the corona. Licking and sucking the head of the penis can work wonders. The shaft of the penis is sensitive, but not as sensitive as the head, corona, or frenulum. The second method of stimulating the man during oral sex involves taking the shaft of the penis into the mouth and licking only the shaft while keeping the penis inside the mouth. This causes many men to experience great pleasure that they have not experienced before. Then the woman moves her head up and down the shaft of the penis only until the man orgasms. This gives a man a different set of sensations during oral sex.

A third technique is for the woman, as she moves up and down the man's penis with her mouth, to move her head to the left side and then to the right. This adds variety to the oral sex. It produces a different set of sensations than when the woman's head was not moving from side to side as it moved up and down the man's penis. For a variation of this technique, the woman can also focus on the head of the penis only. She can move her mouth up and down while moving it from side to side just on the head of the man's penis. This will cause the man to experience intense pleasure at the head of his penis.

A fourth method is for the woman to use her hands in conjunction with her mouth. While the woman's mouth is focusing on licking and sucking the head of the penis, the woman can move her hands up and down the shaft of the man's penis for a combination of hand and blow job. The woman should make sure her hands and his penis are wet so that her hands glide easily up and down. The woman should keep up a steady rhythm with her mouth and hands. Another variation to this technique is for the man to put his penis inside the woman's mouth. Then the woman can encircle the base of the man's penis with her thumb and middle finger. Then as she moves her mouth up and down the man's penis, she should let her fingers follow. The woman should have lubrication, like saliva or a water-based lubricant, placed on her hand and the penis. This technique will cause the man to feel that he is deeper in the woman's mouth because more of his penis is being stimulated. Therefore, it will cause him to experience greater pleasure and excitement.

A fifth method is for the man to insert his penis in the woman's mouth. He should insert it as far as he can while the woman is still comfortable. Then the woman should stroke and massage the penis with her tongue as she moves her mouth up and down the shaft of the man's penis. When the woman's tongue reaches the frenulum, the woman should linger a little bit there before moving on and her tongue should move a little bit more faster, doing a few strokes before moving on. Then when her lips reach the frenulum, she should apply a little more pressure with her lips on the frenulum. Another variation to this technique is for the woman not to lick the penis with her tongue as she moves up and down his penis with her mouth. Rather, she should create suction while moving her mouth up the shaft of the penis on the backward stroke. This creates great pleasure for most men, causing them to want more.

A sixth method in fellatio is for the man to insert his penis in the woman's mouth and then for the woman to slide her mouth down the shaft of the man's penis to the base of the penis. Next she slides her mouth up the shaft of the penis to the point just below the corona. There the woman can apply more pressure with her lips and with a light suction, pull her lips over the corona and head creating a snapping sound. The woman can do this several times.

A seventh fellatio technique is for the woman to open her mouth and for the man to slide his penis inside the woman's mouth. The woman should then slide her tongue under his penis and push it up and down. When the woman does that she should make sure that her tongue does not touch her teeth. The woman could breathe warm air through her mouth as she lifts his penis with her tongue to add variety in the sensations. An eighth fellatio technique is for the man to place his penis in the woman's mouth. The woman applies light pressure with her lips while covering her teeth with her lips. Then the woman moves her head from side to side, allowing the penis to move from one cheek to the other. These two techniques won't make the man orgasm but will add variety to the couple's oral sex experience and bring both of them pleasure.

A ninth technique that has been made famous by the pornographic industry is deep throating. However, most women cannot do it. Deep throating requires the woman to take the whole penis into her mouth and down her throat as far as she can when moving her head up and down the penis. It is a good idea to try it when the whole penis is very wet and the woman's mouth is very wet. This gives tremendous pleasure to the man. However, a woman has to learn how to turn off her gag reflex. It is difficult for most women to overcome their gag reflex. Some women are able to suppress their natural gag reflex by relaxing and breathing through the nose. However, if the woman starts to gag during fellatio, the man should stop right away because the next natural reflex is vomiting, and no one wants to even think about that happening during oral sex. The woman and man have to be careful when using this technique because the tissues in the back of the throat are delicate and easily injured. The woman may find that she has a sore throat the day after deep throating. She should try gargling with warm, salty water.

When the woman takes the man's penis into her mouth during oral sex, she should watch her teeth. Most men hate the feel of the teeth against their penis. The most important tool for giving head is the woman's tongue, but the lips are very important, too. The lips spend most of their time covering the woman's teeth to protect the man's penis. So when performing fellatio on the man, the woman should make sure that her lips cover her teeth. She should make sure that her teeth do not scrape the man's penis. The woman should never bite the man's penis. Fellatio involves the use of the woman's lips, tongue, cheeks, and upper palate. The woman should practice with a cucumber beforehand so that she knows how far to insert the penis before she starts to gag. The first few times a woman performs fellatio, she will have very sore lips the day after. This is because it takes practice for the woman to figure out just how to cover the teeth and how much pressure to put on the lips.

During any time when the man's penis is inside the woman's mouth and the woman is performing fellatio on him, the woman could stroke or gently cup his scrotum. She could also massage the perineum, which is between his scrotum and anus. She could also stroke his chest, nipples, thighs, or any other body part that she finds pleasurable. She can also touch gently around his anus or slowly slide a lubricated finger inside his anus. She should do that only if she knows that the man likes anal contact during fellatio. She should also stay in tune with her partner. She should look him in the eyes if she can. She should read his body language, and take cues from his responses to find out what feels best and what does not work. She should not stop every minute and ask if she is doing a good job. If the man seems to be enjoying what she is doing then she should keep going.

When the man gets close to ejaculating, the woman should keep doing what the man seems to enjoy the most. Most of the time, the man will tell the woman when he is close to orgasm, or he will be thrusting, moving his hips, or moaning in a way to let her know. At that point, the woman should keep up the rhythm in the place that he seems to enjoy the most. Sometimes if the man is very excited, he may try to guide the head of the woman in a rhythm he likes. If that is okay with the woman, then that is fine. But if he is too rough, the woman should tell him not to move her head. Also, sometimes a man will start to thrust the penis deeply into the mouth of the woman as he becomes more excited. Some will even place their hands on the head of the woman and hold it down to try to get the penis deeper into her mouth. If this makes the woman uncomfortable she should let the man know. The woman can also place her hand at the base of the penis to control how deeply the penis can enter her mouth. Sometimes, in the heat of action, a woman may take the penis deep so inside her mouth that she begins to gag. The man should not think that this is because she finds him disgusting. Rather, he should know that this is a reflex action when something goes way down her throat. The man should know that she cannot help herself. Many women worry that they will gag if they take their partner deep into their mouth or throat. The woman can generally control the depth of the penis in her mouth by using her jaw muscle and clamping down on the penis with her lips and not her teeth.

During fellatio most men orgasm from the rhythm of the sucking on the head of the penis only, the rhythm of sucking on the shaft of the penis only, the rhythm of sucking on both the head and shaft of the penis only, or the combined sucking of the head of the penis with hand stimulation of the shaft of the penis. When the woman is stimulating the man's penis she should not be surprised if the man's penis becomes soft. It happens. If the man seems to be enjoying what the woman is doing, even if the penis becomes soft, the woman should keep doing what she is doing. It won't be long before his erection returns. Also, to add variety during fellatio, the woman can put ice in her mouth before performing fellatio, which will give a different set of sensations to the man during oral sex. Or she can drink something hot before performing fellatio, which will give the man a different set of sensations during fellatio.

The woman should figure out where the man is going to ejaculate. She should ease up after orgasm. After orgasm a man's penis may be so sensitive that he does not want it touched. The woman can touch him in any other place on his body, she can cuddle with him, or she can kiss him on the mouth. After waiting for a while, the couple can resume having sex if they want.

The woman should remember that every man is different and likes different things. The best way to find out what the man likes is to ask him. Some men find it difficult to describe in words what turns them on during fellatio. If this is the case, the man should tell the woman his likes or dislikes while she is performing fellatio on him. Every time she performs an action on him, he can tell her whether he likes it or not. Also, the woman can observe his verbal and nonverbal cues, and it will become obvious to her what he really enjoys. Being able to tell what her partner enjoys during fellatio and doing it is what makes a woman an amazing oral lover.

Spit or Swallow

A woman should alone come to the decision about whether she wants to swallow the man's semen or spit it out. Nobody should interfere with her decision because it is she that is doing the swallowing. Several issues are involved in reaching the decision. The first issue is the composition of the semen, and if it is harmful. The semen is very rich in nutrients, including vitamins, minerals, sugars, and proteins. All these components of the semen nourish and energize the sperm and help protect it from the acidic environment of the vagina. If the semen is swallowed, one ejaculation has only 10 to 50 calories. If it is swallowed, it has no harmful effect on the woman. The second issue involved is the taste of the semen. Some women like the taste of the semen, while other women do not. Some women have described its taste like bleach. Others have described the taste like salt water. Some women have described the taste as bitter, while others have described the taste as sugary. The answer, in regards to the taste of the semen, is that it is different with each man and that it is influenced by what he eats.

The third issue is the transmission of sexually transmitted diseases. If a woman has semen in her mouth or swallows it, there is the risk of contracting sexually transmitted diseases including HIV (the virus that causes AIDS). The only time that she should not worry about sexually transmitted diseases during fellatio is if she knows for certain the man is disease-free or if she practices safer oral sex. The fourth issue is pleasing the man. Some men feel better having the mouth-on-penis contact while they are having an orgasm (and ejaculating) from oral sex. Some men also feel more accepted or even more loved if their partner swallows their semen. The woman should find out if it matters to her man if he ejaculates in her mouth and whether it matters to him if she swallows. The fifth issue is intimacy. The couple sometimes feels more intimate if the woman swallows. The woman should see whether her man feels more intimate if she swallows. She should also consider whether she feels more intimate with her man if she swallows.

Once the woman has considered all the issues involved, she should make her decision. She should make sure that the decision that she makes is what she wants and that she is not putting herself at risk of any disease. She should make her decision based on what she thinks is best for her health and happiness. The man should be respectful of the woman's decision and not put pressure on her, since she is the one doing the swallowing.

It should be noted that some women will swallow their partner's semen at certain times and at other times they will not. That is perfectly normal. Just as at certain times a woman likes to eat cake and at other times she does not for no reason except that she does not feel like it. Likewise, a woman at certain times will swallow a man's semen because she feels like it, and at other times she will not because she does not feel like it. The woman should do what she feels like doing and not feel obligated that she always has to swallow the semen. If she swallows because she feels obligated to, that will build resentment in the woman and make her disdain fellatio. The man has to understand that it is normal for the woman to have different preferences towards swallowing his semen at different times and be respectful of that.

If the woman decides not to swallow then she has several options. The first option is she can have the man ejaculate in her mouth and she can spit it out. If the man ejaculates in her mouth, she should be certain he is disease-free. She should do that because a woman can get certain sexually transmitted diseases from the semen in her mouth, even if she does not swallow. The second option is she can tell the man to let her know when he is about to come so that she stops stimulating his penis with her mouth, and so that she brings him to climax with her hand.

Cunnilingus Positions

There are many positions for cunnilingus. One popular position is for the woman to lie on her back with her legs straight. Then the man lies on his stomach between her legs and places his mouth on her clitoris or vagina. The man's legs are straight in this position. The woman can relax every part of her body in this position and let the man bring her to climax. Another variation of this position is for the woman to lie on her back with her legs straight. Then between the woman's legs, the man, facing the woman's face, can kneel on his knees and then bend over his upper body to the woman's clitoris or vagina and place his mouth on either of them. The man should remain in a kneeling position with his knees on the floor. As a way to change the sensations in this position, the woman can place pillows under hips. This allows a better range of motion for the man and allows the woman to position her hips so that she can spread them more openly. The woman can adjust how open she is by adjusting the distance between both of her thighs. She can also use her hands to pull up on the outer labia to assist her partner. If a woman has a hypersensitive clitoris that cannot tolerate strong direct contact, then she should have her legs together.

An alternative to this position is for the woman to lie on her back with both legs straight and the man, while between both of her legs, to kneel facing the woman's face. Then he is to bend his upper body towards her clitoris or vagina until his face reaches the woman's clitoris or vagina. The woman can place one of her legs over his shoulder with a slight twist of her hips. This allows the man to access a variety of the woman's sensitive spots without much effort. Another modification of this position is for the woman to lie on her back and keep her legs straight. In between the woman's legs, the man is to kneel on his knees while still facing her face. The man is to keep his back upright. Then with his hands he should take the woman's legs and put them on his shoulders. This will cause the woman's clitoris and vagina to become closer to his mouth. Then with the man still in the upright position, he should move his head to her vagina or clitoris.

Another popular oral sex position is for the woman to sit on the edge of the chair or bed and for the man to kneel in front of her while facing her face. The man stays upright in the kneeling position and moves his head towards her clitoris. Another popular position is for the man to lie on his back with his legs straight. Then the woman, facing the man's face, is to straddle his face with her knees. The woman should have her clitoris and vagina close to the man's mouth so that he can reach them while his head is still resting on the floor. The woman remains in an upright kneeling position, just relaxes, and lets the man bring her to orgasm. The man, while still relaxed and with his head resting against the floor, can stimulate the woman's clitoris or vagina. In this position the man can also relax every part of his body except his tongue. For variety, the couple can do this position except they can have the woman face the man's feet. This allows the man to easily play with the woman's breasts while he is stimulating her clitoris with his tongue, which tends to relax her more.

Most women enjoy the feeling of their partner holding them tightly around the waist while performing oral sex on them. The couple should experiment to find the position that feels best for them. Each couple is different and will prefer a different set of positions. In all these positions the man can stroke the clitoris and vagina using upward strokes or downward strokes. Also, the man can use circular motion or side-to-side motion to stroke the clitoris and vagina in any of these positions.

Cunnilingus Techniques

The typical tongue is four inches long and weighs a mere two ounces. It is an array of muscles and nerves held together by a membrane covered with thousands of taste buds. It is the most versatile sex organ. It can touch, taste, and lick. The tongue is a perfect instrument for stimulating the woman's clitoris because it is strong, flexible, and soft. For some men, the tongue is the most important sex organ because it enhances their sex life and allows them to bring their partner to orgasm. Unlike the penis, a man never has to worry whether the tongue will perform when he needs it to. Unlike the penis, the tongue is equally effective when hard or soft. Most men think their penises are the most important organ for sex. But in reality, if women were forced to choose between the man's tongue or penis for sex, most women would prefer the tongue.

Does the man's tongue receive pleasure during oral sex? Merely rubbing the tongue is not gratifying on its own. No man goes around stroking his own tongue for pleasure. The man's brain has to be aroused so that the man's tongue receives pleasure when it is rubbed. So during cunnilingus, the man's tongue feels erotic pleasure because the brain is aroused as the man's tongue strokes the woman's genital area.

Good cunnilingus begins slowly and should not be rushed. The man should not immediately rush to attack the woman's clitoris. The man should begin by kissing, nibbling, and licking the woman's inner thighs, lower abdomen, and perineum. Then he should plant kisses on the woman's labia majora, labia minora, and mons. Then he should spread the woman's labia apart and lick and suck each lip gently, one at a time. When the man feels the woman is ready for more, he should lick her slowly from her vagina up to and over the top of her clitoris and back down again. The hood of the clitoris should remain on the clitoris as this is done. He can perform as many strokes as he likes, varying the movement of his tongue to keep it interesting.

When the man feels the woman is ready to be stimulated to orgasm, he can use several methods. One method for a man to stimulate the woman to orgasm is to stimulate the clitoris indirectly. He can do so by moving his tongue on it from side to side or up and down. He can also move his tongue in circles around it or on it. The hood should remain on the clitoris as this is done. He should do so until the woman orgasms. Feather light tongue-twirling on top of the clitoris itself can be sensational. So can flicking the tip of the tongue from side to side immediately beneath the clitoris.

Some women like direct stimulation of their clitoris. Therefore, they enjoy having the hood pulled back to completely expose the clitoris during oral sex. There are three ways that a clitoral hood can be lifted. The first option is for the man to use the index and middle fingers of both hands, puts upward pressure on the inside of the outer labia and lifts the entire area. The second option is for the man to pull the woman's pubic hair and use an upward pressure toward her head. This will move everything up and create a more taut, open area for the man's mouth. The third option is for the woman to hold herself open using both hands. She can use her fingers to spread and hold her labia back to better expose her clitoris and vagina opening. Once the hood is lifted the man can stimulate the clitoris directly. The second method for a man to stimulate the woman to orgasm involves stimulating the clitoris directly. To start, the man should place his lips on the clitoris and do light suctions. The man's sucking on the clitoris can be exciting for most women. Then the man should move his tongue slowly around the woman's clitoris. Then the man can lick the glans of the clitoris directly, with the hood pulled back, in order to stimulate the clitoris directly. He would do so until the woman orgasms. For some women, direct clitoral stimulation of the glans may be too much. The third method for a man to stimulate the woman to orgasm would be much more appropriate. The third method involves the man licking along the shaft of the clitoris only. Women that do not like direct stimulation of the glans might get the most pleasure from this method. The man could also lick the sides of the clitoris and focus on the woman's labia in order not to stimulate the clitoris glans directly.

The man can use his fingers to stroke and tug the woman's inner labia as he licks her clitoris. The man should not get stuck on the clitoris because the whole vagina is sensitive. The fourth method for a man to stimulate the woman to orgasm involves the vagina. The man can insert the tongue inside the woman's vagina and move it in and out. The man should do so until the woman orgasms. Also, he can do this, while he is manually stimulating the clitoris with his hand for more intense pleasure. When the man inserts the tongue as far as he can into the woman's vagina it can be a real turn on to the woman. Also, the vaginal opening is very sensitive. So when the man is doing this method he can lick and suck the vaginal opening to add a variety of pleasurable sensations. The fifth method for the man to stimulate the woman to orgasm involves the man placing his thumb inside the vagina of the woman and pressuring the bottom of the vaginal entry within the first two inches while stimulating her clitoris with his mouth. This arouses and excites the woman greatly. For a variation, if the woman has a G-spot, the man can also give the woman's vagina some attention by inserting a finger or two into her vagina and massaging her G-spot while his mouth is stimulating her clitoris. Another variation of this method is for the man to put his finger or two fingers inside the woman's vagina and slowly move them in and out while stimulating the woman's clitoris with his mouth. This will drive the woman wild. Women usually prefer penetration of the vagina while the clitoris is being stimulated.

Many men make the mistake of assuming that the clitoris is just like a penis. That is a mistake because it is much more sensitive. As a matter of fact, the clitoris is very delicate. Whatever the man does he should keep it light and gentle unless his partner requests that he does otherwise. Every woman's clitoral sensitivity differs, so the man should occasionally check with the woman for feedback. He should keep his tongue moist because a dry tongue can be abrasive. He should not jump from one method of movement to another too quickly. He should try one method for a while to see how the woman responds to it before he goes on to the next method. Some women like the man to move his tongue in small repetitive motions, whereas other women want variety. The woman may like the man to use his tongue in broad general strokes in the beginning, and then as she becomes excited she may want the man to zero in on her clitoris and concentrate on that spot. The secret to good cunnilingus is to focus on the places where the woman enjoys stimulation the most and not move around too much. However, a man should not overdo it and stimulate a certain spot so much that the pleasure decreases and the spot becomes numb. The man should check with the woman and ask her if she would like him to change the location of the spot being stimulated when he is in doubt.

Women do not like it when the man goes fast or rough during cunnilingus. This ends up rushing the woman, which will totally disrupt the buildup of sensation and cause her to feel less pleasure. The slower and gentler the man goes in cunnilingus, the faster the woman will orgasm. In order for a woman to orgasm, she needs to have a buildup of sensation. The speed of movement of the man's tongue should build the sensation up slowly and gradually. Then as the woman begins to approach orgasm, the man should keep the same pace and not speed up. The man should quicken or slow the movement of his tongue during cunnilingus depending on what he sees and feels is pleasurable to the woman during oral sex. However, the movement should remain slow and gentle. How quickly the woman orgasms depends on how relaxed and comfortable she is. An indication of a woman's arousal during cunnilingus may be if she arches her back and goes up on her shoulders. During cunnilingus, some women are afraid that they are not going to orgasm and experience anxiety. The man needs to help his partner and let her know that it is perfectly okay not to orgasm. That will relieve her stress and make her more likely to orgasm.

If the man's tongue gets tired, he should curve it up against the outside of his upper lip. This way he can relax his tongue and not break the sensation of softness and heat the woman is enjoying as he is performing cunnilingus on her. Then the man, using the chin, could pressure the bottom of the vaginal entry within the first two inches. This arouses many women. The man can do so until his tongue is rested and he is ready to resume cunnilingus again.

There is a powerful link of arousal between most females' breasts and their vagina. By stimulating a woman's breasts while stimulating her clitoris or vagina, a man can intensify her pleasure greatly. During oral sex, the man can also use his hands to stimulate the woman's whole body. He can touch her inner thighs, butt, or other parts of her body while performing oral sex. This will gratify a woman a lot. He can also touch gently around her anus and slowly slide a lubricated finger inside her anus and back out again as he performs oral sex on her. He can do that several times. Many women find the stimulation of the anus very pleasurable while receiving oral sex. Usually, a woman gets great pleasure if the man kisses her vagina the same way he kisses her lips, in a big soft, wet and warm kiss.

The woman can use nonverbal communication during cunnilingus. She can move her hips to guide the man's tongue and lips to her most sensitive spots. She can moan, groan, sigh, or call out the man's name as signs that she is enjoying what he is doing and that she wants him to continue. The woman can also put her hands on the back of the man's head and use her hands to direct his head to her most sensitive positions. Likewise, if the woman desires a G-spot massage during oral sex, she could guide one or two of the man's fingers to her G-spot and start moving them at the pace and direction she likes.

Communication is the key to good oral sex. If the woman knows what pleases her, she should let her man know. She should not hesitate to tell her partner. If the man is new to cunnilingus, then the woman should tell him what she likes and she should give him clues as they go along. As in any sexual activity, if anything the man does is painful, the woman should let him know. The key to being an amazing oral lover is for the man to realize that every woman likes something different. The man should talk to the woman to find out what she likes by asking her the proper questions. Then he should pay attention to the way she moves her body during cunnilingus to let him know what she likes the most.

Sometimes a woman may like oral sex, but prefers to have it only as a prelude to intercourse. She may stop the man before she achieves orgasm from the oral stimulation, so that they begin having intercourse. The man should be flattered and not disappointed, because he got her so turned on that she did not want to continue oral sex but wanted to have intercourse. The man should never think that he was not good enough at oral sex and that is why she wanted to change to intercourse. In fact it is probably the opposite.

The 69 Position

The 69 position is the position that both the man and woman assume in order to perform oral sex simultaneously on each other. The man and woman assume the 69 position by lying side by side with their heads at each other's genitals. Another variation of the 69 position is for the man and woman to lie on top of each other (the man or woman can be on top), with their heads at each other's genitals. The couple can have the woman on top at one time and then another time they can have the man on top since each instance produces a different set of sexual sensations to both partners. The most comfortable 69 position is often when the couple is lying side by side with their heads at each other's genitals. The 69 position got its name because of the artistic shape created by the two bodies in that position.

This position allows the couple to get turned on by giving and receiving oral sex at the same time. It is intensely intimate and requires a large degree of trust for both partners. It can also be deeply satisfying to both partners. As with any sex act, it is fun for most people because it offers a variation in sex.

Some people do not like the 69 position because they find it distracting to focus on giving their partner oral pleasure while they are receiving oral pleasure. They want to focus only on receiving their own pleasure because they cannot concentrate enough to give oral sex and receive it at the same time. Also, some people prefer receiving fellatio or cunnilingus separately on the grounds that if they focus entirely on themselves rather than on their partner, their sexual sensations will be more intense. Also, if they are performing oral sex on their partner without receiving oral sex at the same time, they can concentrate solely on giving optimum pleasure to their partner. If this is the case, the man and woman can remain in the 69 position, but take turns receiving oral sex. That way, both partners can enjoy the 69 position without distraction.

Danger from Cunnilingus

A man should never blow air into the woman's vagina because it could cause an embolism. An embolism is an air bubble that enters the woman's bloodstream, which could be deadly. A pregnant woman is particularly susceptible to these embolisms because the veins of her uterus are dilated in order to get more blood to the baby.

Safer Oral Sex—Cunnilingus

Many people do not practice safer sex during cunnilingus because they do not think that the risk of contracting a sexually transmitted disease or HIV (the virus that causes AIDS) is that great during cunnilingus. It is a myth that sexually transmitted diseases cannot be transmitted during cunnilingus. Vaginal secretions may carry bacteria and viruses, including HIV. In order for the man to get HIV from oral sex, HIV infected blood or vaginal secretions need to get into a cut in his mouth, a canker sore in his mouth, or any part where his gums are open, like from brushing teeth. As you can imagine, that is possible. So it is possible for a man to get infected with HIV from cunnilingus.

Also during cunnilingus, the danger of getting a sexually transmitted disease other than HIV does not have to happen by secretions getting into the man's bloodstream. In some cases, such as with herpes, all that has to happen is that the man's skin has to come in contact with herpes-infected skin. Some people have herpes on their mouth and some have it on their genital area. That means that in the case of herpes, the man can get it during cunnilingus if his mouth comes in contact with herpes infected skin on the woman's genital area.

Also, it is possible for the woman to get herpes during cunnilingus. If the man has herpes-infected skin on his mouth (oral herpes), he can transmit the herpes to the woman if his herpes infected skin comes in contact with the skin of her genital area. The woman could have genital herpes as a result of that.

Therefore, unless the man and woman are absolutely certain that their partner has no sexually transmitted infection, they must practice safer oral sex during cunnilingus. A man should use a dental dam when he performs cunnilingus on the woman. Or he can cut a condom or rubber glove and use it like a dental dam. Dental dams are thin sheets of latex designed for use by dentists which can be laid over the woman's whole vulva during sex. They are often sold in drugstores and are displayed near the condoms. The man should have the dental dam cover the woman's whole vulva during oral sex in order to practice safer oral sex. The dental dam, if used properly, should prevent the spread of sexually transmitted diseases, including HIV, during cunnilingus. The man can place a drop of water-based lubricant on the side of the dental dam that will be touching the woman to increase her pleasure. The man can use flavored dental dams to make the oral sex more interesting. If the dental dam is unflavored, the man can add fat free food products like jelly, syrup, or honey to the surface to give it a flavor. He should not use any products with fat because they may damage the latex and make the dental dam less efficient in preventing the spread of sexually transmitted diseases.

Safer oral sex practices are particularly important if the man is practicing oral sex on the woman during her period. It is important because the man most likely will make direct contact with blood. Safer oral sex practices are also especially important if the man is practicing oral sex on his woman and she has a vaginal infection with discharge. It might not sound too appealing to have oral sex on a piece of latex because the man and woman will be sacrificing some sensations. But it is worth it because both partners ensure their health is well and have peace of mind that they are healthy as a result of their safer oral sex practices.

Safer Oral Sex—Fellatio

Many people assume that the risk of contracting a sexually transmitted disease, including HIV, is not great from fellatio. Therefore, many people do not practice safer oral sex during fellatio. It is a myth that sexually transmitted diseases, including HIV, cannot be transmitted during fellatio. Although the risk of getting HIV and other sexually transmitted diseases during fellatio is less than during intercourse, the risk is still there. As a matter of fact, fellatio is one of the most efficient ways of transmitting the HIV virus and other sexually transmitted diseases because always the semen and sometimes the blood are involved. The blood and semen are the two bodily fluids with the highest concentrations of HIV and sexually transmitted disease. During fellatio, the woman is definitely exposed to the semen and sometimes to the blood. The semen and sometimes the blood could get into a cut in the woman's mouth, a canker sore, or any part where the woman's gums are open, like from brushing teeth.

During fellatio, sexually transmitted diseases can be transmitted between both partners without semen or blood being involved. In some cases, as with herpes, all that has to happen is for the infected skin on the man's genital area to come in contact with the skin on the mouth of the woman. This causes the herpes virus to be transmitted to the woman's mouth. Some people have herpes on their mouth, known as oral herpes, while others have herpes on their genital area, known as genital herpes. In this case the man has genital herpes and can give the woman oral herpes if she performs fellatio on him.

However, a man can also get sexually transmitted diseases from the woman during fellatio without any semen or blood being involved. If the woman has oral herpes and her infected skin comes in contact with his genital area, then she could transmit herpes to the man's genital area. The man would then have genital herpes.

Therefore, unless both partners are absolutely certain that their partner has no sexually transmitted infection, then both partners should practice safer oral sex during fellatio. Safer oral sex during fellatio involves the man using a latex condom. The latex condom, if used properly by the man, should be effective in preventing the spread of sexually transmitted diseases, including HIV. Spermicide usually tastes horrible, so the man should not use spermicide with a condom. To make the fellatio more interesting, the man can use flavored latex condoms. If the condoms are not flavored, the man can add fat free food products like jelly, syrup, or honey to the surface of the unflavored condom. Food products with fat should not be used because they damage the latex and make the condom inefficient in preventing the spread of sexually transmitted diseases. Edible condoms do not protect against sexually transmitted diseases. It might not seem too attractive to have oral sex performed on a latex condom, since both partners will be sacrificing some sensations. However, it is worth it because both partners ensure that they remain healthy and they both have peace of mind that they are healthy because they practiced safer oral sex during fellatio.

Chapter 12

Anal Sex

Most people are embarrassed to talk about anal sex and few will even admit that they indulge in it. However, many people have indulged in anal sex. Many people have indulged in anal sex because they have curiosity and interest in experiencing it. Many people love anal sex, while others hate it. Most women have tried anal sex at least once, usually because their partner had suggested it. Many heterosexual couples find anal sex completely natural, extremely sensual, and exciting. Some people who have never tried anal sex are intrigued by the thought of trying it. Some people enjoy anal sex simply because it feels good to them. The men that enjoy anal sex claim that when they penetrate the woman's anus with their penis, it feels like a tighter fit than a vagina. The women that enjoy anal sex enjoy it because the anus contains many nerve endings that are stimulated during anal sex. The anus has numerous nerve endings, just like the vagina or the penis. So the anus has a vast and usually untapped potential for pleasure. It is naturally sexual, so a person should not be surprised or ashamed if it seems erotically responsive. Pressure and fullness in the rectum feel good to some women, just like the fullness in the vagina. Deep anal penetration can stimulate the woman's G-spot. Many women enjoy anal sex because they claim the sexual feelings can be intense during it.

For some people anal sex is appealing because of the psychological thrill rather than the physical pleasure. Some people are thrilled to do something that is considered to be unconventional or taboo. They are excited to explore what is perceived as forbidden territory. For some people, anal sex is appealing because they do not have to worry about pregnancy as a result of it. Some people use anal sex during a woman's period as a way of avoiding menstrual blood while engaging in a form of sex. Anal intercourse is used by some women to maintain their virginity, while still providing pleasure to their partner and themselves. Many heterosexual couples participate in and enjoy anal sex because it is simply another option for sexual gratification.

Anatomy of the Anus

It is important to understand the anatomy of the anus and rectum in order to get a better understanding of anal sex. If the buttocks are spread, the opening to the anus would be visible. The skin surrounding the anus opening is darker in color and contains sweat and oil secreting glands. It also contains hair. Beyond the anus opening there is the anus, a tube that is about 1 ½ inches long. It has no hair and no glands. It does not produce any secretions for lubrication. But the anus and the surrounding skin contain many nerve endings and are therefore very sensitive to touch and stretching.

Inside the anus there are the external and internal sphincters that hold the tube closed until a person is ready to release waste. The internal and external sphincters are two rings of muscle. A person has control over his external sphincter muscle and can tighten and release it. But the internal sphincter muscle is not under the voluntary control of the person. Rather, the internal sphincter muscle is involuntarily controlled by the body and will tighten automatically whenever something is pushed into the anus. Although the anus appears small and tight, it is capable of stretching enough to accommodate any penis size.

The rectum is at the top of the anus. The rectum is the lower part of the large intestine. The rectum is around another 5 to 9 inches, and takes a sharp curve forward in the direction of the stomach. It has several turns. It contains few nerves and is therefore much less sensitive than the anus. However, some people enjoy the feeling of fullness that is created when an object is placed in the rectum. The tissue of the rectum is delicate and is easily damaged by sharp objects. If force is used to enter the rectum, damage to the tissue can result. So a person should be careful when dealing with rectum tissue. The vagina lies in front of the rectum and can be stimulated through the thin anterior wall of the rectum.

Misconceptions Regarding Anal Sex

Of all the sexual practices, anal sex seems to be the most misunderstood. Myths and misconceptions abound about it. One common misconception is that the anus is a very tight hole and that if the male partner inserts his penis in the woman's anus, it would hurt the woman and cause her pain. That is not true since the stool is wider than a finger and it does not hurt when it comes out. The anus can stretch just like the vagina. The vagina can enlarge enough to accommodate a ten-pound, twenty-inch-long baby. The average penis is just six inches with a diameter of a little more than two inches, so the anus can handle it.

Anal sex does not have to equal pain. The high concentration of nerve endings in the anus mean that mistreatment during anal sex can be painful. But it also means that with careful treatment, anal sex can be pleasurable. Anal sex needs to be done slowly and carefully or it can hurt. When anal sex is done properly, slowly with lots of lubrication, it is 100 percent pain free. The lubrication should be on both the condom, which is on the penis, and on the anus. If the man is not wearing a condom, the lubrication should be on the penis. The man should enter the woman's anus slowly and thrust slowly. If force is used to enter the anus, injury to anal tissue might result. Vigorous thrusting especially without enough lubrication won't just hurt; it will also tear the lining of the anus and could tear the condom, which is dangerous. The tearing of the condom is dangerous since it may put both people at risk of being infected with sexually transmitted diseases. Anal sex can become painless once a couple is used to it and they settle into a pace that they both enjoy. Both people can get to the point where they enjoy anal sex as much as any of the other sexual variations.

A second misconception is that there are negative aftereffects from anal sex. There are no negative aftereffects from anal sex. The anus is resilient and pliable and will return to its normal shape, no matter what is done to it during anal sex. Anal sex has no negative aftereffect on the sphincter muscles. Anal sex might actually tone the sphincter muscles, just as exercise tones any muscle group. Anal sex is exercise for the sphincter muscles, and it will strengthen them, and not weaken them. A third misconception is that anal sex does not bring pleasure to the woman. That is not true, since some women can have orgasms from anal stimulation alone. Deep anal penetration can stimulate the woman's G-spot. Pressure and fullness in the rectum because of the man's penis feels good to some women, just like the fullness in the vagina. A fourth misconception is that anal sex has to be enjoyed by everyone. Every person is different and has his or her own preferences. It is perfectly normal for some people to like anal sex, while others do not. If a person tries anal sex and does not like it, then he or she should not do it anymore.

A fifth misconception is that anal sex is unclean. Some people incorrectly believe that a person comes in contact with feces during anal sex. That is not true. The rectum and anus are relatively clean, since they are not storage areas for feces. Rather, waste passes through them. The feces are stored deeper inside the colon. To ensure that no dirt exists in the anal area, a woman should take a shower before anal sex. Some people, although not necessary, use an enema to make sure that the lower rectum is free of waste before anal sex.

Etiquette

A person should never force or pressure anyone to engage in anal sex. If one of the partners does not want to engage in anal sex, then the other partner should be respectful of his or her decision and should engage in other sexual activities. The other partner should accept that it really does not appeal to his or her partner. Sometimes one partner will feel uncomfortable with the idea but will agree to give it a try. If this is the case, the other partner should agree to stop as soon as his or her partner wants to stop. This will help build trust between both partners. It often helps for the reluctant partner to talk about his or her anxieties towards anal sex. The other partner should offer reassurance to the reluctant partner in regards to the reluctant partner's anxieties. At all times, a person should remember that he or she is in control of what he or she does sexually and should never allow anyone to force him or her to do anything that is not appealing.

Anal Sex Positions

There are many positions that can be used for anal intercourse. A couple should experiment and find the one that is most comfortable for them. The best position for rear entry is for the woman to be standing with her back bent forward and her shoulders touching a table. There should be pillows underneath the shoulders. The man should stand straight behind her so that his penis is behind her anus. This position gives the man good access to the woman's anus. Another anal sex position has the woman lying straight on the bed on her chest and stomach and then the man could lie on top of her with his penis entering her anus. A third anal sex position has the woman lying on her back with her legs rolled forward as close as possible to her chest with a pillow under her hips. She can hold her forearms under her thighs to increase the curve of her body and give the man more access to the anus. Her legs should be spread apart as far as possible. Then the man can lie on top of her and insert his penis inside her anus. A fourth anal sex position has the woman lying on her side while the man lies on his side behind her and penetrates her anus with his penis. A fifth anal sex position has the woman on her knees and hands. The palm of her hands should be on the floor so that her weight is spread out among her knees and hands. Then the man kneels behind her and places his penis inside her anus. This position gives the man the deepest penetration. While some people often imagine anal sex as taking place with the man inserting his penis in the woman's anus from behind, that is not the only position that works. Sometimes, especially for the first time, anal sex can be more comfortable if the man lies straight on his back, while the woman is on top squatting over the penis. The woman can lower her anus onto the man's penis and then move her anus up and down on his penis. The penis sometimes slides more easily in this position and the woman can have more control in this position. The woman can control how deep the penis is allowed to go inside the anus and the speed of anal intercourse.

Anal Sex Techniques

In order to have an enjoyable anal sex experience, a couple should adhere to certain techniques. First, the man should make sure that the woman wants to have anal sex. This is important because if she is reluctant to participate, it will be hard for her to relax her muscles, and this will most likely be a tense and not a pleasurable experience. The man can make sure that the woman wants to have anal sex by discussing it with her. Nonoxynol-9 is the most common spermicide that has been shown to irritate the tissue of the rectum, so it should never be used during anal sex. Preparatory foreplay is needed with anal sex just as it is needed with vaginal sex. There are two sphincter muscles in the anus. There is the internal sphincter, which is under involuntary control, and there is the external sphincter, which is under voluntary control. The external sphincter is the one that a person voluntarily relaxes during defecation. The inner sphincter is involuntary and it will clamp shut if something attempts to enter it too fast. The anal sphincter muscles will open, but they require stimulation first. The man should take his time in stimulating them. He should never push or force anything in the woman's anus. Using a lubricant is required for comfortable anal sex. A person can never use too much lubricant during anal sex.

A man can use a well lubricated finger to massage the opening of the woman's anus and the area surrounding it until she becomes more aroused. Then the man can enter the woman's anus with his finger, spreading the lubricant higher into the anus. The man should place a water-based lubricant on the shaft and head of the penis. Once the woman has loosened up, the man should place the penis at the entrance of her anus and apply light pressure, then slowly slide the penis a little further into the anus. The internal sphincter muscle will tighten, resisting the entry of the penis and will make the woman feel as if she needs to have a bowel movement. This is a normal reaction and will pass. The man should never force the penis into the anus or rectum, because it may cause tears or cracks in the delicate tissue of the anus or rectum. Instead, the man should penetrate the anus gently and a little bit at a time, not at once.

The man should keep the penis still until the woman's muscles relax and she is ready to have him proceed with deeper penetration. During the wait the man can massage the area surrounding the anal opening with his hand to help the woman's sphincter muscles relax. Also during the wait, the man can massage the woman's anal area that is closest to the vagina, since that area is a very erogenous area. Then, when the woman's sphincter muscles are relaxed, the man can slowly slide the penis deeper into the rectum, a little at a time. Once the penis is inside the woman, the man can find the stroke and rhythm that works best for both of them. The man should not thrust so rapidly or deeply as he would in the vagina. Rather, the man's thrusts should be shallow and slow. It is important that the man be very gentle during anal sex. If at any time the man or woman feels that the woman's anus has become dry, the man or woman should add more lubrication to the anus. The semen is not irritating to the anus or rectum. Removing the penis from the anus should be done very slowly.

Communication is very important during anal sex. The man should always perform anal sex slowly. He should never thrust rapidly during anal sex. If the woman feels pain, the man should stop what he is doing right away and wait. Then he should proceed only if the woman accepts that he proceeds. On the other hand, if the woman is enjoying what the man is doing, she should share that with him as well. The woman should let him know what she is enjoying during anal sex and what she is not. That way the man knows how to proceed during anal sex. It is important that the woman be in control during anal sex because she is the one on the receiving end, and she is the one that will most likely experience pain if anything goes wrong.

Safer Anal Sex

Receptive anal intercourse is the sexual practice carrying the highest risk of HIV infection among heterosexual women. HIV is estimated to be ten times more easily transmitted to the receiver of anal sex than the giver. This is mainly because, unlike the vagina, the rectum is not naturally lubricated, and penetration causes tiny abrasions in its delicate lining, which opens a direct pathway into the bloodstream. HIV and other sexually transmitted diseases can be transmitted through these tiny tears or abrasions in the rectum during intercourse. If a person does not know his or her partner's HIV status, he or she should avoid anal intercourse entirely, or should practice safer anal sex. Because HIV is most easily transmitted during anal intercourse, many people have been misled to believe that anal sex is always dangerous. In fact, if a couple uses latex condoms and water-based lubrication very effectively, then the risk is reduced greatly. The use of latex condoms on the man's penis prevents the transmission of fluids during anal sex. A couple must always use a condom during anal sex if the HIV status of one of the partners is unknown. On the other hand, if a person is absolutely certain that his or her partner does not have HIV, anal intercourse poses no risk of AIDS transmission. A person cannot get HIV through anal intercourse if neither member of the couple is already infected.

Using a condom during anal sex will protect the man and woman from HIV and most sexually transmitted diseases. However, even with a condom, the human papilloma virus may be transmitted and may cause some types of anal cancer. A woman should let her doctor know that she indulges in anal intercourse and she should routinely ask him or her to check the anus. Anal inspection, anal culture, and the rectal pap smear are similar to the cervical pap smear, and are done sometimes by doctors for women who indulge in anal sex.

Hygiene

The bacteria that inhabit the anus are different from the ones that inhabit the vagina. So in order to prevent vaginal infections, a person should not move a finger, penis, or toy from the anus to the vagina without washing it first. If the penis enters the vagina after having been in the woman's anus, the woman's vagina easily becomes infected. After anal sex, a man should not return to vaginal intercourse until he has washed his penis or changed his condom. Otherwise, the woman's vagina is most likely to be infected.

Finger Stimulation

Some women who do not like anal-penile penetration do enjoy having a finger stimulate their anus. But other women do not like finger stimulation of their anus. So their partner should be respectful of their preference of not liking finger stimulation of the anus. A man can create many sensations for his partner, using his finger in and around the anus. Before the man begins to stimulate his partner's anus with his finger, he should make sure that his fingernails are very short and smooth. This should be done because the tips of the nails can cause a lot of damage to the walls of the anus and rectum. A man can use gloves on his fingers to cover the fingers and nails to protect the anus from damage. During finger stimulation of the anus, there should be a lot of water-based lubricants on the anus and the fingers since the rectum and anus do not produce their own lubrication.

During finger stimulation of the anus, the woman should lie on her back with her knees bent and her legs open while the man kneels between her legs. The man, since he will be performing the finger stimulation, should apply a generous amount of lubricant to his fingers and to the outside of the anus of the woman. The man can gently stroke and massage the opening of the woman's anus. The woman should become aroused. As soon as the woman becomes aroused, the man should lightly press the anal opening with the pad of his finger. If the man notices that the woman is tightening up as a result of the anal sphincter muscles, then he should not force his finger inside. Instead, he should maintain the same pressure until he sees the tightening loosen. Once the tightening loosens he should push his finger in a little further slowly, following the natural course of the anus and rectum. The man, if he likes, can massage or lick the woman's inner thighs, vaginal entrance, vagina, and clitoris, as he waits for the loosening to happen. This will help the loosening to happen. It is very important that the man inserts his finger inside the anus very slowly. His hands should be palm up so that the finger points towards the stomach as it enters. Another way to enter the anus for finger stimulation is to have the woman bear down as if having a bowel movement and then push her bottom towards the man's finger while the man keeps the finger stationary. The woman should stop moving when she feels the finger cannot move because of tightening in the anus. Rather, the woman should wait until she feels loosening in the anus. Then she should move her anus slowly on the man's finger.

When the man's finger is as far as it can reach, the man can begin a slow massage of the front wall of the rectum. The massage should be slow to produce pleasurable sensations and not pain. The massage should have firm strokes. The man may be able to stimulate the sensitive anterior wall of the vagina, where the G-spot is located. The man may also be able to stimulate the G-spot as a result of this massage of the woman's rectum. Some women can experience orgasm as a result of this anal stimulation by the finger of the man. Even if the woman does not experience an orgasm as a result of the finger stimulation of the anus, the woman experiences great pleasure as a result of the sensations that the man's finger creates stimulating the anus, rectum, and area surrounding the anus.

Anal Penetration with Clitoral Stimulation

Many women like being anally penetrated with the man's penis while their clitoris is being stimulated with his fingers. The best position for this to happen is with the woman standing straight and bending her upper body forward until her shoulders are lying on the table. Pillows should be placed under the woman's shoulders. The man should stand straight behind the woman and then penetrate her anus with his penis. As the man thrusts inside her anus, he should move one of his hands to her clitoris. Then he should stimulate the area around her clitoris so that her clitoris is stimulated indirectly with his fingers. Then he could move his fingers and stimulate her clitoral hood, which will stimulate her clitoris indirectly. Then if he knows that she does not mind direct clitoral stimulation, he could stimulate the glans of the clitoris directly, after removing the clitoral hood with one of his fingers. All this clitoral stimulation should happen as the man is thrusting his penis in her anus.

Many women are profoundly turned on by the combination of penile penetration of the anus and stimulation of the clitoris by hand. Many women orgasm as a result of the clitoral stimulation. Another popular position to use during anal penetration and clitoral stimulation is the side-by-side position. The woman should lie down on her side with the man behind her. The man should penetrate her anus with his penis. Then he should move his hand over her body until it is resting near her clitoris. As the man is thrusting his penis inside her anus, the man should stimulate the clitoris with his fingers, either directly or indirectly. He should stimulate the clitoris as he sees fit. Many women get excited and turned on in the side-by-side position while they are being anally penetrated and their clitoris is being stimulated. Many women orgasm in the side-by-side position as a result of the stimulation of the clitoris.

Rimming—Analingus

Analingus is commonly known as rimming. It is the stimulation of the anus with the mouth. Some men and some women like the sensation of a warm, wet tongue against their anus, while others absolutely hate the thought. Therefore, it is best that both partners know each other well and know whether their partner likes rimming. Before rimming, it is important that the person receiving it has the area around his or her anus cleaned with water. Some couples share a bath or shower before any form of anal sex or rimming. The easiest position for rimming is for the receiving partner to be standing with his or her back bent forward and his or her shoulders touching a table. There should be pillows underneath the shoulders. The partner performing the rimming should kneel straight behind the receiving partner so that his or her face is behind the receiving partner's buttocks. This position gives the person performing the rimming very good access to the receiving partner's anus. A second position for rimming is for the receiving partner to be on his or her knees and hands. The palm of his or her hands should be on the floor so that his or her weight is spread out among his or her knees and hands. The person performing the rimming should kneel behind the receiving partner and place his or her face behind his or her buttocks.

The partner performing the rimming should first kiss and lick along the receiving partner's buttocks, moving closer and closer to his or her anus. Then he or she should use his or her tongue to stimulate the opening of the anus and surrounding area by licking it. If the partner performing the rimming has a very strong tongue, then he or she may be able to insert the tongue a short distance into the anus and stimulate it. Bacteria, parasites, hepatitis, and other sexually transmitted diseases can be picked up during rimming. For a person to be safe during rimming, he or she should use a dental dam over the anus.

Things that Make Anal Sex Uncomfortable

There are several things to remember about anal sex that make anal sex uncomfortable. First, it is best to avoid anal sex during pregnancy because the blood vessels surrounding the anus become dilated and more easily damaged. Therefore, tears and abrasions can result more easily in the rectum and anus during pregnancy. Second, some women have hemorrhoids, which make anal sex uncomfortable. Third, the rectum tissue and anal tissue are very delicate and can be easily damaged. The man should make sure that he never forces his penis into the woman's anus or rectum, because it can easily damage the anal and rectum tissues. The man should make sure that he never thrusts rapidly into the anal and rectum area, since it can easily damage the anal and rectum tissues. Rather, he should insert his penis inside the woman's anus slowly, when her anus is relaxed.

Chapter 13

Pre-foreplay

Pre-foreplay is the term used to describe a series of behaviors that occur outside the bedroom that lead to more pleasurable sex. It can start a couple of hours before intercourse, twenty-four hours before intercourse, or even forty-eight hours before intercourse. It is all about how a person treats his or her partner. It involves a person being loving to his or her partner, since this leads to an exciting and more pleasurable sex life. It also involves a person being nurturing and understanding to his or her partner's needs, in and out of the bed. A person being nurturing and understanding to the needs of his or her partner leads to an ecstatic sex life.

Pre-foreplay requires that a person set time and space to be alone with his or her partner. During that time, a person needs to give his or her partner undivided attention and be pleasing to his or her partner. This is a key to relaxing his or her partner and getting the partner in the mood for sex. It makes the partner feel special and turned on. It releases the partner's inhibitions and lets him or her let go. It causes the partner to experience his or her body and its reactions on a completely different level. It makes both people experience a connection between each other, which helps cement the relationship and keep both people together.

Pre-foreplay requires that a person have good manners towards his or her partner and treat his or her partner as his or her equal. Good manners are comprised of being polite, being respectful, and treating the partner as he or she wishes to be treated. If a person takes care of the partner's pleasure and comfort, the partner will be greatly turned on and the sex that ensues will be extremely pleasurable to both people. This is especially true when the man treats the woman like a lady and with great respect. It will drive her mad with sexual desire for the man, and the sex that ensues will be extremely pleasurable for both people.

Pre-foreplay can be done in different ways. One form of pre-foreplay is for the couple to have a candlelight dinner. It allows a person to reconnect with his or her lover after a long day and sets the mood for after-dinner fun. A second form of pre-foreplay is for one person to give his or her partner flowers. It is a very romantic gesture and gets the person in a romantic mood. A person writing and reciting love poems to his or her partner is a third form of pre-foreplay. Many people view it as very romantic. A fourth form of pre-foreplay is for the person to kiss his or her partner away from the bedroom, in a non-sexual setting. It helps build up an anticipation for sex, which leads to pleasurable sex.

A fifth form of pre-foreplay is for a person to tell his or her partner, away from the bedroom, in a non-sexual setting, that he or she loves him or her. Both lovers can stay up all night drinking alcoholic beverages like red wine or whiskey, which is a sixth form of pre-foreplay. A seventh form of pre-foreplay is for the couple to go for moonlight walks on the beach. It is very romantic and puts the couple in a romantic mood. The couple can read romantic stories to each other at bedtime, which is an eighth form of pre-foreplay. Such an act helps build up sexual lust between both partners. A ninth form of pre-foreplay is for the couple to call each other adorable pet names throughout the day. It builds affection between both partners, which leads to extremely delightful sex. A tenth form of pre-foreplay is for the couple to go out to the movies together. It helps the couple to get close to each other. An eleventh form of pre-foreplay is for the couple to tell each other throughout the day what they are going to do in bed in the evening or the next evening. They could tell each other the explicit details of the sexual encounter that they are looking forward to. They could reveal the details in tiny bits throughout the day, and not all at once. This causes greater excitement for the sexual intercourse, which makes the sexual intercourse more pleasurable when it happens. A twelfth way of pre-foreplay is that throughout the day both partners be good mannered, loving, and pleasing to each other. Doing so will cause both people to have great passion to each other, which will result in intensely delightful sex.

Touching

Another form of pre-foreplay that is very important is physical touching in a nonsexual way. When the couple physically touches each other throughout the day in a nonsexual way, and in a nonsexual setting, it makes the couple more in the mood for sex. It increases the lust that both people have towards each other, and eventually leads to a great sexual experience in the bedroom. If a person touches his or her partner in a nonsexual way, it makes the partner feel affection to the person. It shows that the person loves and is concerned about his or her partner. If a couple touches each other in a nonsexual way, it is a form of subtle flirting, and is very exhilarating.

The following are some ways a person can use nonsexual touching during pre-foreplay. One way is for the person, while walking with his or her lover, to put his or her hand around the lover's waist and casually let it slip down to the lover's hip for a second. Then the person brings it back to the waist. A person can also let his or her hand slip up to the partner's back and then bring it back to the waist. A person can do this several times. Such acts increase the sexual passion between both people. A second way is for the person, while sitting next to his or her partner, to place his or her hand on the partner's thigh for a few moments. After a few moments, the person can remove his or her hand. A person can do this several times. Each time a person does it, he or she can put his or her hand on a different area of the partner's thigh. A third way is for the person, while walking, to hold his or her partner's hand. A fourth way is for the person, while sitting next to his or her partner, to hold his or her partner's hand.

A fifth way is for the person, with his or her hand, to caress his or her partner's face from time to time throughout the day. The caress should be just one brief casual caress on the face from time to time. A sixth way, is for the person, with his or her hand, to caress his or her partner's hair from time to time throughout the day. The caress should be just one brief casual caress from time to time. A seventh way is for the person to put his or her hand on the partner's shoulder from time to time while they are walking or while they are sitting next to each other. An eighth way is for the person to hug his or her partner from time to time throughout the day. During the day, both people should take the opportunity to touch each other from time to time, just to indicate that they are happy to be together. All this touching should make both lovers feel more loved and more open to sex. It should drive both lovers wild with passion for each other, which will result in amazing sex.

Talking

Setting the sexual mood using talk hours in advance of the sexual encounter is another form of pre-foreplay. Early in the day, a person can share his or her thoughts with his or her partner about the last sexual experience that they had. This helps put both people in the mood for sex, which results in an extremely pleasurable sex life. The person can share his or her thoughts with his or her partner about what he or she thinks will take place in this upcoming sexual encounter. This results in an extremely pleasurable sexual encounter. The person can share his or her thoughts with his or her partner about an encounter that will happen that same night, the next night, or two nights later. A person can call his or her lover during the day, and tell the lover that he or she has a surprise for him or her that same night or the next night. This will get the lover excited until the encounter occurs.

A person can casually make sexy or romantic comments throughout the day before the sexual encounter. This will add to the partner's sexual anticipation, which results in a pleasurable sexual encounter for both partners. A person does not have to talk dirty to set the mood. Although some people do talk dirty to their partners, and their partners are aroused by such talk. A little verbal teasing and flirting can be an amazing form of pre-foreplay. For example, a person can compliment his or her partner and tell the partner that he or she looks good today. Another example of verbal flirting is for the person to tell the partner that he or she wants to feel the partner's body next to his or her body.

A person can set the sexual mood using talk by telling his or her partner about the positive feelings that he or she has for him or her. A person could tell his or her partner how it feels good for him or her to spend time with his or her partner. A person could tell his or her partner that he or she is glad that they are in each other's lives. A person letting his or her lover know the positive feelings he or she feels towards him or her makes both of them get closer and increases their desire for each other. A person can tell his or her partner during the day how much he or she is lusting for him or her. This works wonders in the sensual imagination of both people.

A person can tell his or her partner about the parts of the partner's body that he or she finds attractive and appealing. A person can do that often and regularly since it will turn the partner on and eventually lead to extremely delightful sex. When a person talks to his or her partner during pre-foreplay, he can do that face to face or over the phone. If the person talks to the partner face to face, then he or she should maintain eye contact with his or her lover to build intimacy and make the talk more pleasurable to both of them. If the person calls his or her lover on the phone, it is very erotic to his or her partner, even though there is no eye contact. Just the fact that the person took time to call his or her partner because he or she was thinking about the partner, turns the partner on.

Benefits of Pre-Foreplay

Pre-foreplay is important since it allows both people to be erotic and loving with each other, which leads to amazing sex. Pre-foreplay allows a person to subtly seduce his or her lover throughout the day, which creates more lust for sex in both people. It excites both partners and increases the sensuousness all day. It starts sexual tension and romance that build up for hours prior to sex. It prepares both lovers for a night of passionate sex. Pre-foreplay makes the sexual experience more sensual and more pleasurable for both people. It brings both people closer and cements the relationship. It makes both people feel connected.

Romance is what keeps the relationship going between a man and woman. It keeps a person falling in love with his or her lover over and over again. Romance is what keeps the sex going between the man and woman. Romance is what makes the sex pleasurable to the greatest extent between the man and woman. Pre-foreplay is an important ingredient for romance and for pleasurable sex. Sure, a person could have sex with his or her partner without setting the proper mood for sex. However, if the mood existing prior to sex is not the proper mood for sex, the sex that follows will not be pleasurable to the greatest extent. For example, if prior to sex the man was tired from work, the woman was tired from taking care of the children, and there was no sexy mood between the two, then the sex that follows will be not pleasurable to the greatest extent. As a matter of fact, a couple might find the sex annoying and boring. However, if prior to sex the man and woman had set a sexy mood between them using pre-foreplay, then the sex that ensues will be very pleasurable to the greatest extent, and will be exciting to both of them.

Pre-Foreplay Important Especially for a Woman

While pre-foreplay is valuable to both partners, it is essential for many women. There is an old cliché that women want romance, while men want sex. The truth is that both men and women want sex, however, women just need more romance than men to awaken their sexual energy and bring it to their genital. Pre-foreplay serves the purpose of providing the romance to the woman that she needs to awaken her sexual energy. It provides arousal for the woman and man long before they reach the bedroom. It ignites their passion for each other and for sex before they fall into bed.

Chapter 14

Dressing for Sex

The way a person dresses before he or she has sex has an effect on the sexual encounter. If a person is dressed up in a way that is attractive, then the sex that ensues will be pleasurable to the greatest extent to both parties. However, if a person is not dressed up in a way that is attractive, then the sex that ensues will not be pleasurable to the greatest extent to both parties. If a person is dressed in an attractive way, then the partner will be attracted to the person and will enjoy having sex with the person to the greatest extent. Also, the person will enjoy the sex to the greatest extent because the partner is enjoying the sex to the greatest extent and is performing well in bed. However, if a person is dressed in an unattractive way, then the partner will not be attracted to the person as much and will not enjoy having sex with the person to the greatest extent. Also, the person will not enjoy the sex to the greatest extent because the partner is not enjoying the sex to the greatest extent and is not performing his or her best in bed. As a matter of fact, a common complaint among many people that are in relationships is that their partner gets sloppy about his or her grooming habits after they get to know each other well. The fact that the partner's grooming habits are sloppy turns a person off and causes a widening in the relationship.

Dressing in an attractive way not only makes the person attractive to the partner, but it also makes the person feel more attractive and sexy, which makes him or her perform better in bed. This leads to a sexual encounter that is pleasurable to the greatest extent to both parties. For a person to turn his or her lover on and to make himself or herself feel sexier, he or she does not have to put on extravagant or unusual outfits. He or she just should try to look his or her best and add a few sexy touches. This chapter contains a few suggestions for women and men on how to dress before sex so that they look their best and be sexually appealing to their partner.

Ways for a Woman to Dress

When a woman dresses for sex she should wear tight clothes that emphasize the curves and contours of her body and draw the eye to the genital area, chest, and buttocks. For example, the woman can wear tight dresses that draw the eye to her chest, buttocks, and the genital area. The woman can also wear tight shirts that squeeze her shoulders, emphasize them, and emphasize her breasts. With the shirt, she could wear a tight skirt that emphasizes her buttocks and genital area. The skirt could be a short skirt that draws attention to her legs. With the shirt, the woman can also wear tight pants that emphasize her genital area and the buttocks. The clothes that the woman wears should be either difficult to take off or extremely easy to slip out of. The fact that the clothes are easy for a woman to slip out of is very erotic and arousing for a man. An example of a way that the woman can dress in easily removable clothes is for the woman to skip the pantyhose by going barelegged and skip the pants or jeans by wearing a soft skirt that is extremely short. She could also wear a blouse or shirt without wearing a bra underneath, which makes her look very seductive and makes her clothes seem to be easily removable. Wearing clothes that are easily removable sends the message "touch me", which is very seductive. Also, the fact that the clothes that the woman is wearing are difficult to take off is arousing to the man because it is teasing to the man that the woman is seductively dressed but extremely difficult to access. For example, if the woman wears a pantyhose and an attractive dress, that might seem erotic to the man because he finds it hard to access the woman's flesh since he has to remove her dress and remove her pantyhose. Another example of hard-to-remove clothes is for the woman to dress in pants. The man will find that arousing because he finds it hard to access the woman's flesh since he has to unbutton her pants and then remove her pants before accessing her flesh. A third example of hard to remove clothing is if the woman is wearing a jacket over her shoulders, since the man has to remove the jacket, then the clothing article beneath the jacket before he can access the flesh.

Romantic clothing that a woman wears should be soft to the touch and easy on the eyes. Another way a woman can dress for sex is by her wearing clothing that shows a little skin, but leaves something to the imagination. For example, long skirts with a slit up the sides, dresses showing most of the back of the woman, or dresses that do not cover the shoulders but cover the breasts downward are very seductive because they leave something to the imagination. Another example of a woman wearing something that shows a little skin but leaves something to the imagination is for her to wear a black or red top that reveals a large portion of her stomach and a large portion of her breasts. She should also wear a short black skirt so that a large portion of her legs are showing.

Other ways for a woman to dress for sex is for her to wear a rubber or leather outfit. If a woman dresses in a shiny black rubber outfit, she will seem very sexy to her man. It is extremely sexy for the woman to wear a rubber outfit since rubber clings to every pore of the woman's skin and squeezes her flesh. Rubber emphasizes the curves and contours of the woman's body. Also, if a woman dresses in a leather outfit, she will seem extremely sexy. A leather outfit gives the woman an attractive look. If a woman wears a tight leather outfit she will seem extremely irresistible since a tight leather outfit will emphasize the curves of her body. Leather is recognized fashion material, and fashion shows for leather are a regular part of the clothing industry. There is a vast range of stunning, close-fitting rubber and leather clothing available. Sometimes one partner can get dressed up in a rubber or leather outfit before sex, and sometimes both partners can get dressed up in a rubber or leather outfit before sex.

The woman should dress in unexpected ways to shock her partner, since the partner finds it erotic that she is dressed in an unexpected way. For example, if the woman normally dresses down in her everyday life, she should try dressing up for sex. Also, if the woman normally dresses up during her everyday life, she should try dressing down for sex. If the woman tends to wear conservative clothes during her everyday life, then should wear provocative clothes for sex. Further, if the woman usually wears provocative clothes during her everyday life, then she should wear conservative clothes for sex.

Lingerie

What a woman wears underneath her clothing can even be more alluring than the clothing that she is wearing. For instance, if a woman wears a lacy bra and matching panties, then when she takes off her clothes, she will look more attractive in her underwear than in the clothes that she was wearing. Also, what a woman wears underneath her clothing can make her feel sexy and attractive. To a man, there is nothing sexier than a woman who feels attractive and sexy. The underwear is the last item of clothing that the woman sheds before sex, so it has an important symbolic value. White underwear conjures up ideas of virginity, purity, and cleanliness, which is a real turn on for many men. Black lacy underwear expresses confidence and sexual assurance and shows the man that the woman wants to take control during the sexual experience. When the underwear is silky and sexy, it can have a great effect of making the woman feel great and making the man long to get his hands on her. Therefore, what a woman wears under her clothes is important to her sex life, since if her underwear makes her attractive to her partner and makes her feel sexy then the sex will be pleasurable to the greatest extent to both parties.

Lingerie improves many couples' sex lives. The man does not have a fetish towards the lingerie, but the garment makes the woman look irresistible. It lets the woman seem racy and adventurous. It makes the woman seem exciting and excites the man. The lingerie pleases the man because the man is visually stimulated, and when he sees the woman wearing the lingerie he becomes sexually aroused. Many married men like their woman to wear lingerie because it resolves the old Madonna/whore dichotomy. The Madonna/whore dichotomy says that the man wants a good girl to marry and be the mother of his children, versus a bad girl that he wants to play with in bed. So if a woman wears the lingerie, she helps resolve the dichotomy for her husband because she is a good girl that is the mother of his children and looks slutty enough to be a bad girl that he can play with in bed. Many men find their woman extremely sexually appealing when their woman wears lingerie in combination with high heels and lots of makeup.

It is important that the woman wears lingerie that makes her comfortable. If the woman is not wearing lingerie that makes her comfortable, then she won't enjoy herself. If the woman does not enjoy herself then the man won't enjoy himself either, and the sex that ensues will not be pleasurable to the greatest extent to both parties. Many stores, including some sex shops, sell erotic lingerie. So a woman has a variety of lingerie available that she can choose to wear.

Shoes

An area of the human body that is overlooked by some women when dressing for sex is the foot. The way the woman's foot appears has a powerful sex appeal with men. Prostitutes in particular are very aware of the foot and its clothing, the shoe. They are aware of them being an erotic symbol of the female body. Prostitutes are very aware of the arousing power of high heel shoes. That is why many prostitutes wear high heel shoes to attract and arouse men. So if a woman wants to dress for sex, she should not forget to wear high heel shoes since they are very seductive to the man. A woman could sometimes wear high black leather boots because the high heels of the boots make the woman's feet seem very seductive, and the black leather on the boots is very attractive and draws attention to the woman's legs and feet.

One way that a woman can dress to sexually arouse the man involuntarily by drawing attention to her feet and legs is to wear sheer black stockings, a short skirt, and tremendously high stiletto heels. The high heels are very erotic to the man when seen on the woman's feet. They attract the man's attention and direct it to the woman's feet. They make the woman's feet seem very attractive. The short skirt is very sexually arousing, and the legs being covered with sheer black stockings are very arousing. The stockings are very arousing because they leave something to the imagination and tease the man since he wants to see the flesh of the legs. The sheer black stockings draw attention to the woman's legs and make them seem sexy. A large number of prostitutes dress this way because they know that it involuntarily sexually arouses the man.

Cosmetics for a Woman to Wear

If a woman wears dark lipstick on her lips, the man will find it very sensual. Dark lips are universally viewed as sensual and attractive. Crimson lipstick, which is a deep purplish red, is very erotic for a woman to wear. Dark eye shadow on a woman is universally viewed as sensual and attractive. If a woman wears dark eye shadow with dark lipstick, she is bound to look more attractive than without cosmetics.

Ways for a Man to Dress

The way for a man to dress for sex is for him to wear what looks good and feels good. In order to dress romantically, he should wear stuff that are nice to the eyes and pleasant to the touch. For example, if a man wears a comfortable, nice looking cotton or cashmere sweater, or even a nice looking, soft T-shirt, it is romantic because it feels good to the touch and is pleasant to the eyes. If a man wears jeans or nice looking polyester pants, it is romantic because it feels good to the touch and is nice to look at. A man can also dress romantically by wearing a nice looking silk, polyester, or cotton shirt. It is romantic because it feels pleasant to the touch and is nice to look at. A man should also wear tight clothes to emphasize certain parts of his body. A man should wear tight shirts that squeeze his shoulders and emphasize them. The tight shirts also emphasize the man's chest. The man should also wear tight pants that emphasize the buttocks and the genital area. By wearing tight clothes, the curves of his body are outlined, which many women find sexy.

When a man dresses in a black, shiny rubber outfit, the woman usually admires his appearance. The woman usually finds it erotic because the rubber clings to every part of the skin and squeezes it tight. A woman also finds it sexy when a man dresses in a leather outfit. A leather outfit usually makes a man better looking to the opposite sex. There is a large variety of rubber and leather outfits for sale at different stores, including some sex shops. Sometimes one or both partners can get dressed up in a rubber or leather outfit before engaging in sex.

Underwear

Men have fewer types of underwear to choose from to wear for their sex partner. However, a man should always remember that what he wears underneath his clothing can be more alluring to the woman than the clothes he had on. A man can wear silk boxer shorts or attractive colored briefs. Silky and attractive underwear can have a wonderful sensual effect, making a man feel great and making his partner long to get her hands on him. Therefore, if a man wears attractive underwear, it will make the sex between the man and the woman extremely pleasurable to the greatest extent.

Dressing in Petals

A person could take fresh petals from long-stemmed red roses and scatter them over the naked body of his or her lover and over his or her own naked body just prior to engaging in intercourse. Then a person can kiss and lick the partner's body around the rose petals, on the stomach, chest, nipples, and thighs. Then the partner can do the same to the person. Finally, both the man and the woman can have intercourse with rose petals between them which provides a very sensuous addition to sex. This provides a very sensuous addition to sex because the petals cling to both bodies due to the sweat generated and leave interesting patterns when the sex is over. Many men and women find the experience highly romantic and erotic.

Smell and Sex

Most people realize that smell has a lot to do with their sex appeal. As a result, men and women spend billions of dollars each year to enhance their sex appeal through sweet smells of perfumes. Odors have the power to arouse a person sexually. A person's sense of smell affects who he or she falls in love with and whether he or she stays in love. If a person loses his or her sense of smell, he or she actually loses his or her sexual function. As proof, most people that lose their sense of smell as a result of heat trauma lose their sexual function as well. This shows how important the sense of smell is to sex. No wonder perfume has been known to some people as sex in a bottle, since by a person improving his or her smell he or she would be more sexually appealing to his or her partner.

Every person smells slightly different and each person has a personal odor print as distinctive as his voice, hands, and intellect. When a person meets someone new whom he or she finds attractive, he or she will also like the smell of the new acquaintance. Then once the person becomes infatuated with his or her new acquaintance, the new acquaintance's smell becomes an aphrodisiac and a continuing stimulant to the love affair. There is an anatomical reason why this happens. The acquaintance's smell is picked up by some of the thousand or so odor receptors that are lumped together in a small patch of tissue in the person's nasal cavity, right behind the bridge of the person's nose. These receptors feed their finds to the person's olfactory bulbs, which process the raw data and send it on to various portions of the brain. One of those places is the limbic system, a primitive region in the brain that controls emotions and sex drive. Therefore, the new acquaintance's odor affects the person's sex drive and emotions when it reaches the limbic system. Among the five senses, smell is unique because it has a nonstop flight to the limbic system. The limbic system is also the seat of long-term memory, which is why a person can remember odors years later, while sights and sounds fade after a few days or weeks.

Anatomically, smell and the emotions overlap in the brain. If a person smells something nice, it is going to make him or her feel better. Perfume smells tend to make both men and women feel better. The smell also makes the woman or man attractive to the opposite sex. Perfumes can also make a person feel calmer, more confident, and therefore sexier. If one person dislikes the other mate's smell, there is trouble and there is no amount of counseling a person can do to make that go away. The way to deal with it is to keep good personal hygiene by showering every day and by using fragrances. The fragrances do not mask a person's odor print, but blend with it. The person comes out with a new odor. Fragrances are useful in enhancing a person's interactions, both at work and at play. Most importantly, perfume enhances the couple's sexual encounter. If a person uses perfume before sex his or her partner will find him or her sexually appealing. This will make the sexual encounter more pleasurable to both people.

Chapter 15

Kissing

Kissing is one of the most intimate and meaningful contacts that human beings can experience together. It brings two people's faces and bodies so close together and makes them tingle all over. With a kiss on the lips the senses of touch, taste and smell are all evoked and these feelings are all combined to produce a strong emotion of affection and excitement in both the giver and receiver of the kiss. Kissing is a real turn on to both the giver and the receiver since it causes the release of endorphins in the human body. Endorphins are chemicals that make a person feel good. Kissing is both physically and emotionally stimulating to both the giver and the receiver. Kissing is the most potent aphrodisiac that a person has at his disposal. In fact kissing can be very sexually arousing. Even though two people might love each other, sexual chemistry will not exist between them if they do not kiss each other or if either partner hates the way the other kisses.

To some people, touching cannot replace kissing in the intensity of arousal that it causes in both partners. There is nothing more appealing to some people than the sensuous power of a kiss. For some people, kissing is more erotic and intimate than intercourse because kissing conveys feelings of love and commitment in a way that intercourse alone does not. For other people, kissing is only a step along the route to intercourse. Kissing is often the first and most important sign to a person that another person is interested in becoming physically intimate. Kissing is usually a prelude to sex.

Kissing is usually the first intimate physical contact a person has with his or her partner and throughout their relationship it continues to be a key part of lovemaking. Kissing is an important aspect of foreplay. Kissing is the number one form of foreplay to get a couple aroused and ready for intercourse. Kissing is often the first intimate physical activity to be lost in a short-term relationship that is suffering or a long-term relationship that has simply lost its spark.

Great kissing is sometimes so good that some lovers can kiss for hours without even wanting to go any further sexually. Just making out without doing anything else can be a sexy idea for people who have decided to wait a while before they have intercourse, or even for couples who have been having intercourse for years but just want a variety in their sex life. Many people believe that a person's ability as a kisser is a good indication of what kind of lover he or she is likely to be. They think that if a person does not know how to use his or her lips, he or she cannot possibly have mastery over his or her other body parts. But a person should not turn away a potential lover because of his or her poor kissing ability, because like anything else kissing can be learned.

Most people kiss for the first time in life when they are in their teen years. But some adults still do not know how to kiss in a sensual way. There are some people and some couples who have never kissed passionately. Their kissing would not be considered stimulating. Rather, their kissing is usually a friendship peck on the lips or on the face. In their kissing they have never used the tongue, or the teeth, and they have not enjoyed full mouth kissing. There are some couples who have stopped kissing passionately and reduced their kissing to a mere friendship peck on the lips or on the face. There are some couples who stop kissing completely. For couples that have never kissed passionately, for couples who have reduced their kissing to a mere peck on the face or mouth, and for couples who have stopped kissing completely, it is fun and rewarding for them to find a new area of stimulation, their mouths.

Kissing is important to a relationship. Without kissing, many relationships suffer and usually end. Kissing is important in sex because without kissing many couples have an unsatisfied sex life and their relationship usually ends because of it. Kissing is very important, so a person should take his or her time when kissing and be conscious of how he or she kisses his or her partner. A person should put his or her heart in the kissing. In fact, in some cultures kissing is so important that it is taught. For example, the Kama Sutra in the Indian culture recognizes kissing as important and as an art that has diverse forms that are taught. In this book, kissing techniques have been described because kissing is a very important form of foreplay and is very important for a successful relationship and for a fulfilling sex life.

Kissing Techniques

Before both people kiss they should both cuddle up and get very close and comfortable. To be really wonderful, kissing mandates the full participation of both people and it must be reciprocal, with each person participating and responding to the actions of the other. For kissing to be truly pleasurable, both people should be completely involved in it. Both people should not be nervous or anxious before they kiss. If they are, then they should let those nervous feelings go away as much as they can before they kiss. The best and most pleasurable kisses happen when both people feel at ease. Most kisses are variations of two different types of kisses. One type of kissing is kissing with a closed mouth, and the other type of kissing is kissing with an open mouth.

Kisses should initially begin with the mouths of both people being closed or only slightly parted. The muscles of the faces and mouths of both people must be relaxed. The lips of both people should not be tightly pursed since tightly pursed lips are not kissable and make a person seem like a novice in kissing. The lips of both people should be relaxed. The kisses should be initially soft and gentle. A person should begin by lightly brushing his or her lips across his or her partner's lips, while at the same time planting soft gentle kisses against his or her partner's lips. The partner should reciprocate whatever the person is doing. A person can add variety to the kissing by gently kissing his or her partner's cheeks, nose, brows, eyelids, ears, or neck from time to time, while still maintaining most of the kissing action on the lips of his or her partner. A person can also add variety to the kissing by varying the pressure of the kissing by making the kisses either firmer or softer. A person can also add variety to the kissing by varying the length of time that his or her lips are touching his or her partner.

After a while, when both people have had enough of the kisses on the lips, they can move on to a different type of mouth stimulation. Then a person can allow his or her tongue to trace just the inside of his or her partner's lips, starting from the corner of the partner's lower lip to the opposite side of the lower lip. Then a person can move his or her tongue across the upper lip of his or her partner, starting from one corner of the upper lip to the other corner of the upper lip. The partner can just do nothing as the person does that, or the partner can reciprocate and do whatever the person is doing at the same time. Usually it is more pleasurable if the partner reciprocates everything the person is doing.

The person can then take his or her partner's lower lip into his or her mouth and explore the outer and inner surface of it with his or her tongue and suck very gently on it. At the same time the partner can take the person's upper lip into his or her mouth and explore the outer and inner surface of it with his or her tongue and suck very gently on it. Then they both can reverse roles.

Then they can start with open mouth kissing known as French kissing. Both people open their mouths and place them on each other with their lips gently pressed together, but not too tightly. Then they go further by allowing their tongues to enter each other's mouths. Both people's tongues should flirt, chase, and explore each other. Both people should use their tongues to explore each other's teeth and gums also. Both people can even use their tongues to explore the inside of each other's cheeks. Then both people can take turns having one person slowly suck on the tongue of the other. It is important that the tongue sucking be done slowly, because it is most pleasurable when done slowly. Then both people can kiss open-mouthed spontaneously and let their whole mouth get into the act. This will allow both people to experience a great amount of passion and arousal. When a kiss becomes more passionate and sensual, the promise of things to come is also heightened. French kissing should be gentle. A person can end the kiss by withdrawing his or her mouth from his or her partner. Then he or she can kiss the partner another French kiss, and another, as many as both of them like. To add variation to the French kissing, a person can kiss the partner from time to time on his or her neck, face, or ears.

French kissing is widely known. A good French kiss can last for a long time, sometimes hours. French kissing sounds exotic, but in reality most people indulge in this kind of kissing regularly. Both people should keep their mouths and tongues relaxed and not tense them up during French kissing. No one should try to force his or her tongue deeply into the mouth of the other or down the throat of the other. If one of the two people forces his or her tongue deeply into his or her partner's mouth, the partner should pull away and start again. This will cause the person forcing his or her tongue deeply into the partner's mouth to get the message.

During kissing, both people should put their hands in a comfortable place, maybe on their partner's back or shoulders. Both people should get passionate in the kissing, but they should not get carried away. Neither one of the couple should open his or her mouth too wide while kissing, because no one wants a person's entire mouth between his or her lips. Besides, if a person opens his or her mouth too wide, then when he or she pulls away from the kiss, there is a great possibility that he or she will drool or drip saliva. Also, if a person opens his or her mouth too wide, then when he or she pulls away from the kiss, there is a great possibility that his or her partner will have their face from nose to chin wet. Also, before kissing it is a good idea that both people swallow so that there is less saliva in the mouth during kissing. All forms of kissing and mouth stimulation should be done slowly, because both people have the most pleasure when the kissing and mouth stimulation is done slowly. If a person kisses his or her partner well and kisses the partner the way that the partner likes, then most likely the partner is going to melt in the person's arms. This is one way that a person communicates his or her love and intimacy to his or her partner. Great kissers, like great lovers, are sensitive to their partner's feelings and responses during kissing.

The most seductive way for a person to kiss his or her partner is for the person while standing in front of the partner to cradle the partner's head and neck with his or her hands so the partner's head relaxes into the person's hands. A person puts both hands behind the back of the partner's head so that part of his or her arms is behind the partner's neck. That way the person's hands support the partner's head and neck so that the partner can relax into the person's hands. Another way for a person to kiss his or her partner is for a person to have his or her partner against the wall, and the person leans his or her body into the partner's body and they kiss. The male or female can be leaning against the wall. Usually it is the female that leans against the wall, but it does not have to be that way. It is a nice variation to have the man against the wall and to have the woman lean against him. A third way to kiss is for a person to turn up the face of the partner by holding his or her head with one hand and his or her chin with the other hand then kissing. This is a gentle kiss expressing feelings of tenderness.

There is a subtle difference between kissing and being kissed. Just because a person is a male, does not mean he always has to be the kisser. The male should also try being the one kissed, and the woman should also try being the kisser. This introduces a variation in kissing, which makes kissing more interesting and more pleasurable to both parties. Most of the time both partners should be actively involved in the kissing process, however from time to time it is fun and pleasurable if one person takes total control of the whole kissing process, guiding the entire kiss while the other person is passively receiving pleasure. It is even more fun when the woman is the one taking total control of the whole kissing process, guiding the entire kiss. It is more fun because the woman usually is the passive one, and by her taking control she is doing something that she usually does not do.

Kissing does not have to be only on the face and mouth. As a matter of fact, kissing is very arousing during foreplay and sex when it is done on other parts of the partner's body. A person can use his or her lips to kiss his or her partner all over his or her body, including his or her shoulders, arms, inner thighs, back of the knees, and armpits. Some areas of the body are more sensitive to the softness of a kiss than others. The inner thighs and armpits are very sensitive for many people when kissed and bring them great pleasure when kissed. When a person kisses his or her partner on different parts of the body, the partner feels a different set of pleasurable sensations because different parts of his or her body are kissed. Women usually like their breasts to be kissed, especially their nipples. Many women and men like their genital area to be kissed. For many people, if their partner kisses their genital area, it is a special act of acceptance and one of the most powerful aphrodisiacs. When a person is treating his or her partner to an all over the body kissing session, he or she should not forget to use his or her tongue and hands from time to time, to increase the partner's pleasure. A little stroking and licking, along with a lot of kissing, will intensify the passion of the person's kiss and increase the partner's pleasure.

Remember that people's preferences change. At times a person wants French kissing, while at other times he or she does not want it, but wants only dry kissing. There might be no rational reason for his or her change in preferences, but the only explanation is that the person just felt for dry kissing and not French kissing at the time. Also, it is important to remember that each person has his or her own unique brand of kissing. One person might like a certain type of mouth stimulation and kissing, while another might not like the same type of kissing and mouth stimulation. The kind of kisses that turned a person's previous lover on might not turn a person's current lover on. So it is important for a person to cater his or her kissing techniques to his or her partner's preferences. In this section, a variety of kissing techniques were described. Some people might like all of these techniques, while others might not. So it is important that a person uses the kissing techniques that his or her partner likes. One way to find out the kissing techniques that the partner likes is to ask the partner what kissing techniques he or she likes. Another way is to observe him or her during kissing, to see from his or her body language what he or she likes.

Ways to Keep Kissing a Vital Part of the Relationship

Both men and women, especially in long standing marriages or relationships, tend to forget the importance and pleasure of the little thing called kissing. In a long term relationship it is natural to forget about how wonderful kissing can be. People tend to overlook the skillful kissing that used to really make things happen. As a result, some couples stop kissing completely, while at other times some couples limit their kissing only to when one of them wants to have sex. When lovers gradually forget to kiss each other except when they want sex, kissing begins to seem more like a demand for sex rather than an expression of love. A kiss becomes a sign that one of them wants to have sex now. It is important that a person does not stop kissing his or her partner completely, nor limit his or her kissing to when he or she wants to have sex. This is important so that both people can experience the joy of kissing and other sensuous touches and feel loved and not taken for granted sexually. It is important in a relationship that kissing not only be a prelude to sex, but also to be innocent and flirtatious at times.

There are certain ways to keep kissing a vital part of the relationship. One way is for a person to be aware of how he or she is flavoring his or her kisses. Smoking, drinking alcohol, or eating spicy food, garlic, or onions prior to kissing can leave a disagreeable taste in a person's mouth. It is important that a person keeps his or her mouth with a pleasant taste, since a mouth with a disagreeable taste will produce badly flavored kisses which will cause the partner to shy away from kissing the person. Sometimes a person is not aware that he or she gives off badly flavored kisses, and his or her partner is too shy to mention it. This usually leads both partners to shun from kissing each other, which usually will cause the relationship and the sex to suffer. It is not uncommon for some relationships to be wrecked as a result of a person's bad-tasting mouth. It is not uncommon for the pleasure during sex to suffer as a result of a person's bad-tasting mouth. A bad-tasting mouth of a person will cause the kissing to stop or decrease greatly between a couple, which usually leads to a less pleasurable sex life and a less pleasurable relationship. If a person has a partner that has a bad taste in his or her mouth, he or she should let the partner know and should advise him or her as to how to keep the mouth with a good taste in it. In order to keep the mouth tasting pleasantly, a person should drink plenty of water prior to kissing. A person should also brush his or her teeth, if possible, prior to kissing. If all else fails, a person should suck on a mint or other treat before kissing. Breath fresheners provide a short term solution, but are not a substitute for a clean mouth.

Another way to keep kissing as a vital part of the relationship is for a person to make it a point that when he or she kisses, to gaze into his or her partner's eyes. Sometimes one or both people close their eyes during kissing. It is important that both people during kissing keep their eyes open, so that they look into each other's eyes, which produces extremely intense intimate and romantic feelings in both of them. When such feelings are produced during kissing, kissing tends to remain a vital part of the relationship. However, if during kissing one person closes his or her eyes, then each one of the couple will feel less intense intimate and romantic feelings. This will decrease the likelihood that kissing will be a vital part of the relationship.

A third way to keep kissing as a vital part of the relationship is for a couple to exchange words of affection during kissing. This makes both of them feel great affection towards each other during kissing. This will make it more likely that the couple will continue to kiss each other regularly. A fourth way to keep kissing as a vital part of the relationship is for both people to feel the lips of each other and to feel the sensations that are produced during kissing. Many people take kissing for granted and do not dwell on the sensations produced during kissing, nor on the feel of their partner's lips during kissing. Rather, they kiss each other while ignoring the sensations and feelings produced because they take them for granted. The lips are very dense with nerves, and therefore are very sensitive and produce a large amount of sensations. Therefore, if both people during kissing concentrate on the sensations produced, the kiss will be electrifying for both of them and kissing is more likely to remain a regular part of their relationship.

Keep Kissing Safe

Kissing can bring great joy but like some pleasurable things, there are risks involved. Both partners should not kiss each other on the lips if either of them has a cold sore near or on his or her lips. They should not even give each other a quick peck on the lips if either of them has a cold sore near or on his or her lips. This is because the herpes virus can be transmitted during kissing of any kind. Also, a person should not kiss his or her partner on the lips if either of them has mononucleosis (kissing disease), hepatitis, the common cold, or flu because these diseases can be transmitted while kissing an infected partner on the lips.

Difference Between Men and Women in Kissing

Usually women love to kiss more than men. The most common complaint among women regarding kissing is that they do not get enough of it. A man usually regards kissing only as a step towards intercourse. While a woman usually regards kissing as an important act that shows love and passion. A woman does not like it if a man kisses her only when he wants to have sex. A woman likes it when a man kisses her to show love and concern. She likes it when a man kisses her just for the sake of kissing her, without expecting sex afterwards, because it makes her feel loved and wanted. If a man only kisses his woman when he wants sex, then kissing will be a demand for sex on the woman, and will not be pleasurable for both the man and woman. The woman will not feel loved and will not feel that her man cares for her. The sex that ensues will not be pleasurable to the greatest extent. Therefore, a man and a woman should kiss each other regularly just for the sake of kissing, without expecting sex afterwards, so that both people feel love and intimacy between them. If both people feel love and intimacy between them, then the sex between them becomes pleasurable to the greatest extent, and most important of all the woman feels loved and cared for. The woman also, is more open to sex and more responsive to her man during sex, as a result of feelings of love and intimacy between them.

Also, during foreplay kissing is very important to a woman because it usually gets her ready for sex. A common complaint among women is that men do not kiss them enough during foreplay to get them ready for sex. When a man does not kiss the woman enough during foreplay and rushes to intercourse, the woman will not enjoy sex to the greatest extent. She will feel something is lacking during intercourse. However, when a man kisses the woman enough during foreplay, the sex that follows will be pleasurable to the greatest extent. During foreplay it is a good idea for the man to ask the woman if she has had enough kisses before he proceeds to intercourse, because that is the only way that a man can tell that the woman has had enough kisses.

Chapter 16

Foreplay

Most people divide sex into two stages. The first stage is foreplay, followed by the second stage: intercourse. In most sports the players usually spend some time warming up until they feel ready for the real game. Likewise, for sex, the man and woman usually spend some time warming up until they feel ready for intercourse. When the man and woman spend time warming up for intercourse it is called foreplay. As a matter of fact, in order for a couple to have great pleasurable sex, they have to have great pleasurable foreplay. This is especially true for women because they can barely enjoy intercourse without first having foreplay. Foreplay is important to a couple because it relaxes both of them and gets both of them ready for sex. Foreplay is especially important for a woman because a typical woman will not get turned on and will not experience an orgasm if she is not relaxed. Foreplay especially allows the woman that has difficulty experiencing an orgasm to let go so that the man can bring her to orgasm and to the heights of pleasure.

Fabulous foreplay is all about enticing and exciting both the mind and body. Foreplay is the sweet skin to skin seduction of sex before intercourse. Kissing, hugging, snuggling, licking, and touching are what make up foreplay and are a necessary and often very satisfying part of lovemaking. These are important because they let both partners relax. What enhances a couple's sex life the most is lots and lots of foreplay. The couple that has lots of foreplay before actually having sex has incredible orgasms. Usually both members of the couple that has lots of foreplay experience incredible orgasms. Foreplay is important because it makes sex a totally different experience for both the man and the woman.

Foreplay is a must. Setting time aside for foreplay before sex is a must. It is important to set aside time for foreplay before sex because foreplay sets both the man and woman in the mood for sex. Foreplay creates an anticipation for sex in both the man and woman. Foreplay builds up arousal. This is important because arousal makes sex fun and is a really delicious part of sex. More than anything else, arousal is what drives good sex. Arousal is what a person feels when he or she starts appreciating his or her partner's sexiness during foreplay.

Although foreplay usually makes sex more pleasurable for both the woman and the man, it is usually more important to the woman. It is more important to the woman because the man can experience an orgasm without sufficient foreplay, while a woman cannot experience an orgasm without sufficient foreplay. As a matter of fact many women fake orgasm because men do not perform sufficient foreplay before intercourse. Some people find foreplay at times more enjoyable than sex.

Usually a man is ready for sex after a minute or two of foreplay. However, a woman is usually ready for sex after 20 minutes of foreplay. It is important that the woman get sufficient foreplay, usually 20 minutes, before sex in order for her to enjoy the sexual encounter and orgasm.

Foreplay is Important to the Woman

One thing about foreplay is that men usually tend to neglect the fact that it often takes women longer to get in the mood for sex than it takes them. Most men tend to make the mistake of initiating sex as soon as they have an erection without having done sufficient foreplay. They succumb to what may be an evolutionary urge to spread their DNA as quickly and as often as possible. Most men touch the woman only when they are initiating sex. They do not spend enough time touching and showing affection as foreplay to get the woman ready for sex. To them, touching and showing affection means that the woman is ready for sex, when the woman in reality wants more affection, touching, hugging, and kissing.

Men do not realize that women need intimacy prior to sex, because they use sex to gain intimacy. Women need more foreplay than men because they need an emotional connection with a man before they are willing to have sex. While most men usually do not need an emotional connection with a woman before they have sex. Women want more foreplay than men because foreplay tends to show the woman that the man is attracted to her for personal and emotional reasons than a mere carnal desire. However, most men do not care if the woman is attracted to them for a mere carnal desire.

Men are more visually stimulated than women. A good deal of the man's arousal is by visual stimulation rather than by touch or tenderness. That is why a man can be hot and ready for sex when the woman is not yet. The woman needs physical affection to get aroused, but the man has already been aroused visually by her. Therefore, the man is ahead of the woman on the arousal curve and does not need as much foreplay or any in order to start having sex and in order to experience an orgasm. A woman needs to be romanced a little before sex. Women seem to require more overall, non-genital, whole body touching before escalating things to intercourse. Gentle touching is evidence to the woman that the man cares about her as a person. She needs that before she can become aroused.

The most common complaint of women for lack of pleasure during sex is the lack of tenderness and intimacy during sex. Intimacy during sex for a woman is usually attained through foreplay. Women desire more holding, touching, caressing, snuggling, and kissing before intercourse than men. Women want more romance involved with the sexual encounter than men do. For example, women like sipping champagne in front of a fireplace with her man and hearing from him that she is the most amazing woman he has ever met. Then she might enjoy dancing with her man followed by having him undress her and himself before they have intercourse. On the other hand, most men just want a little foreplay, like a little kissing and touching, and they are ready for sex. When foreplay is lacking for the woman, she does not feel loved, appreciated, desired, and secure enough to relax and enjoy sex. When foreplay is lacking for the woman the woman does not feel intimate with the man. On the other hand, the man feels intimate with the woman when he has sex with her regardless of whether they had any foreplay or a little foreplay before sex. Women tend to want a romance novel in bed, which is a substantial amount of foreplay before sex, while men tend to want a pornographic movie in bed, which is little or no foreplay before sex.

One important fact that most men do not realize is that more foreplay will also increase a man's pleasure during sex. An erection results because more blood is entering the penis than is going out of the penis. The pulsations of an orgasm feel great in part because the volume of blood in the penis is beginning to normalize. The longer the buildup of blood in the penis as a result of foreplay, the more blood to evacuate during orgasm, the longer the orgasm, and the greater the pleasure during an orgasm. Also, more foreplay will make a man's erection larger and thicker, making the encounter more pleasurable to both people.

Another important fact that most men do not realize is that foreplay is important for a woman not just for non-physical reasons. It is important to a woman for physical reasons also. Foreplay is important to a woman because it lets her become aroused, which causes her vagina to become longer and wider and generate more lubrication. This is important because if a woman has intercourse before she is adequately aroused, the vagina would not have become longer and wider, and the penis will thrust against the cervix, uterus and ovaries of the woman, causing discomfort. The pain that results is usually sharp but may have a burning quality. If a woman has intercourse before she is aroused she would not have lubricated her vagina well. Lubrication is important for the woman and man during sex because it will facilitate a smoother entrance for the penis and smoother movement for the penis and the vagina. Without adequate lubrication the sex will be painful for both the man and the woman. It is very important for the woman and man to spend time on foreplay before sex for physical reasons, because without adequate foreplay the sex will be painful for the woman.

A woman should not allow herself to be rushed into intercourse before she has received adequate foreplay and is ready for sex. Most women need and desire more foreplay than men to become sufficiently aroused before intercourse. When sex begins and ends according to the man's erection the woman feels unsatisfied physically and emotionally. Usually, if the man enters the woman as soon as he has an erection, the woman may feel uncomfortable physically and emotionally, since she is not ready physically or emotionally to handle the penetration. Also, the sex may be painful for the woman and orgasm may be unlikely. A woman needs more foreplay so that she becomes adequately aroused, so that the sex is not painful but pleasurable, and so that the chances of orgasm are very high.

Men should be aware that vaginal lubrication or vaginal wetness is not a reliable indicator of whether or not a woman is turned on. Older women often have trouble producing adequate vaginal lubrication for sex. Also, female lubrication is linked to female sex hormone levels and fluctuations in these hormones along with many other factors can sometimes make it difficult for a woman to get wet naturally, even if she is sexually aroused. So during foreplay, if the man has spent enough time on foreplay and sees or feels that the woman is not lubricated enough, he should not feel that he has not aroused her enough during foreplay. He should not feel that he did a bad job during foreplay. Rather, he should understand that he did a good job of arousing her during foreplay but that there are other factors like her hormones or her age that are not letting her be lubricated enough even though she is very aroused. The couple could compensate for the woman's lack of natural lubrication by using a water-based lubricant.

Non-Physical Foreplay Techniques

There are tried and proven ways for a person to help his or her partner loosen up during foreplay so that the sex becomes more pleasurable. The first way is for the person to let his or her partner know that he or she likes the partner's body and finds it attractive. A person will not relax and let himself or herself experience pleasurable sex if he or she feels self-conscious or bad about his or her body. Most people, both men and women, question their attractiveness and often have negative feelings about their body image. Even people with bodies like models are self-conscious about their bodies and have negative feelings about their bodies. The person should try to make his or her partner feel good about his or her body and comfortable with his or her body. The second way is for the person, during foreplay, to try to make his or her partner feel special. A person can do that by taking his or her partner's pleasure and comfort into consideration and treating his or her partner the way that the partner wants to be treated. A person should give his or her partner his or her undivided attention, which is a key in relaxing his or her partner and getting his or her partner in the mood for sex. Quite simply, if a person makes his or her partner feel that he or she has gone out of his or her way to treat his or her partner special, the partner will most likely have pleasurable sex. Women are most likely to have an orgasm if they feel that the man has gone out of his way to treat them special.

The third way is for a person to make his or her partner comfortable mentally and physically. A person can do that by providing a good, safe, and enjoyable environment for a sexual encounter. A person can make the room that the couple is going to have sex in inviting for his or her partner by keeping it tidy. The person can keep the room tidy by putting away all clothes in the room, always using fresh sheets and making sure the bed is made. A person should do that because many people are turned off by an unclean or untidy room, and this translates into them being not comfortable and happy during the sexual experience. A person can use the lighting in the room to make it more romantic. A person can dim the lights in the room or use candles to provide lighting in the room that is romantic. Dim lighting is seductive for both members of the couple. Dim lighting is easy on the skin, making it look warmer, smoother, younger, and purer. A person can play some music in the background to make the atmosphere more relaxing and seductive. If the music is played in a low volume in the background it can have a calming, soothing effect. Usually music that has a slow beat or rhythm can be used because it calms the nerves and helps contribute to a romantic atmosphere. If a person plays his or her partner's favorite recordings it would be a plus. A person can also put a small decorative fountain that fits easily on top of a table or bookshelf. The fountain produces a sound of trickling water in the background that helps to create a romantic atmosphere and increases the couple's sexual appetite. Also, the sight of trickling water in the background can be relaxing and helps the couple increase their sexual appetite.

The room should be kept warm. The room should not be cold because if the skin gets cold it tenses unpleasantly and touch is then experienced less pleasurably. A cold room will interfere with having pleasurable sex. Both partners will not feel comfortable making love in a cold room and this discomfort will decrease their ability to enjoy sex and their ability to orgasm. A room should not be kept hot, either, because if it is hot then both partners will be hot and sweaty and will not be comfortable making love. This will decrease their ability to enjoy sex and their ability to orgasm. The room should be kept warm so that both people feel comfortable being naked and making love. If the answering machine is in hearing distance of the bedroom a person should turn off the volume. If there is a phone near the bed a person should turn off the ringer. There is no greater mood shatterer than a ringing phone. The person should minimize interruptions so that he or she makes the room a haven for intimacy. A person should strive to make the room that the couple has sex in an oasis for his or her partner. If a person makes the room into an oasis it will show his or her partner that he cares about him or her and that will usually turn his or her partner on.

The fourth way is for a person to set aside enough time for foreplay by planning for it. Just as a person sets aside time for the workout at the gym or for a car tune up, the person needs to set aside time for foreplay, romance, and relaxation. A person should spend enough time with his or her partner during foreplay since it gets both of them sexually excited. The fifth way is for a person to make sure that his or her partner is not burdened with stress or high expectations about the outcome of the foreplay or the sexual encounter. A person can do that by letting his or her partner know that he or she should not worry about the outcome of the foreplay or the sexual encounter. A person can let his or her partner know that as long as they enjoy themselves during foreplay and the sexual encounter, that is what is important, regardless of the outcome. The sixth way is a person can make sure that when both people come to enjoy foreplay that neither of them is tired and low on energy. It is important that neither member of the couple be tired because if one of them is tired, then he or she will lack sexual desire and the foreplay and intercourse would not be pleasurable for both of them.

Undressing For Sex

Undressing for sex can be a form of foreplay. When the time comes for both people to undress before engaging in sex they have the chance to tantalize each other. They can undress for sex by undressing each other or by stripping for each other. Men and women are usually turned on when their partners undress. When undressing each other, a man and woman can take turns removing a clothing article from their partner slowly and erotically until they are both naked. This can make the sexual desire of both partners increase before intercourse. Usually, they start with the shirt or dress, then the shoes, socks, pants or skirt, and then the underwear.

Sometimes a person likes to have his or her partner undress before his or her eyes slowly in a seductive way by removing one clothing article at a time. The person likes to sit and relax as he or she watches the partner remove his or her clothing. The partner could also remove his or her clothing while moving his or her body in a sensual, teasing way. A person likes his or her partner to strip before his or her eyes because he or she views it as erotic. The fact that the partner is taking off his or her clothing slowly, one clothing article at a time, is very teasing to the person since he or she wants to see the partner totally naked as soon as possible. Teasing is a natural part of love play and it makes love play more pleasurable. Usually men like to have their partner strip before their eyes more than women do. While stripping, sometimes the partner can add some sexy music to help him or her get into the rhythm. While stripping, the partner can dance around the person, emphasizing his or her chest, buttocks, and legs. While dancing, the partner might also want to put his or her foot on the person's thigh and rub it in an erotic way. While taking off his or her clothes the partner might want to tease the person by slipping his or her shirt off a little and then putting it back on before completely removing it slowly and seductively. Then he or she can unfasten the pants then refasten it again before completely removing it. If the partner is a woman the woman can take off the skirt or dress a little and then put it back on before completely removing it. When the partner takes off each article of clothing he or she should gently toss it in the lover's direction. Once the partner is down to his or her undergarments he or she can be more seductive with the way he or she removes them. Before completely removing the underwear, the partner can lower his or her underwear, but then slide it back on. If the partner is a woman, before she completely removes the bra, she can drop her bra strap then put it back on. When all the clothes are off the partner can move around nude. He or she can roll his or her hips seductively. He or she can touch his or her body everywhere, even his or her genital area. This will drive the person wild with lust for his or her partner. Then the naked partner can take a seat and wait for the person to start stripping.

Showering Together

Another method of foreplay is for a person to help his or her partner shower or take a bath. Many people have fallen in love with their partner and married them because their partner bathed or showered them. Helping the partner shower or take a bath is seductive because the person is taking care of his or her partner and thinking of him or her. Every partner in the world wants to know in his or her heart that the person he or she is with can and will take care of him or her physically and emotionally, and every partner wants to feel special and appreciated.

Also, the man and woman should shower or bathe together as a form of foreplay so that there is no body odor that will be offensive to either person during foreplay. The fact that there is no body odor will make the foreplay more enjoyable. When both the man and woman shower or bathe together it is a totally erotic experience. It is amazing how easily a soapy hand can slide over nipples, between thighs, and around and between the curves of the buttocks. It can feel great to soap each other up, exploring each other all over. It is very erotic for the man and woman to shampoo each other's heads. While shampooing each other they can carry out a luxurious head massage, applying deep circular pressure with fingertips at the temples, the hairline, and all over the scalp. A person feels very erotic rubbing his or her soaking wet body against his or her lover's body. A person likes the feeling of his or her mouth filling up with water as he or she kisses his or her lover under the shower. The shower or the bath is a great place for sexual play. Both the man and woman experience great pleasure by having a handheld showerhead placed between their legs. It puts them in a new state of relaxed and energized bliss. A person can use the flow of water from the showerhead to stimulate different parts of the partner's body.

Bathing together can be a totally romantic experience if the right mood is set with bubbles and candles. In a bath, both people can take turns enjoying leaning back and relaxing in the other person's arms. Once out of the shower or bath a person can give his or her partner a massage. The partner wants attention.

Touch

Touch is an essential part of foreplay. Foreplay is not complete unless there is touching between both the man and the woman. Touching releases a hormone that increases affection, sexual responsiveness, and sexual sensitivity. The hormone is oxytocin. Touching increases the production of sex hormones and decreases stress. Touching keeps couples together, since it leads to strong emotional bonds. The skin is a very large erogenous zone, and it should be stimulated during foreplay to produce erotic feelings in both partners. Touching is one of the best ways to stimulate the skin.

Touch is the best method for a person to use to relax his or her partner before sex. A person can use touch to arouse his or her partner sexually during foreplay before sex. A person can tell if his or her partner is relaxing as a result of touch by looking for different signals. One signal he or she can look for is if the partner's breathing changes and becomes deeper and slower. Another signal he or she can look for is if the partner's body doesn't seem to be tense. Being touched is important for a woman because, unlike the man, she cannot experience an orgasm unless she is totally relaxed.

Both partners should touch each other during foreplay to show each other love and concern. Both partners feel more loved and greater pleasure during foreplay and sex as a result of being touched. Both partners should touch each other's whole body during foreplay to intensify the pleasure during foreplay and during sex. Many women complain that their man does not touch them enough during foreplay. They claim that he touches them only when he is initiating sex. When a man touches the woman only to initiate sex touch begins to seem more like a demand rather than an expression of love. It is important for the man to provide sensuous touching during foreplay without initiating or demanding sex, just for the woman to make sure that the man is not taking her for granted sexually. When the woman feels more loved she is more open to sex and more likely to experience an orgasm. A woman enjoys and sometimes relies on touching to get her wet and ready for penetration and orgasm. When a man touches the woman, the woman should make sure that he touches her whole body and that he overlooks no surface. She should do that so that he gets a sense of how and where she likes to be touched, since every woman is different. Women tend to like the whole body to be touched so that they become aroused, while men do not care if the whole body is touched in order to become aroused. Women tend to have a problem with lack of touch from the man during foreplay, while the man, it seems, never has a problem with lack of touch during foreplay. This is because the woman takes longer than the man to become sexually aroused and ready for sex.

Touching is essential for a relationship to last, and is emotionally satisfying for both the man and the woman. Touching decreases the frustrations and anger that one partner might have for another. Touching and being touched results in the release of oxytocin, which increases affection and bonding between the couple. Touching and being touched results in a sense of wellbeing as a result of oxytocin and endorphins being released. Touching decreases the stress level, blood pressure, and pulse rate of the provider and the receiver of touch. The more the man and woman touch each other the more they both want to be touched.

Sometimes a person does not know or is not sure what he or she wants in regards to touching. This might be because of lack of sexual experience, or because he or she grew up in a sexually repressed household where it was not okay to talk about sex. Also, sometimes a person does not know what is pleasurable in regards to touching because the previous partners that he or she had did not know everything in regards to what is pleasurable during touching. So a person does not know what is pleasurable in regards to touching until the partner touches him or her and experiments with him or her. So the partner doing the touching should ask the person to let him or her know what he or she is enjoying during the touching sessions. The partner should note the areas that the person enjoys being stroked and concentrate on those areas when touching. The person could also move the hands of the partner doing the touching to the spots that the person wants stimulated. The person could also move the hand of the partner doing the touching in the way that the person wants him or her to move it during the touching.

Touching can be done in a variety of ways. One way to touch is percussion, which is light tapping movement with the fingers or the palm of the hand. Another way to touch is kneading, which is to pick up and squeeze the skin and underlying tissue between the thumbs and fingers. Kneading is wonderful in the area of the body with large muscles like the back, upper arms, thighs, and buttocks. A third way to touch is to pinch the skin carefully and lovingly. A fourth and most common way to touch is to stroke and caress the skin. The caressing of the skin can be done in an up-and-down motion, side-to-side motion, or in a circular motion. A person can touch his or her partner using his or her fingers or thumbs.

A person should touch his or her partner gently and slowly. This causes the partner to experience pleasure to the greatest degree. The slower and gentler the touch, the more pleasurable the sensation that is provoked in the partner touched. If a person touches his or her partner rapidly, the sensations will not be very pleasurable. If the touching is done extremely fast, it might even irritate the partner and cause discomfort. However, a person can touch his or her partner in a fast motion from time to time. He or she could do so even though the sensations are not very pleasurable because it is something different. The fact that it is something different makes it very exciting and extremely pleasurable, even though the sensations produced are not very pleasurable. When the person does it from time to time he or she should do it fast, but not extremely fast, because if it is done extremely fast, it will irritate the partner and cause discomfort. Even though the gentle pressure of the stroke is very erotic and sensual and produces pleasure to the greatest degree, the stroke can sometimes have a lot of pressure. Strokes with a lot of pressure can be used to release major tension in any area of the body. They also improve circulation and relax muscles. A person should keep a steady rhythm during a sensual massage. A person should not use sporadic jerky motions because that will take away from the pleasure of the massage.

Head

A person usually can start by touching his or her partner's head. The majority of people like to have their head touched and massaged. The person can massage his or her partner's head from the back to the top and then to the sides. The person can massage his or her partner's head with one hand or both. The person can use a gentle circular motion as he or she moves his or her hand from the back to the top and then to the sides of his or her partner's head. The person can also use a gentle straight up-and-down motion as he or she moves his or her hand from the back to the top and then to the sides of his or her partner's head.

The majority of people that have hair like having their hair touched and played with by their partner during foreplay. The person can run his or her fingertips or a hairbrush through his or her partner's hair gently and steadily. The person should brush the entire head, not just the back of the head of his or her partner. The person should gently play with his or her partner's hair at the base of the neck, lift it, and kiss underneath it.

Face

Face touching is a very gentle and intimate gesture. The key to making it as sensual as possible is to increase the intensity of eye contact between both partners. The person should use the back of his or her hand or his or her finger to touch his or her partner's face. The person should move slowly and lightly over his or her partner's face since the face is very sensitive and a very erogenous zone. Usually it is more exciting and erotic for the person to use a finger or two to touch the face instead of using the back of his or her hand. Using the fingertip of a finger or two, a person can touch his or her partner's entire face slowly and gently. Such an action is very seductive and erotic during foreplay. Many people enjoy having their lips touched by their partner's finger or fingers.

Ears

A person should stroke the partner's rim of the ear and the back of the earlobe slowly and softly with a finger. A person should touch these two areas lightly and slowly in order to arouse his or her partner. Many people like to have the rim of the ear and the back of the earlobe licked and kissed by their partner. They find it sexually exciting and delightful. Many people become aroused when their partner's tongue goes into their ear. Some do not enjoy it.

Neck and Shoulders

The top of the neck and shoulders take a lot of strain and reflect any tension that a person is experiencing. Touching and massaging the top of the neck and the shoulders relieves them of any tension. The neck and shoulders are erogenous zones that, if touched the right way, can create goose bumps and shivers all over the body. It is best to use a circular motion rather than a straight up-and-down motion when stroking this area. A person can stroke this area with the palms of his or her hands, fingers, or tongue. The skin in this area is very sensitive and thin, so a person does not need to use a lot of pressure. A small area on the neck if stimulated through touch can cause the partner's entire body to react and shiver all over. The sides of the neck from the base of the earlobes to the top of the neck are the most sensitive areas on the body. If a person stimulates these areas on his or her partner using touch, the partner will feel very excited and aroused. Stimulating the shoulder blades can relax a person greatly. The person can start from his or her partner's top of the neck, move down the back of the neck and continue across the partner's shoulders, licking or lightly touching using the tips of his or her fingers in circular motion.

Back

The whole back is an erogenous zone. It is packed with numerous nerve endings. Stimulating these nerve endings produces a large amount of pleasure. If a person strokes his or her partner's back, the pleasurable sensations produced in the back will move throughout the whole body. The whole body of the partner will feel better. Also, the back generally holds a lot of tension, so massaging the back can ease the tension and spread a sense of relaxation throughout the rest of the body. A person can gently stroke the whole back area in a circular motion with the tips of his or her fingers or with the palm of his or her hand. A person can move his or her hands up and down his or her partner's back in a circular motion. Also, a person can move his or her hands up and down his or her partner's back in a straight motion. A person can alternate between using the palm of his or her hand, or the tips of his or his fingers to produce a variety of sensations. A person should touch his or her partner's back gently and slowly.

A person, using a finger, can stroke the partner's tailbone or the bottom of the spine, since it is highly erotic if touched. A person can concentrate on the small dimples on the back of his or her partner when stroking the back since they are very sensitive. A person can stimulate the spinal cord of his or her partner by stroking it from the top to the bottom and then from the bottom to the top. If a person strokes, kisses, or licks the spinal cord of his or her partner, it will send sensuous shivers throughout the partner's body. A person can lick his or her partner's back using his or her tongue softly and slowly. A person can lick the whole back area, from top to bottom and then from bottom to top. Using the tongue to stimulate the back will produce a variety of sensations that are different from the sensations produced when using the finger tips or the palm of the hand. However, the finger tips seem to be most often, used during the touching of the back during foreplay.

Buttocks

A person can stroke his or her partner's buttocks slowly and lightly, which can be very seductive and arousing. A person can use his or her fingertips or the palm of his or her hand to stroke his or her partner's buttocks. A person can move his or her finger tips or the palm of his or her hand in a circular motion or in a straight up-and-down motion to stroke his or her partner's buttocks. If a person stimulates his or her partner's buttocks, that will arouse and stimulate the genital area of the partner. Stimulating the buttocks is very erotic because the buttocks have many nerve endings. The areas where the buttocks meet the upper thighs are very sensitive. The buttocks muscles are often neglected but they can be quite tense and in need of attention and relaxation.

Breasts

Women's breasts are usually a major part of lovemaking and sexual play. Most women love to be touched on their breasts. To most women it is very pleasurable. They love to have their breasts cradled, sucked, and played with. Also, males enjoy kissing, licking, and stroking the woman's breasts. When a man kisses, licks, or strokes the woman's breasts the woman greatly enjoys it and is very aroused by it. Some women, a very small percentage, can even reach orgasm purely through stimulation of their breasts.

One way a man can touch the woman's breasts is by doing the following: with one or two of his fingertips on each breast, he can start touching the breasts from the bottom and gently move towards the nipples. The man should not touch the nipples at this point. Rather, when he reaches the nipples he should move his fingers back down again towards the bottom of the breasts. A person can do this several times and change the location on each breast each time. After doing this several times then the man can put a finger on each nipple and then massage the nipples in a circular motion. If the man goes straight to the nipples without massaging the breasts, it is not as pleasurable as gradually moving to the nipples because the stimulation is not built up gradually. However, if the man goes straight to the nipples without massaging the breasts, it is still pleasurable and could be done.

The man can massage the woman's breasts using his fingers or the palm of his or her hand. He can move his hand or fingers up and down or sideways to stimulate the breasts. The man can also move his hand or fingers in a circular motion to stimulate the breasts. The majority of ladies do not enjoy intense pinching of their nipples. The majority of ladies do not like their breasts being tightly squeezed.

A man can lick the woman's breast from bottom to top and then top to bottom. A man can also lick the woman's breast from side to side. A man can kiss the woman's breast from bottom to top and then top to bottom. A man can also kiss the woman's breast from side to side. A man can suck on the breast of the woman by putting his mouth on her breast anywhere. Then he could suck air in, which will create a pleasurable feeling for the woman on her breast.

During sex play, a man's gentle dalliance over a woman's breasts can also send sexual signals that tingle all the way down to the woman's vagina. It is a good idea to stimulate a woman's breasts during foreplay because it creates sexual excitement for the woman and gets her vagina aroused and anticipating sex. Also, some women have frequently stimulated their own breast or breasts during masturbation, which shows that to most women there is a connection between breast stimulation and sexual pleasure. However, it is important to note that every woman experiences a change in hormone levels from time to time. These changes could be before the woman's period, during the woman's period, during the first days of pregnancy, or as the woman enters menopause. As a result of these changes, the woman's breasts may be so tender that the thought of someone touching them makes her cringe. So if at times a woman does not want the man to touch her breasts he should not be surprised.

Men's breasts are mistakenly believed to be not sensitive because they are less prominent than those of the woman. In reality, men's breasts are sensitive to touch and can create great excitement when touched during foreplay. A woman can lick the man's breasts from top to bottom and from bottom to top. A woman can kiss the man's breasts. A woman can also move her fingertip or fingertips in a circular motion on the man's breasts. This will create great delight for the man and have him ready for sex.

Nipples

There is a connection between a woman's nipples and her vagina when she gets aroused. Stimulating a woman's nipples will often stimulate the vagina at the same time, or at least start an itch in the vagina that demands to be scratched. The woman's nipples contain many nerves. Stimulating a woman's nipples gets the woman anticipating sex and lets her start lubricating. Some women, although rare, can orgasm from nipple stimulation alone. That proves that there is a connection between nipple stimulation and pleasurable sex.

The nipples become hard and erect when the woman is sexually aroused. One way for the man to arouse a woman's nipples is by licking them with his tongue. He can lick the nipples either from top to bottom or bottom to top. A second way for the man to arouse a woman's nipples is touch each nipple with one or two fingertips. Then he can move his fingertip or fingertips in a circular motion on the nipple. The man should move his fingertip or fingertips lightly and gently not putting too much pressure. A third way for a man to arouse a woman's nipples is for him to place his mouth on her nipples and suck air in. This will cause a suction of air that will produce pleasurable feelings. The more the woman's nipples become engorged with blood due to the stimulation by the man, the more sensitive they become and the more sensitive the breasts become. This leads to a more pleasurable sexual encounter.

Many people think nipple stimulation is just for women. The fact that the man's nipples are less prominent than the woman's nipples has led to the mistaken belief that the man's nipples are not sensitive. Many men have sexually sensitive nipples. Many men find that their nipples even get erect when aroused. Sex researcher Alfred Kinsey during his research discovered a few men who could reach orgasm through nipple stimulation alone. Although most men do not experience an orgasm from nipple stimulation alone, most men experience great pleasure from having their nipples stimulated by their woman. Stimulating the man's nipples most often gets him in the mood for sex. As a result of nipple stimulation most men experience greater pleasure during foreplay and during sex.

One way to arouse the man's nipples is to touch each nipple with one or two fingertips. The woman then should move the fingertip or fingertips in a circular motion that is gentle and slow. This should get the man's nipples aroused and excited. A second way to arouse the man's nipples is for the woman to lick them from top to bottom or bottom to top. A third way for the woman to arouse the man's nipples is to put her mouth on his nipple and suck on each one. This usually creates a warm and pleasurable feeling for the man.

Navel

Some people love to have their partner stimulate their belly button using a tongue or finger. A person can stimulate his or her partner's belly button with a tongue by licking the belly button. A person can stimulate his or her partner's belly button with a finger by stroking it with one of his or her finger tips in a circular motion. A person can kiss his or her partner's navel, since many people find it arousing. Some people put champagne or other beverages in their partner's belly button and then lick it. They use the belly button as a repository for champagne or other beverages. The belly button is close to a very erogenous zone, the genital area. Any stimulation to the belly button will spread stimulation to the genital area.

Arms and Hands

It is important that the person touches the arms and hands of his or her partner. Both arms and hands should be touched equally. Touching the arms and hands is a way to stimulate the nerve endings there. A person can stimulate the arms and hands of his or her partner by using his or her fingertips or the palms of his or her hands. A person can move the fingertips or the palms of the hands, in a circular motion or in an up-and-down movement. A person can lick the arms and hands of his or her partner using an up to down movement, and then a down to up movement. A person can kiss the arms and hands of his or her partner from top to bottom and then from bottom to top. Many people find such an action very seductive. A person can suck on his or her partner's fingertips, since many people find it romantic. The stimulation of the nerves in the arms and hands spreads excitement to other nerves in the body, which makes foreplay and sex more pleasurable.

Legs

It is important that the person touches the legs of his or her partner. Both legs need to be touched equally. When it comes to touching the legs a person can use more pressure because the skin is thicker. Touching the legs is a great way to enliven the nerve endings in the legs. While touching the legs a person can also concentrate on stimulating the inner thighs of his or her partner because the inner thighs are very sensitive. If a person touches the partner there it is exciting because it creates a sense of anticipation that the lover's hands will wander to the genital area. The places where the inner thighs meet the pubic area are very sensitive areas for many people. A person can stimulate the legs of his or her partner by using his or her fingertips or the palms of his or her hands. A person can move the fingertips or the palms of the hands in a circular motion or in an up-and-down movement. A person can lick or kiss the partner's legs, especially the inner thighs, using an up-to-down movement, and then a down-to-up movement. This is very erotic to both people. When the partner's legs are stimulated and enlivened through touch the sex and foreplay become more delightful and pleasurable. The sex and foreplay become more pleasurable because the partner's nerves are excited in the partner's legs which spread the excitement to other nerves in other parts of the body.

Feet

Feet have long been associated with sex in both men and women. Toes tend to curl involuntarily during orgasm. In fact the feet are so rich in nerve endings that some people receive great pleasure from foot caresses alone. Many men and women enjoy having their feet held and caressed by their partner during sexual intercourse, after intercourse, or before intercourse. Touching the feet during foreplay is very important. It is very important because it releases the tension of tiny muscles and ligaments holding the little bones in place. This is important because when a person is relaxed the foreplay and sex becomes a lot more pleasurable.

The foot is one of the most sensitive parts of the human body. A foot massage can do more than just relieve physical stress. The surface of the foot's skin contains neural receptors that affect heart rate, blood flow, and hormone flow. Stimulating these receptors releases endorphins, which are natural painkillers that are structurally similar to morphine. They are similar to morphine and also trigger a sense of wellbeing like morphine. A foot massage is very sensual. A person can turn his or her partner on just through a foot massage.

A person can use the thumbs to massage the partner's feet. On one foot at a time with both thumbs, it is best to use small circular strokes from the heel up to the toes and then from the toes to the heel. It is important that a person be gentle and slow when touching his or her partner's feet. The person can release his or her partner's toe pressure by gently pulling each toe in an upward motion using the thumb and index finger. In order for a person to produce a variety of sensations, he or she can use one or two fingertips on each foot to massage the heel up to the toes and then back again from the toes to the heel. He or she can do so in a circular motion, in an up-and-down motion, or in a side-to-side motion. In order for a person to create a different set of sensations, he or she can use the palm of the hand to massage from the heel up to the toes and then back from the toes to the heel. He or she could do so in a circular motion. This will make the partner very relaxed.

A person should massage three inches along both sides of the bone running from the back of the heel up toward the calf of the leg. A person should massage that area using a thumb. He or she should move the thumb in a circular motion from the back of the heel up toward the calf. This is important because there is a lot of tension in that area from standing, and the person massaging this area will lead to the partner being relaxed. This will in turn lead the partner to experience more pleasurable sex. If a person massages the partner's whole foot, that will reduce his or her partner's anxiety and clear his or her mind. The foot massage is very erotic because the foot contains a number of erotic trigger points, which, when pressed, will create sensations in a person's genital area. The foot massage is the best thing to get a person relaxed and in a mood anticipating sex.

Anus

The anus is the opening to the rectum and exit for the bowels. The anus has hundreds of nerves and some people find their anus being stroked quite arousing. A person can stroke the anus by inserting his or her finger inside the partner's anus and move it in and out, while moving it around the anus opening. The anus does not produce its own lubrication so a person needs to lubricate his or her finger to ease the insertion of the finger inside the anus. Also, a person should wash the finger after taking it out of the anus so that certain bacteria are not spread. The anus and the area surrounding the anus are the most sensitive areas of the human body. Gently caressing the skin surrounding the anus opening with a finger can send some people into ecstasy.

Perineum

The perineum in a man is the region between the scrotum and the anus. The perineum in the woman is the area between the posterior vulva junction and the anus. In other words, the perineum is the span of skin between the genital and anus of the man or woman. This is a very sensitive area to touch and provides considerable erotic pleasure when stimulated. Stimulating this area through touch can get a person ready for sex. This is especially true for women. If the man stimulates this area for a woman by touching it, the woman is most likely to lubricate, relax, and be in the mood for sex. The woman is more likely to orgasm during sex as a result of physical stimulation of this area before sex. A person can stimulate the perineum of his or her partner by licking it. A second way that a person can stimulate the perineum of his or her partner is by moving his or her fingertips in a circular motion on the perineum from top to bottom and from bottom to top.

Genital Area

During touching it is important to delay going to the partner's genital area until it is the last spot left to be touched. The key to amazing foreplay is for a person to travel along his or her partner's body caressing it while at the same time staying away from the genital area. A person should not go to the genital area and start touching it until he or she has caressed all of the rest of the body because by doing so there is a gradual buildup of sexual arousal that contributes to more pleasurable sex. The person should enjoy the feel of the body beneath his or her fingertips as he or she works his or her way to the genital area from the perineum. The person should be delighted with the smoothness of the skin under his or her fingertips. The person using his or her fingertips could do smooth, gentle, soft strokes in a circular fashion on the naked flesh, gradually working his or her way from the perineum to the genital area.

The female genital massage is very interesting. Most women do not want the man going close to the clitoris until they are very stimulated. Once the woman is stimulated the woman prefers that the man to start with a soft barely touching tapping on the clitoral hood using one of his fingertips. Then she loves soft and gentle continuous touching directly on the clitoral hood and the area surrounding it using his fingertips. The clitoral hood in both previous instances should be covering the clitoris. The fingertips should be moistened so that the touching is pleasurable both to the man and the woman. A woman's clitoris has the greatest concentration of nerve endings in the body and it is because of this intense sensitivity that it must be touched with real care and real understanding.

The more the clitoris is engorged with blood because of stimulation, the more pleasurable the foreplay and sex will be for the woman. Therefore, after stimulating the clitoris while it is still covered with the clitoral hood, the man should circle around the clitoris on the genital area with his fingertip or fingertips to draw energy to it and help prepare it for direct stimulation. Then the man can remove the clitoral hood with one hand and with the other hand use his fingertip to stroke the less sensitive base and sides of the clitoris. Then he can gently stroke the extremely sensitive glans of the clitoris with his fingertip. For some women direct stimulation of the glans is always too intense, so a man needs to look at nonverbal and verbal cues in deciding whether to continue direct stimulation of the glans. When the man is massaging the woman's genital area he should do his best just to stimulate the area, but not give the woman an orgasm. He should stimulate the genital area so that the area is aroused, so that the sex becomes more pleasurable.

The man could also fondle the woman's general pubic area with his hand. Then he could use his hand to stimulate the outer labia. He could try different strokes of varying pressure and see what feels best for the woman when he is stimulating her outer labia. Then the man can use his hand to stimulate the woman's inner labia. He could try different strokes of varying pressure and see what feels best for the woman when he is stimulating her inner labia. Then the man could explore the vaginal entrance with his hand by stroking it with his fingers. He could move his fingers in and out of the vaginal entrance and around the vaginal entrance. Once he locates the area of the vaginal entrance that gives the best and most pleasurable sensations, then he could concentrate on stroking that area so that he gives the woman pleasurable sensations. But when he strokes that area he should make sure that he strokes enough only to produce pleasurable sensations and get the area stimulated but not to give the woman an orgasm.

The male genital massage is also very interesting. The woman should start by moving her hand over the man's testicles very gently and slowly. She should feel his testicles very softly as she moves her hand. Then she should put her hand on top of the man's penis, while keeping the hand open, without grabbing the penis. Then with an open hand she could stroke the penis softly in an up-and-down motion. Then when the penis has become a little erect she can put one hand on each side of the penis shaft. The index finger and the thumb on each hand should surround the penis. Then she could slide both hands in opposite directions at the same time as if she was trying to twist the penis in half. Then she could slide both hands back again to their original position. She can do this several times until she has the genital area stimulated. Then she could grasp the penis with one hand. Then with the other hand she could rub the palm of her hand over the head of the penis.

The frenulum is the skin just below the head of the penis on the underside of the penis. It is above the shaft of the penis. It is where the head and shaft meet. It is the most sensitive part of the penis. The woman could grasp the penis with one hand and with the other hand she could put her thumb on the frenulum and rub it. This will give the man great pleasure. The woman can put her thumb on the underside of the shaft of the penis, and rub it in an up-and-down motion. This also makes the man feel ecstatic. When the woman is massaging the man's genital area, she should do her best just to stimulate the area, but not give the man an orgasm. She should stimulate the genital area so that the area is aroused, so that the sex becomes more pleasurable. It is important to remember that the main point of the genital massage for both the man and woman is to get both people aroused and ready for intercourse. It is not done to get either the man or woman to orgasm.

Body to Body Massage

Both partners should spread lots of massage oil over their chest, abdomen, and the front of the legs and arms. Then one of the partners should lie down on his or her back with his or her legs straight. The second partner should lie down on top of him or her. Both partners should have their chest and abdomen against each other. The partner on top should move his or her body up and down and side to side while touching his or her partner. The partner on the bottom should remain still as the partner on top does that. Then the partner on top can get off his or her partner and let the partner on the bottom lie down on his or her stomach with his or her legs spread out straight. Then the partner can once again lie down on him or her with the top partner's abdomen and chest against the bottom partner's back. Then the partner on top should move his or her body up and down and side to side over the expanse of the bottom partner's back, buttocks, and legs. The partner on the bottom should remain still as the partner on top does that. Both partners can then reverse roles and do the whole process again.

Note

Erogenous zones are the parts of the human body that feel particularly sensual when stimulated. Every person's erogenous zones are different. The part of the body that might feel sensual to one person when stimulated, might feel ticklish to another person when stimulated, and might have no sensation when stimulated for a third person. Many people are erotically responsive in all sorts of other less obvious locations like the lower abdomen, upper abdomen, chest, throat, and under the armpits. The only way for a person to find out what other parts of the body become eroticized when the partner is aroused is to slowly, carefully, and gently go in search of them with the fingertips or tongue. A person can always try new approaches to touching, like gently stroking feathers or sensual materials over his or her partner's body. A person can try these new approaches to touching because these new approaches may create different pleasurable sensations in the partner. These new approaches to touching increase the variety that a person has at his or her disposal in touching his or her partner. Using scented oil or baby powder during touching can amplify the sensations.

Sensual Materials

A person can incorporate sensual materials into his or her touching sessions. The top materials that have extremely sensual textures are velvet, satin, silk, feathers, fur, leather, rubber, and vinyl. A person can touch his or her partner using any of these materials. If a person touches his or her partner with either of these materials it adds variety to the touching and makes it more pleasurable. When a person touches his or her partner with one type of sensual material and then another type of sensual material, the partner feels a different set of sensations every time he or she is touched with different material. The sensations that a partner feels when he or she is touched with fur are different than the sensations that a partner feels when he or she is touched with silk. A person can use any of the sensual materials as a blindfold on his or her partner. A blindfold adds to feelings of anticipation and excitement during foreplay and during sex.

One of the most exotic touching is with a feather. Feathers look nice, skim lightly across the skin, and tickle the recipient into wriggling submission. A person can use a group of feathers together, or just one feather to stimulate his or her partner's body. A person can use a feather or group of feathers to tickle every inch of his or her partner's skin, using light rapid movements. A person can touch with the feather or feathers all the body areas except the genital area, leaving it until last. This will cause the partner to wonder when the person will touch the genital area. The person should keep his or her partner waiting for as long as possible in anticipation as to when he or she will touch the genital area. The anticipation will serve to heighten the pleasure of the bodily touching, and when the person finally touches the partner's genital area with the feather or feathers, the partner will feel great pleasure.

Kissing

Kissing is the number one form of foreplay to get a couple aroused and ready for intercourse. The mouth, lips, and tongue are among a person's most erogenous zones.

Stimulating a person's mouth can stimulate his or her whole body and has a direct effect of arousing his or her genital area. For some people kissing is more erotic and intimate than intercourse because kissing conveys feelings of love and commitment in a way that intercourse alone does not. Kissing is important during foreplay because it usually gets a woman ready for sex. Without enough kissing during foreplay, the sex will be less pleasurable for the woman. Kissing is an important act that shows love and passion. It makes a couple feel love and intimacy between them. For details on different kissing techniques the chapter on Kissing should be read.

Food During Foreplay

Many people think that combining food and sex is very sexy. Both eating and sex are two of life's greatest sensual pleasures, and combining them provides a lot of sensual pleasure. Another form of foreplay is for both the man and woman to be naked in bed and each one take turns feeding the other in bed. Many people enjoy being fed in bed by their partner. They find it sexually stimulating. Also, many people enjoy feeding their partner in bed they find it exciting. The usual food that is used is grapes, strawberries, and plums. They are used because if a person drops them it does not create a mess. Nuts, olives and pickles are sometimes used because they can be easily carried in the hand of each partner. Strawberry dipped in chocolate or in sugar is used because it is delicious, although it can create a mess if dropped. Raw oysters can be used because eating them in bed can be quite erotic since they resemble the female genitalia. They also contain a lot of zinc, an important mineral that increases male potency. A bowl of strawberries, grapes, or apple slices dipped in honey can be used because they are very delicious and help a person get aroused when eaten. Also, the man and woman can take turns letting their partner drink from the glass in their hand. Both partners find that erotic. Beverages like wine, champagne, and cool water are usually used.

Another kind of food game that could be used as foreplay is to have the partner's body decorated with stripes of honey and whipped cream using a paintbrush. Once the partner is covered in the food, the person can lick his or her body from the neck down to the toes. A person could also, put on his or her partner food such as jams, cake decorations, syrups, and a variety of creams and lick them off his or her body. A person could take fruit like grapes, cherries, strawberry, figs, sliced plums, and sliced peaches, crush them against his or her partner's body and massage them into his or her skin. Then the person can lick the partner's body and the crushed fruit also. A person could also dribble a beverage such as champagne over his or her partner's body and then lick the partner's body and lick the beverage along with it. These types of food games are popular and erotic because it is not the food that is the sex trigger but the manner in which the food is eaten. These food games are erotic since a person is eating food in a manner that suggests that he or she would rather be eating his or her partner. As a result his or her partner acquires a large appetite for sex. Another appealing aspect of these food games is the forbidden factor. Most children are taught to keep clean while eating, and during these food games a person is being messy by putting food on his or her lover's body which is exciting since he or she is doing something that is forbidden.

Another type of food game to play is one involving ice. One type of ice game to play is to rub an ice cube all over the partner's body. The shock of extreme cold starts adrenaline flowing promoting feelings of anticipation and excitement. These feelings will make the sex more pleasurable. A person should make sure that if he or she ever puts any food in the vagina it should be easily and completely removed. A person should avoid putting honey, whipped cream, and chocolate sauce inside the vagina since they are difficult to remove and will increase a woman's risk of vaginal infection. Some people get pleasure from eating food during foreplay because they are unconsciously motivated during foreplay to recreate very early and primitive bonds of love and sensuality they experienced when they were infants, especially during breast feeding.

Both people sitting naked in a room and eating together prior to sex is a form of foreplay. What a person eats prior to sex can set the tone for the entire evening and make the difference between good sex and great sex. The right foods for a person to eat prior to sex should be light and stimulating to the taste buds. Foods like grilled or baked fish and chicken, fruits, and vegetables are healthy foods that are light and stimulating to the taste buds. The chicken and fish should be prepared with the right seasonings that bring out the best flavors of the food. Foods that are high in fat should be avoided because they decrease testosterone levels and decrease libido. Too much alcohol, wine, and champagne should be avoided prior to sex because they will interfere with a person's sexual performance and enjoyment. A person should not drink more than two glasses of alcohol during the evening.

Eating a variety of healthy foods is essential for a great sex life, because everything a person eats or drinks affects his or her motivation and desire for sex, his or her ability to respond to sexual stimulation, and the intensity of his or her response. For a healthy sex life a person should regularly eat grilled or baked fish and chicken, fruits, and vegetables, and should avoid foods that are high in fat. Such a diet provides vitamins, minerals, and nutrients that are necessary for optimal health. People who have a high fat diet have a higher chance of getting clogged arteries. Men who have a high fat diet have a larger chance of becoming impotent because the clogged arteries impede blood flow to the penis just as they impede blood flow to the heart. A person should also try to include garlic in his or her diet since it stirs his or her sexual appetite. It also improves a person's blood circulation and decreases his or her blood pressure so that a person has good blood flow to his or her genitals. As a result it makes a person's performance during sex better.

Sharing Fantasies During Foreplay

Both lovers can share sexual fantasies as a form of foreplay. They can tell each other about their sexual fantasies that are unrealistic or realistic. An example of an unrealistic sexual fantasy is for the man or woman to imagine that he or she is on a remote island cut off from civilization, with ten or twenty members of the opposite sex that want to have sex with him or her. Some unrealistic fantasies like the one just described cannot be acted out. However there are some unrealistic fantasies that can be acted out. Examples of some of these unrealistic fantasies that can be role played are pirate captain / galley wench, pizza boy / bored housewife who lost her purse, Conan / Red Sonia, Prince Charming / rescued princess, detective / suspect, the cat burglar / sexually bored owner of the house, etc. Each partner would play a part in acting out the fantasy. They could dress for the part or just act out the part in their regular clothes. They could pretend that they are dressed in clothes that they are not dressed in and that they are in a certain location that they are not in. For example, when playing pirate captain / galley wench, the man could pretend that he is dressed like a pirate although he is dressed in his regular clothes and he could pretend that he is on a boat in the ocean while in reality he is in his bedroom. In addition to sharing their unrealistic fantasies a couple could sometimes act them out as a form of foreplay to add excitement to the sexual encounter.

The couple can also tell each other about their sexual fantasies that are realistic. For example, a person can tell his or her partner that they are in the hotel room in Jamaica close to the beach. In the hotel room they are making passionate love for three consecutive days and not leaving the room. They order room service every time they need a meal. The person describing the fantasy could tell his or her partner of the different sexual acts and foreplay techniques that he or she would do in such a setting. This is a very realistic fantasy that could be easily acted out. Another example of a realistic sexual fantasy that a person could tell his or her partner is that the man is at a bar and a woman that is dressed up seductively comes and flirts with him. Then they would both go to a motel and make passionate love. This is a realistic sexual fantasy because both the man and woman can act it out in reality by going to the bar, meeting and acting as if they were strangers. The woman would dress up seductively in a way that she does not usually dress. There is nothing unrealistic about it.

The advantage of realistic sexual fantasies is that they can be acted out as if they are really happening. This brings a great amount of satisfaction and pleasure to the man and woman. The couple could share realistic fantasies with each other during foreplay and sometimes act them out as a form of foreplay to add excitement to the sexual encounter. Some people are turned on by acting out fantasies of uncontrollable lust. So in order to act out these fantasies, the man and woman could wear old clothes and rip them off each other during sex. It is important when telling the other partner about the different realistic and unrealistic fantasies not to concentrate only on the setting, but also to describe the different sexual acts and foreplay acts that will take place in such an encounter. It is not a good idea to just say at the end of the fantasy that they just had sex. This book provides a multitude of sexual techniques that can be described at the end of a sexual fantasy.

A word of caution: a person should not exchange sexual fantasies with his or her partner about him or her having intercourse with a real person in their lives, since such an action could lead to jealousy on the part of the listening partner. It could cause the listening partner to feel inadequate and have resentment to the other partner. It could lead to hostility between the couple and to their eventual breakup. It could also lead to a poor sex life.

Lack of Foreplay Not Just the Man's Fault

Typically, especially in some women's magazines, the whole subject of lack of foreplay is portrayed as a problem caused almost entirely by men. The men are portrayed as too impatient, too clumsy, too selfish, and too orgasm-oriented. But the way that they are portrayed is not accurate. Men are neither clumsy, nor selfish, nor orgasm-oriented. Men are also concerned about giving pleasure or pleasing their woman in the true sense of the word. Men are a lot more sensitive than they are usually portrayed.

Women are as much at fault for the problem of lack of foreplay as men are because they do not communicate their needs. Many women still have a great deal of difficulty in communicating what they want and need during foreplay, and if the man does not know what she wants for foreplay his chances of satisfying her are greatly reduced. Many women just assume that the man knows when she is ready for penetration, but the truth is that the man does not know. This is because vaginal lubrication is a much subtler sign of arousal than an erection and it is much more easily misinterpreted than a robust erection. Women do not realize that men are upset that women do not seem to understand that men really want to please them. A man would rather have a woman move his hand, mouth or other part of his body to where she wants it than to have her lie back and think of something else. A woman should not expect that the man is going to know what she wants during foreplay and then get mad when he does not do it. Rather, a woman should tell the man explicitly what she wants during foreplay. As a matter of fact, she can go further and move his hand, mouth, or other part of his body to where she wants it and tell him how she wants him to touch her.

Communication During Foreplay

Casually making compliments before sex is a form of foreplay. It adds to the delight of the experience. For example, a person can tell his or her partner that he or she looks beautiful or handsome tonight. Furthermore, saying sexy or romantic comments before sex is a form of foreplay. It makes the experience more pleasurable. An example would be for a person to tell his or her partner that he or she wants the partner to be next to him or her to feel his or her body. Another example of a romantic or sexy comment is for a person to tell his or her partner that he or she wants to feel his or her partner's touch all over his or her body.

It adds great pleasure to the foreplay experience for a person to talk his or her positive feelings to his or her partner. A person can tell his or her lover numerous positive things, one of which is that it feels good that his or her partner is in his or her life. As a matter of fact both people should tell each other that they feel good that they are together every time they have foreplay because it makes such a big difference in the foreplay experience and the sexual experience. Both people should let each other know their feelings towards each other, since it increases intimacy and desire between the couple. Every person during foreplay likes to hear that his or her partner likes him or her or loves him or her. Such a comment increases intimacy and passion between a couple during foreplay and sex.

If a couple sits in their bed and tell each other what they want to do sexually tonight or what they would want done to them sexually tonight, that is a form of foreplay also. Each person should talk honestly with his or her partner, telling him or her about his or her sexual and foreplay needs and desires. Sometimes a partner's technique is not exactly compatible with the person's needs or desires and the person is reluctant to say anything because he or she does not want the partner to be hurt emotionally. The person should remember that the partner was not born knowing exactly how to satisfy during foreplay or during sex. The person should also know that he or she should take responsibility for his or her own foreplay pleasure and sexual pleasure. Taking responsibility means communicating with the other party what is pleasurable during foreplay and sex. A partner should not be resentful if the person tells him or her what to do during foreplay, since a man or a woman wants something different from one sexual encounter to another, during the same encounter, and from minute to minute. This is because a man or a woman's taste changes from minute to minute during foreplay and during sex.

A few chosen words from the man to the woman during foreplay usually get her absolutely excited and helps her with her lubrication. A few chosen words from the woman to the man during foreplay usually get the man very aroused and wanting to be inside the woman. All the time that a person is saying sexy things, he or she should maintain eye contact with his or her lover to show sincerity.

Chapter 17

Sex Positions

There are six main sex positions. They are as follows: man on top, side by side, rear entry, standing, sitting, and woman on top. The rest of the sex positions are a variation of these main six. The reason these positions were included in a chapter by itself is to inform the reader of the different ways he or she can have sex with his or her partner. The biggest determining factor for choosing a position is the preference a person and his or her partner have for a certain position. It is important to note that some of the positions in pornographic movies are not at all pleasurable for the ladies. A person should not feel inadequate if there are some positions he or she has not heard of. A person should not feel inadequate, that he or she does not use many positions in one sexual session. As a matter of fact, couples typically use two or three positions during one lovemaking session, moving from one position to another before completion, whether completion is orgasm or not. However, the major determining factor in the number of positions to use is to do what works best for both members of the couple in terms of pleasure.

However, a person might wonder why so many sexual positions have been included in this chapter, even though typically a couple uses just two or three positions during one session of sex. The answer is any activity, even an enjoyable one like sex, can become boring. If a person watches a great movie that most people liked and that was his or her favorite, day after day, as much as he or she loves it now he or she would eventually be bored by it. If a person eats his or her favorite dish every day, he or she would get bored of it and eventually detest eating it. If a person listens to his or her favorite song every day, eventually he or she would get bored of it. Sex is no different. If a person behaves exactly the same way every time he or she has sex (by using the same two or three positions), eventually this enjoyable activity will become boring. Therefore, a large variety of positions have been included in this chapter. Also, many couples, after they become used to each other in bed, want to explore new ways of enjoying each other. This variety of positions will fulfill this need.

An enjoyable experience for a couple would be to read this chapter carefully, and then practice each night several different positions without entry. Both could be in the nude, fully clothed, in underwear, or wearing what they wear to sleep. After they have tried all these positions, they might categorize the positions into what was comfortable for both of them, what they would like to try during intercourse, what was not very comfortable for both of them, and what they would not like to try during intercourse.

A sexual encounter to the couple is a time of harmony, moving, enjoying each other's bodies, and pleasing each other. In that process the couple is likely to change from one position to another. When the positions flow naturally out of the couple's enjoyment of being together, it is pleasurable. When the positions do not flow naturally they are less pleasurable. Sex is like dancing, so a couple should think of positions in sequence that do not involve a lot of climbing over legs or turning the sexual partner around. The couple should choose a variety of positions to keep things interesting. Variety in all forms of sexual intimacy is encouraged to increase pleasure. However, a person should not think that there is something wrong with him or her and his or her lover because they prefer using just one position, or because they prefer the old standard position of the man on top of the woman. It is important to do what is comfortable and what works best for both people in terms of pleasure.

A couple should develop an attitude of openness and freedom between both of them during their sex sessions so that both of them let the choice of position grow out of the feelings of the moment. A couple should not be overly concerned with the question of which position to use during sex. Rather they should let it happen spontaneously. As long as the couple practices the positions ahead of the sexual encounter and discusses which ones were pleasurable for both of them, then during their sexual encounter, which positions to use will evolve out of the feelings of the moment. The key to enjoying different sexual positions is simply to try different positions without forcing their bodies into new positions that are not right for them.

Different positions produce different sensations. A person does not have to like them all. A person does not have to repeat them all. A person can find the positions that he or she and his or her partner really love and expand on them while deleting from their future experiences the positions that were not so great. There is no right or wrong way to have sex. A couple should just do what feels natural and pleasurable. They should figure out what is pleasurable for both of them while having fun. The couple will know that they are doing sex right if they are having pleasure from it. They will know that they are doing sex wrong if they do not have pleasure from it. However, changing positions too frequently during a sexual encounter can be distracting and disruptive to the flow of lovemaking.

The couple should try the different positions with a great deal of gentleness, patience, ease, and relaxation. Doing so will most likely create a positive beginning for great sex. Some women feel that ladies do not move too much when they are having sex. This attitude has its roots from Victorian times when women were told not to move at all during intercourse and that the action was up to the man. They were told if the woman stays still and does not move during intercourse, there is a great chance that she will orgasm. The truth is that sex is like a dance between two partners who alternate the lead role, each contributing to the final masterpiece. The woman and man should feel free to move during intercourse. As a matter of fact, both man and woman should equally move during intercourse. So while picking a position or a sequence of positions during your practice session, as mentioned before, choose a position or a series of positions where both of you would move equally during the sexual encounter.

Before getting into any of these positions, the couple should remember to enjoy plenty of foreplay. While in these positions, both the man and woman should vary the speed of their movements for sensational sex. The man or woman should vary the depth of penetration of the man's penis for sensational sex while in these positions. Also, for a real erotic experience and to add variety to the sexual experience, the couple could sometimes try changing from one position to the next without withdrawing the penis.

The Man on Top Position—(Missionary Position)

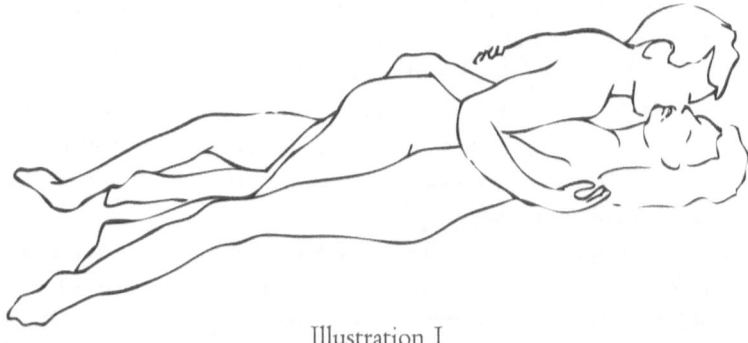

Illustration I

The missionary position is a position for sexual intercourse in which the couple lies face to face with the male on top. It is also known as the man on top position. This position got its name as the missionary position by Pacific Islanders who spied on their local European missionaries making love. They were amused to see that the man was always on top and found the missionaries' movements unvarying and limited. To them, that was amusing because they were accustomed to a more outdoor, physical life. Hence they were more athletic and able to sustain more energetic forms of intercourse. It is the most traditional of all the sexual positions, yet it is not at all boring or old fashioned. It is the most commonly used position in the world. In 1948, sex researcher Alfred Kinsey discovered that 70 percent of Americans had never had sex any other way.

The reason it is so popular is because it seems to be the most basic, and most people get into this position naturally even though it is not their favorite position. People get into this position naturally because it conserves the most energy and is the most comfortable for the couple. Also, it is very romantic and satisfies a couple's craving for intimacy during sex because it provides close face-to-face contact and allows for lots of eye contact during sex. It allows a person to see what his or her partner looks like as the partner reaches orgasm. It lets both partners sense and feel each other better and feel more connected to each other. This position is also desired by many because it offers both partners the opportunity to kiss, hug, and touch each other during sex. In this position, the man can reach the woman's body to touch her in many places, including her breasts, and she can touch and rub his body in many places including his head, shoulders, back, and buttocks. This position is very romantic and intimate because it allows both partners to murmur into each other's ear sweet and sexy comments while having sex.

This position is used by couples when the man likes to dominate the woman in bed and when the woman likes to be taken by the man. This position allows the man to be in control of the thrusting and do most of the work. This may seem unfair by some but it is worth it to many men because the man gets more stimulation in this position and finds it easier to reach orgasm in this position than in many other positions. Meanwhile, the woman can lie back and enjoy the feeling of being made love to. But she does not have to be passive and will increase her enjoyment by actively participating in the sexual encounter. She can actively participate by kissing the man all over the body, by licking different parts of his body, by touching different parts of his body, by staring into his eyes and by telling him sweet and sexy comments. Most men like this position because they can control the depth of penetration as well as the speed of the thrust according to how close the couple is to orgasm.

Another advantage of this position is that it is ideal for a woman to get pregnant, since in this position the vagina is like an upright cup and tends to retain semen. On the other hand, it is not always a comfortable position for women once they are pregnant, especially if they are far along in their pregnancy. It is not comfortable for couples in which the man is obese, since if the man is much heavier than the woman he tends to squash her. Although this position is comfortable for the couple, it tends to make the man get tired after a short period of time since he is supporting his weight with his smallest and weakest muscles, which are the muscles of the back and shoulders. Also, men who suffer from premature ejaculation and men who want to last longer in bed to bring their woman to orgasm may find this position to be difficult for them to hold off ejaculating before they want to because it often feels so good that they do not want to stop. For most men, controlling ejaculation is easier with the woman on top than with the man on top.

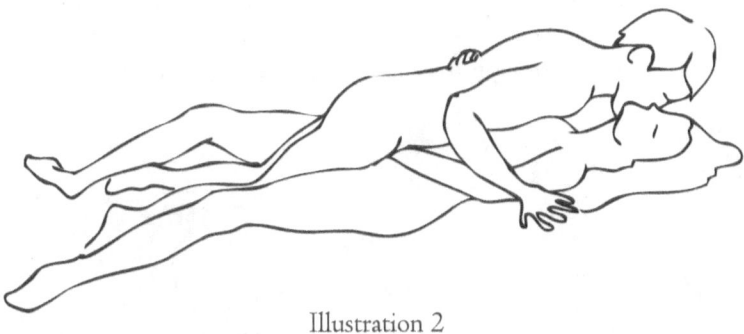

Illustration 2

In the missionary position the woman lies on her back with her legs spread apart either with slightly bent knees or with straight legs and the man gets on top of her. Either the man or the woman guides the man's penis into the woman's vagina.

The man can lie directly on top of the woman, or he can lift his torso and chest up, supporting his weight on his arms. When the penis is fully inserted, the man should lower and close his legs. He can keep both of his legs straight in between the woman's legs, or he can place one leg in between the woman's legs and the other on the outside of the woman's legs. Each way will give a different sensation. The man has most of the control of the pace and rhythm of thrusting.

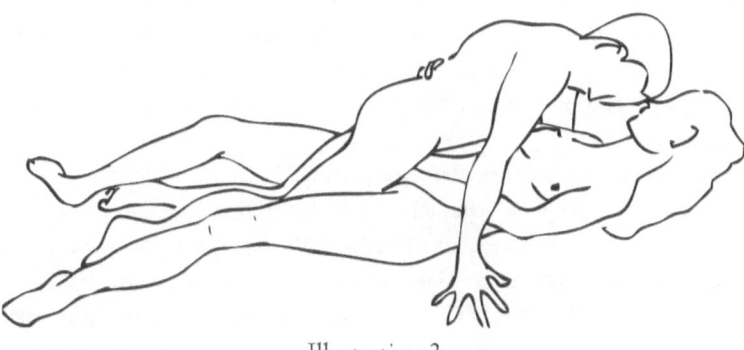

Illustration 3

In the missionary position, no matter how big a man's penis is, it is nowhere near the clitoris. In the missionary position, the entire penis is buried deeply within the moist and warm vagina. Penetration in this position is not deep, but a woman will experience slight stimulation of her clitoris as the penis passes over her vulva on the way to her vagina. There is more friction on the penis than on the clitoris, creating a different pleasurable sensation for the man. During thrusting, the penis receives intense stimulation and this results in the man experiencing pelvic muscle contractions, orgasm, and ejaculation.

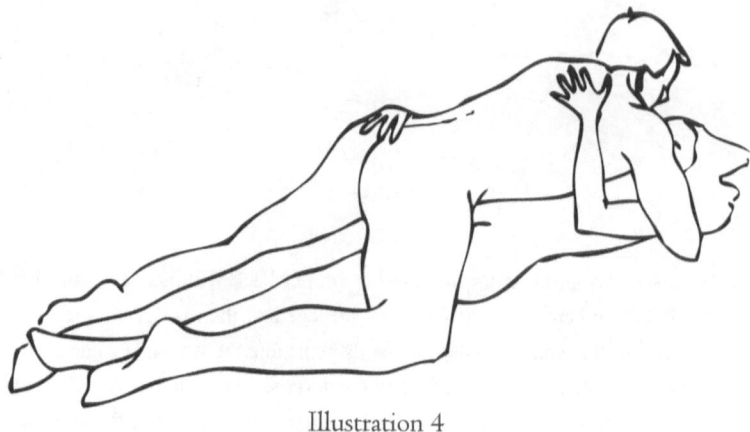

Illustration 4

Another variation of the missionary position is for the woman to put her legs straight out in front of her and closed together [Illustration 4, above]. This time, the man will mount and enter the vagina from on top instead of in between her legs. This offers an intense method of holding the labia minora and labia majora bunched firmly against the penis so that they gain maximum stimulation. This also narrows the vaginal opening and increases the friction on the man's penis. This position also tends to increase the stimulation on the woman's clitoris. Using this position, the man will experience more intense and possibly quicker orgasms. The woman might experience an orgasm using this position.

Another variation of the missionary position is for the woman to pull her legs toward her chest [see Illustration 5, opposite]. The further back she can pull her knees, the deeper the penetration and the greater pleasure for both partners. The man can wedge his arms behind her raised knees. This allows the woman to rest her legs in the crooks of his arms instead of straining to keep them aloft on her own. The man then relaxes, letting his weight down onto his elbows and placing his chest pleasingly along the woman's body, giving an intense feeling of closeness.

The missionary position is usually the worst for stimulating the G-spot with the penis, since the G-spot is usually entirely bypassed as the man's penis presses against

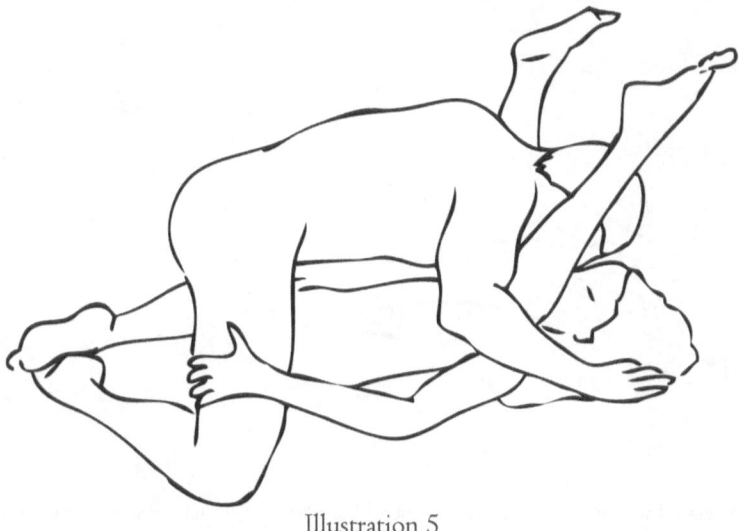

Illustration 5

the back wall of the woman's vagina. However, there is another variation to the missionary position to stimulate the G-spot. In order to stimulate the front vaginal wall and the G-spot, since the G-spot is located over there, a man in the missionary position should arch his back and have his head tilted up away from his partner [see Illustration 6, below]. Then when the man thrusts inside of the vagina his penis will most likely stimulate the front vaginal wall and the G-spot. If a woman has a sensitive G-spot then she is most likely to have a G-spot orgasm. The man should endeavor to point his penis up and tilt his sacrum.

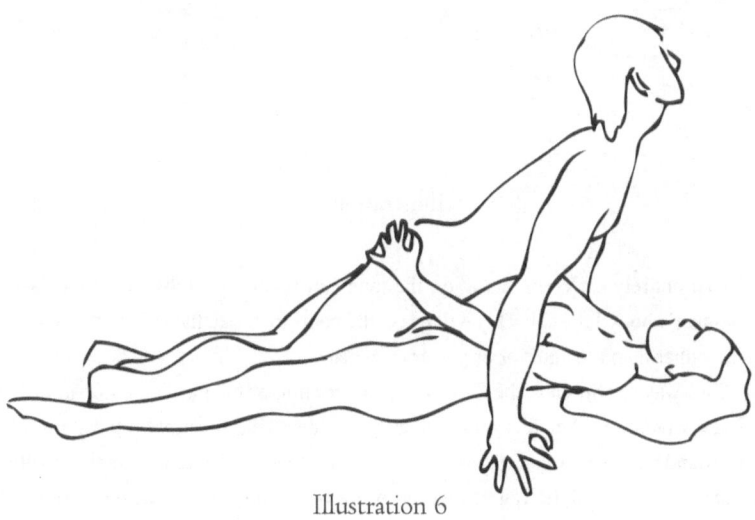

Illustration 6

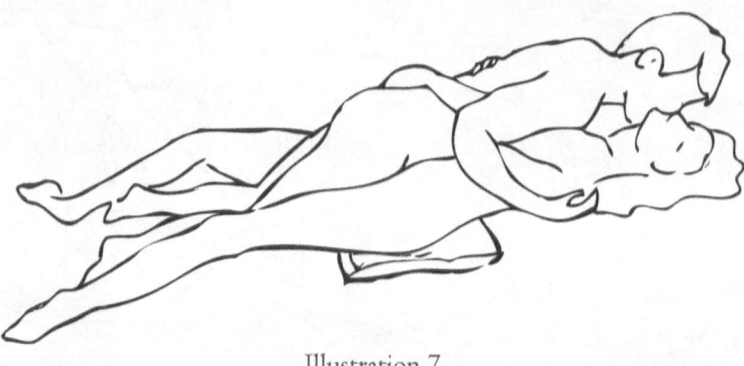

Illustration 7

A second way to stimulate the G-spot with a variation of the missionary position is to have a woman place a pillow under her buttocks [above], which changes the angle that the penis enters the vagina. This causes the penis to enter the vagina deeper and at an angle that presses against the front wall of the vagina. Placing a pillow under the woman's buttocks will increase the stimulation of the clitoris, because placing the pillow under the woman's buttocks thrusts the woman's pelvis further forward, increasing the exposure of the woman's clitoris to the man's penis.

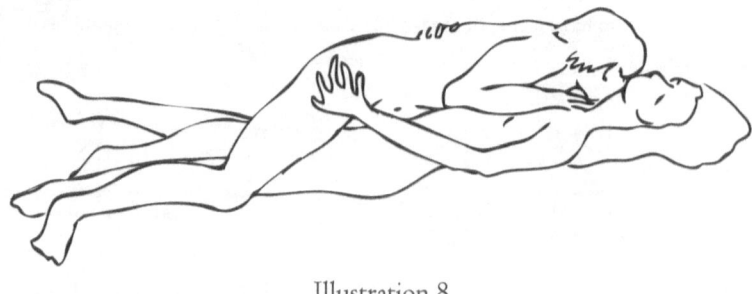

Illustration 8

For an entirely different sensation the man can rotate his body 45 degrees across the woman's body [above]. This will cause the penis to stroke the side of the woman's vagina rather than the anterior or posterior walls.

A third way to stimulate the G-spot with a variation of the missionary position is to have the woman put her feet on the man's shoulders [see Illustration 9, opposite] or even around his neck [Illustration 10]. The clitoris receives no attention in this position, but the anterior wall of the vagina and cervix are well stimulated. Since the G-spot is on the anterior wall of the vagina the G-spot is usually stimulated in this position.

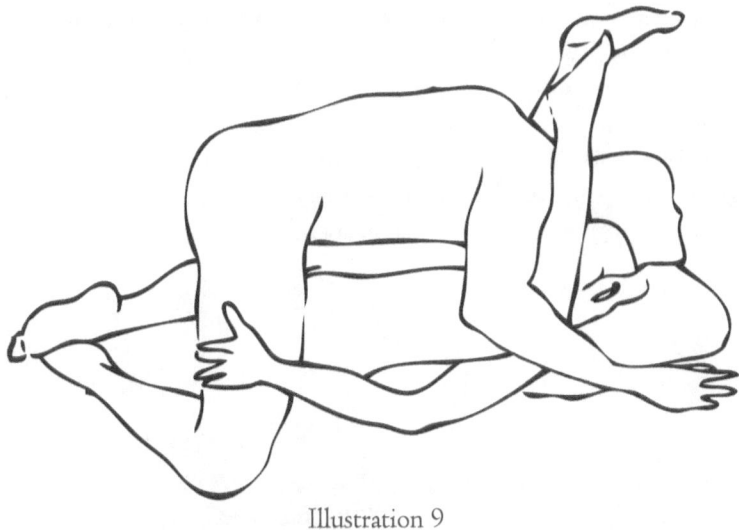

Illustration 9

This position is great for women who love very deep penetration and longer thrusting. It allows the man to stay inside the woman's body and offers him total sensation of the penis. It provides more stimulation for both the man and woman. But because the penetration is so deep some women will find this position uncomfortable, especially during ovulation and just before the menses. Also, in this position the man should take powerful strokes very gently because some women have an oversensitive cervix at the end of the vagina, and slamming into it can shock and bruise rather than delight.

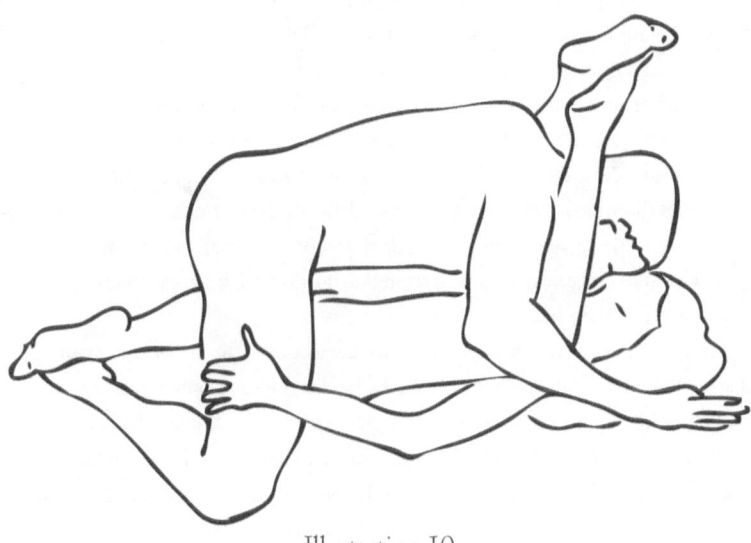

Illustration 10

When initiating this position the man should enter slowly until a comfortable thrusting angle is found. This position is especially good for a man with a small penis or for a woman with a large vagina. In this position the man can put the pillow under the buttocks of the woman if he desires deeper penetration. When having sex in this position the man should try to make contact with the G-spot as much as possible. A man or woman can manually stimulate the woman's clitoris in this position as the man thrusts, thus giving the woman a full body orgasm.

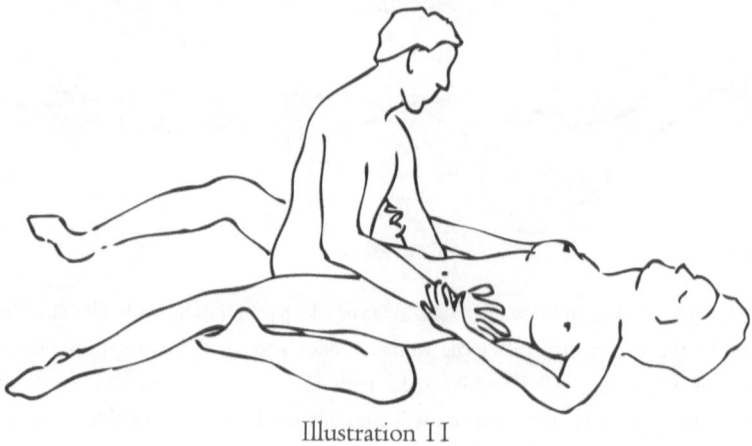

Illustration 11

Another variation of the missionary position is for the woman to lie on her back with legs straight and spread apart and the man to remain upright on his knees in between the woman's legs [above]. Then the woman should place her legs over his thighs so that he is lifting her pelvis up a little. This time the man does not lie on top of the woman. Instead the man should commence thrusting his penis into her vagina. While the depth of penetration is improved because of this position, just the placement of the man's penis against the front wall of the woman's vagina is the key to the success of this position. Just about a few minutes of the man thrusting his penis against the front wall of the woman's vagina and the woman will be tearing the sheets off the bed because of ecstasy, provided that she has a sensitive G-spot. A man or woman can manually stimulate the woman's clitoris in this position as the man thrusts, thus giving the woman a full body orgasm.

A variation of the missionary position is for the woman to lie on her back with a pillow under her hips and for the man to lie over her so that he can easily thrust in her vagina. The pillow creates a nice and relaxing spot for the woman's back and makes it easier for the man to thrust vigorously and still remain inside. The pillow allows the man to thrust deeper into the vagina and thrust at an angle that will hit the vaginal upper wall and G-spot. The woman should then have her legs wrapped over the man's hips so she can control the motion and open herself to more penetration [see Illustration 12, opposite].

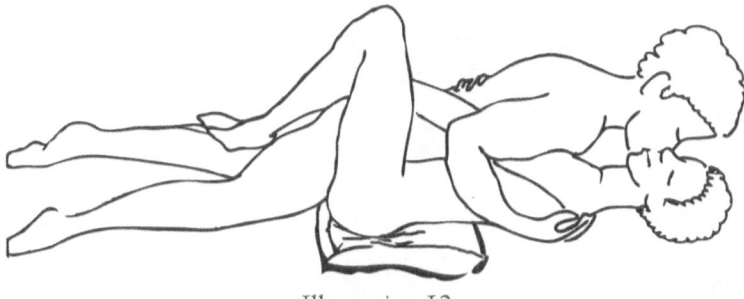

Illustration 12

This position allows the woman to take a more active role in lovemaking, by helping to control the tempo and depth of the man's thrusts. By the woman bringing her pelvis higher than her upper torso the woman is aligning her body so her clitoris and G-spot get incredible stimulation. This can lead a woman to orgasm. The fact that the woman is playing a role in controlling the tempo and depth of the man's thrusts makes this position a position that creates great passion, intimacy, and pleasure between the couple.

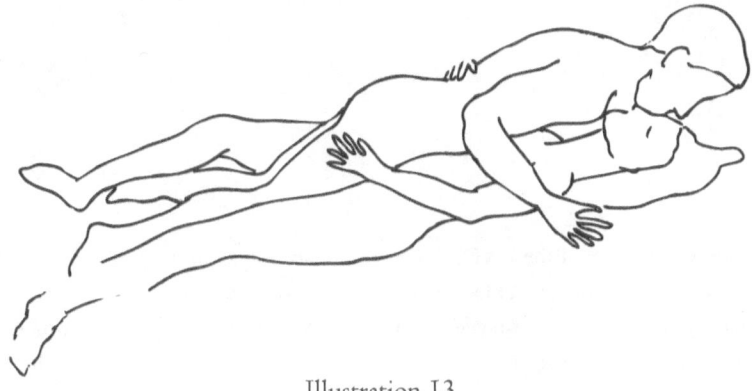

Illustration 13

The Coital Alignment Technique or CAT is a new twist on the missionary position [above]. The couple should begin with the typical missionary position, with the woman lying flat on the ground on her back with her legs spread apart and the man on top of her. After the man has inserted his penis, he moves his pelvis forward so that his pelvis overrides the woman's pelvis. In this position the base of the man's penis is pushed up against the woman's clitoris. The pelvic movement is not the typical in and out thrusting, but more of a rocking motion. The woman remains still, and the man does a rocking motion up towards her face and down towards her feet. The base of the man's penis is in contact with the woman's clitoris at all times. In this way, the man is maintaining contact with the woman's clitoris with the added stimulation of penetration. If a man is deep enough inside the woman and maintains constant contact between her clitoris and the base of his penis, a woman can achieve an orgasm if a rocking motion is maintained. The typical thrusting in and out of the traditional male superior position does not maintain enough constant contact with the clitoral area to have most women orgasm.

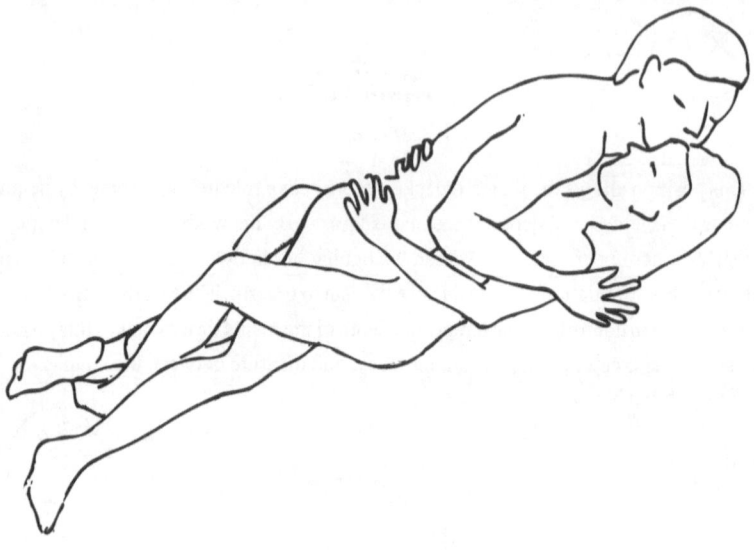

Illustration 14

Another variation of the CAT position is for the woman to wrap her legs around the man's thighs with her ankles resting on his calves [above]. Then the man starts doing a slow, rocking up-and-down motion, not in-and-out strokes. He does the rocking motion while maintaining full body contact and continuous pressure on the clitoris. The pattern of movement and stimulation must be held constant throughout the entire build up and release of the orgasm. This technique is an interesting addition to the different sex positions. It is also very erotic, intimate, and sensual. Another variation to the Coital Alignment Technique is for the man to put the shaft of the penis against the woman's clitoral area without having the penis penetrate the vagina [see Illustration 15, opposite]. Instead of thrusting the man should move his pelvis in a rocking motion up and down. By the man keeping the shaft of his penis in constant contact with the woman's clitoris, the woman is most likely to orgasm. The man also orgasms from the stimulation of his penis.

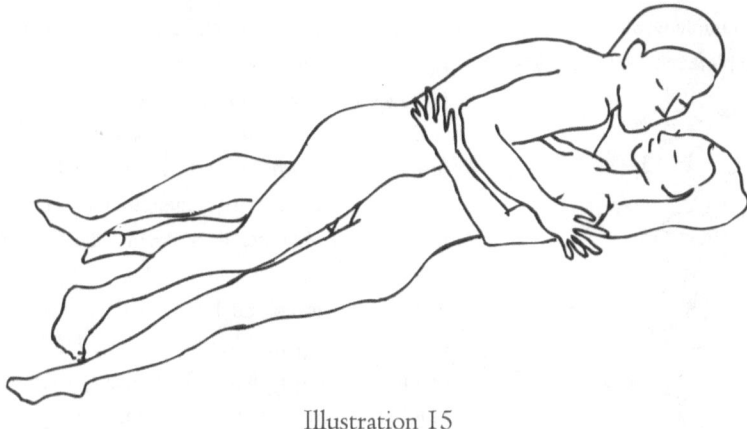

Illustration 15

Standing Positions

The standing position is often a highly erotic sex position. However, standing face to face while having sex is actually one of the more difficult sexual positions to achieve. It is difficult because the man and woman need to be the proper height in order for them to have sex in the standing position. Usually the shorter of the two partners needs to find a way to be just the right level. The shorter of the two partners needs to step on something to gain a little height. If the shorter of the two is a woman and she anticipates an encounter with a standing position she could try wearing something sexy and show up wearing really high heels that bring her to the right level. Many people have the notion that the shower and pool are good settings for the standing position.

In the standing position the person and his or her partner stand facing each other. One of them places his or her back against a wall. The woman spreads her legs and guides the penis into her vagina. Penetration is shallow but the clitoris is stimulated as the penis enters the vagina. If the woman closes her legs the stimulation of the clitoris is very intense. Just both people holding each other face to face and pelvis to pelvis when they are having sex is very sensual, especially if they are both naked. However, when a couple is in the standing position face to face their hands are usually busy trying to hold each other in the proper position; therefore, this is not the best position for a couple to caress or touch each other.

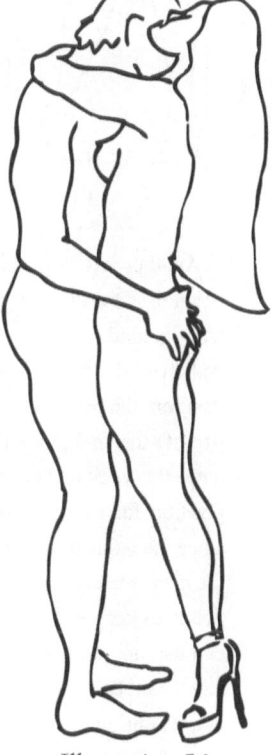

Illustration 16

If a couple wants a quickie, the simplest form to try is for both people to stand without complete removal of clothes. This requires very little space, can be done in a hurry, and provides very pleasurable and hot sex.

Every slight variation of the standing position provides a specific set of feelings and special eroticism. The depth of penetration is increased if the woman has her back against the wall, the man supports her buttocks with his hands, and she wraps her legs around his pelvis [left]. Holding up the female partner during sex is a huge labor of love, and most men will not manage for very long. A man may be surprised by the strength that passion can temporarily give him but he should not overestimate it. Instinctively a woman wants to get as close as possible to her man during intercourse. The woman, while in the standing position, can wrap her legs around his pelvis. This draws the man closer to her, tightens her leg muscles, and energizes her pelvis. This is another variation of the standing position. This position is very exciting for the couple to have sex in.

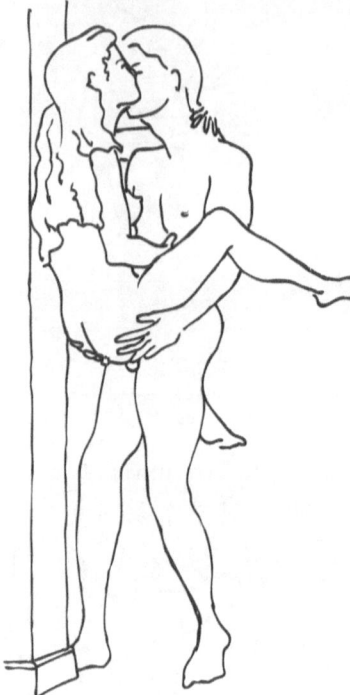

Illustration 17

Another exciting variation of the standing position is for the man to penetrate the woman from behind as she leans her hands against a wall [right]. In this variation of the standing position, the height difference is easier to compensate for. In this position the penis can easily enter the vagina. This position is not the best position for caressing or touching each other, since the woman has her hands on the wall and the man is using his hands to hold the woman's pelvis to keep her in place. However, the man can use one hand to hold the woman in place and the other hand he can use it to stimulate her clitoris during intercourse. Doing this will most likely bring the woman to orgasm.

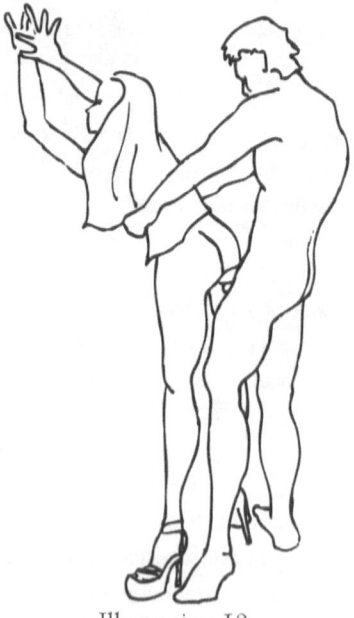

Illustration 18

The standing position works better when the lady is in a lying position. The reason is that the man can then use the strongest muscles in his body, the thigh muscles and the buttocks muscles, to his advantage. Also, this position allows the man to penetrate the woman as deeply as possible. The woman lies on her back on a bed or a table and then the man can lift her feet with his hands as he is standing facing her [right]. Then he can insert his penis inside the vagina and begin thrusting. The woman can stimulate her clitoris with her hand in this position as the man thrusts increasing her sexual pleasure.

Another variation of the standing position that is usually associated with hot steamy encounters is for the woman to lie down on her back on a bed or table and for the man to stand up straight [see Illustration 20, below]. Then the man should hold on to the woman's hips and place the back of her heels on his shoulders. The woman can also, lock her heels over his shoulders [Illustration 21]. Whether the woman's heels are on his shoulders or are locked over his shoulders, this position does get most women to orgasm if they have a sensitive G-spot because the man's penis is stimulating the woman's G-spot area. In this position the man or woman can be manually stimulating the woman's clitoris. If the man or woman stimulates the clitoris while having intercourse in this position, the woman will most likely have a full body orgasm.

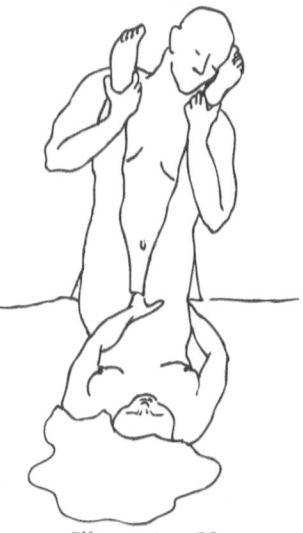

Illustration 19

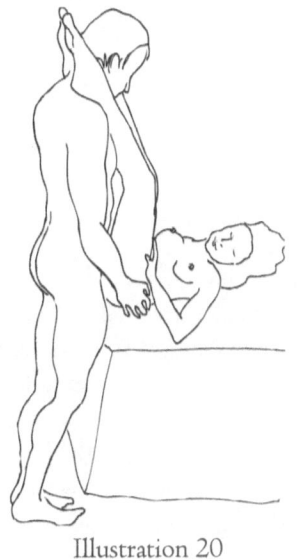

Illustration 20

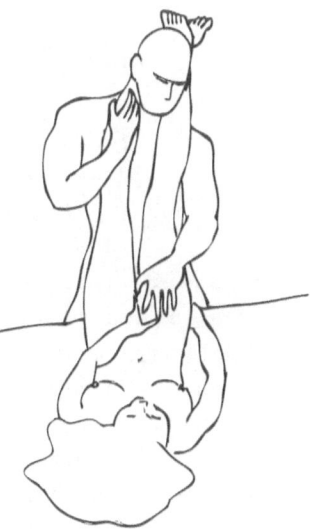

Illustration 21

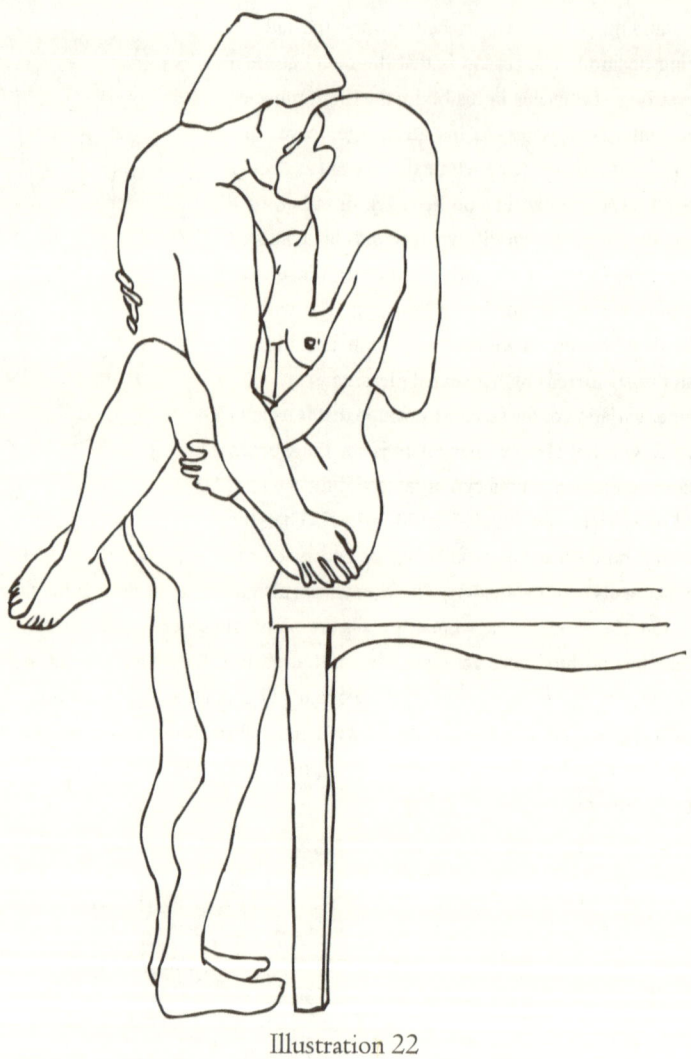

Illustration 22

A common variation of the standing up position is to have the woman sit on a table or on a sink facing the man while the man is upright. Then the man while still upright he can penetrate her vagina with his penis. The woman can wrap her legs around his pelvis while still in the sitting position [above] or she can leave her legs dangling towards the floor [Illustration 23, opposite]. If the woman wraps her legs around his pelvis, this will allow for deeper penetration. This position, whether the woman's legs are wrapped around his pelvis or just dangling is very erotic and sensual. In this position the man or the woman can stimulate the clitoris with his or her hand for added stimulation.

A way to spice up the standing up position is to have the woman stand up straight against the wall, facing the man. Then she can have one leg bent and resting on the chair with the sole of her foot, while the other leg is straight as she stands [see Illustration 24, below]. This lets her open her vagina a little more and envelop the man even further. This leads to greater pleasure during sex. Stimulation of the clitoris manually by the man or the woman during sex in this position will lead to greater pleasure. A second way is to have the woman, facing away from the man, stand with one leg straight, while the other leg is bent and resting on the chair with the sole of her foot. Then the man while standing upright can penetrate her from behind [Illustration 25]. For deeper penetration, the woman can bend her head and upper body forward. Stimulation of the clitoris manually by the man or the woman during sex in this position will lead to greater pleasure.

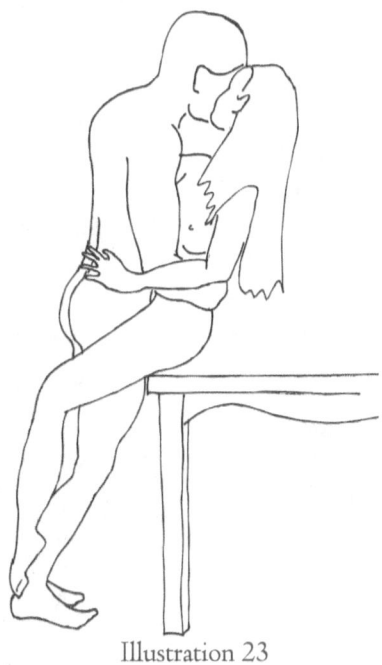

Illustration 23

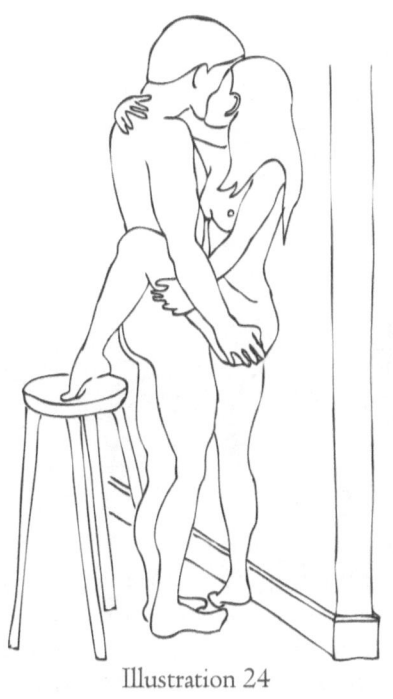

Illustration 24

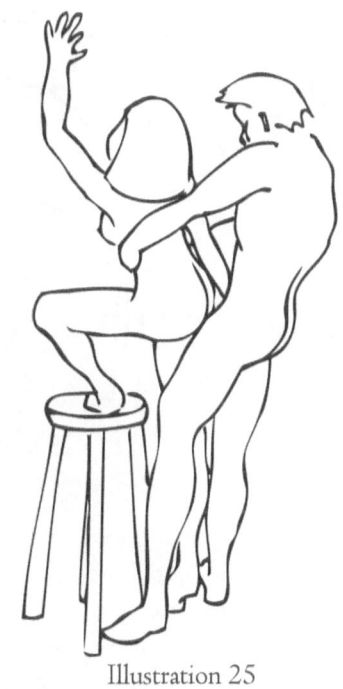

Illustration 25

Sitting Position

Sex in the sitting position does not always give as much pleasure and sensation as the missionary position or the woman on top position. However, sex in the sitting position is practiced by many couples because it is casual and can be extremely erotic, as well as great fun. Sex in the sitting position is fun for a change of pace. It gives a couple a break from their routine. Sex in the sitting position is good for a pregnant woman. Sex in the sitting position is ideal for a quickie when there is not a lot of time for sex. Sex in the sitting position can be very tiring, so a person should not be surprised if halfway through one of the partners needs to change positions.

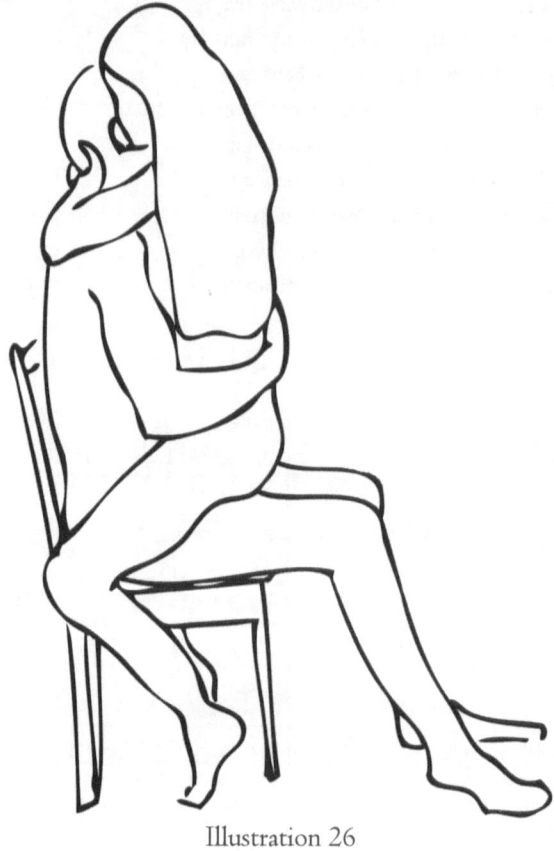

Illustration 26

The first seated position involves having the man sit in the chair with both feet resting on the floor [above]. Then the woman sits on top of him, facing him, with each of her legs resting on each side of the chair. The man then holds the woman's buttocks and pushes her closer to him so that his penis penetrates her vagina. In this position the man can move his upper body energetically. He can reach out easily to kiss and caress the woman's upper body, especially her face, neck, shoulders, and breasts. He can easily caress her buttocks and back with his hands. The man can easily nibble on the woman's nipples in this position. Since the woman is on top, she can control the angle of the thrust by leaning back or by varying the distance from her partner. The woman can also control the speed of penetration by moving as fast or as slow as she wants. The man can assist the woman's movements with his hands against her back or her buttocks. This usually makes the woman feel more aroused and excited because she is in control in this position. This position is very intimate and erotic since both partners are squeezed up against each other's body and are face to face. In this position the woman can stimulate her clitoris manually during sex for added pleasure.

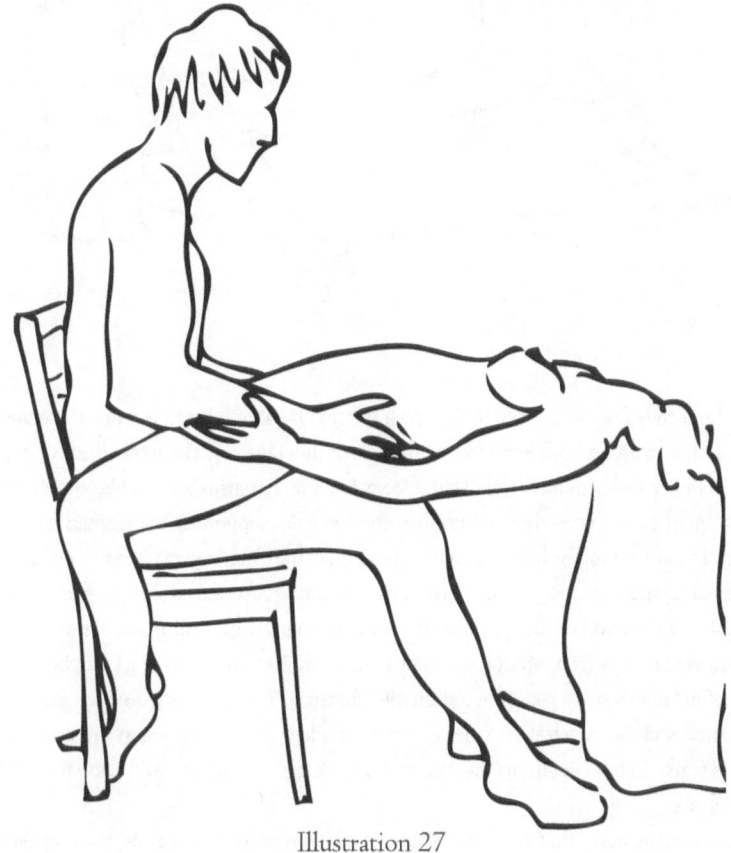

Illustration 27

A variation of this position is to have the woman, while in this position, arch her back until her back is touching the man's knees and legs and her head is tilted back [above]. While she is leaning back in this dramatic fashion, making herself supremely open and vulnerable to his thrusting, he supports her body by having his hands on her back or on her upper back and shoulders. Manual stimulation of the clitoris by the woman in this position during sex will add more pleasure to the encounter.

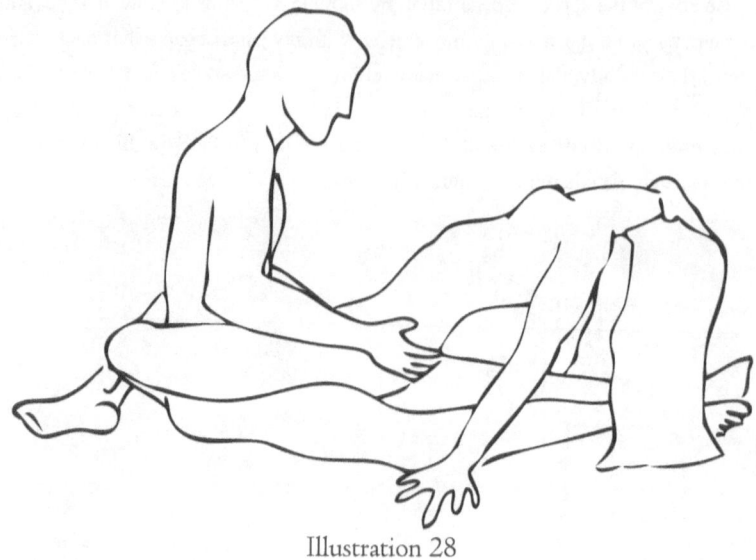

Illustration 28

Another version of the face to face position that is more relaxed is when the man sits on the floor with his both legs straight in front of him [above]. The woman sits on top of him with her feet around his waist and leans back on her arms and on his legs. Each of the woman's arms is resting on the floor on each side, supporting the woman's weight. When she sits on top of him she has his penis penetrate her vagina. She can control the speed of the penetration, and its rhythm by moving as fast and as slow as she wants.

Another variation of this position is for the woman, while still in the same position, to unwrap her legs from around the man's waist and have them resting straight on each side of the man's body [see Illustration 29, opposite]. This position provides a different sensation and the penetration is less deep than when the woman's legs are around the man's waist. In both positions the man or the woman can manually stimulate the clitoris during sex.

A sitting position that is more exciting to a woman is to have the man sit on the floor with both his legs straight in front of him. The woman then sits on top of the man facing him, with each of her legs on each side of his back, and with the soles of her feet resting on the floor. The woman then hugs the man around the neck and the man hugs the woman around the lower back [Illustration 30, opposite].

Sex Positions

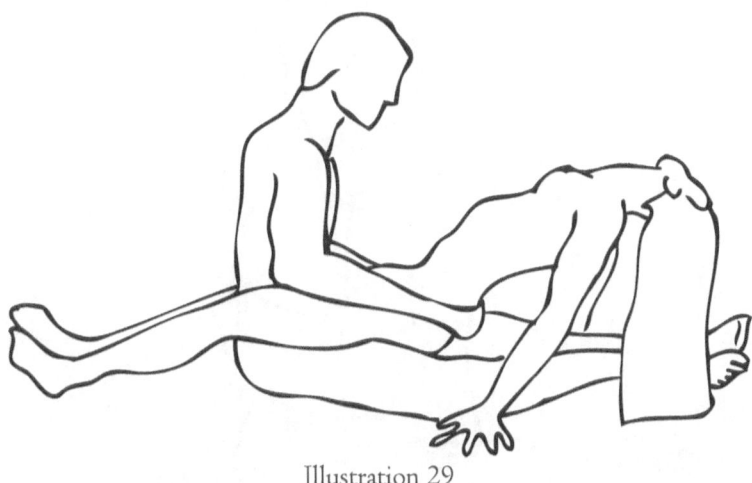

Illustration 29

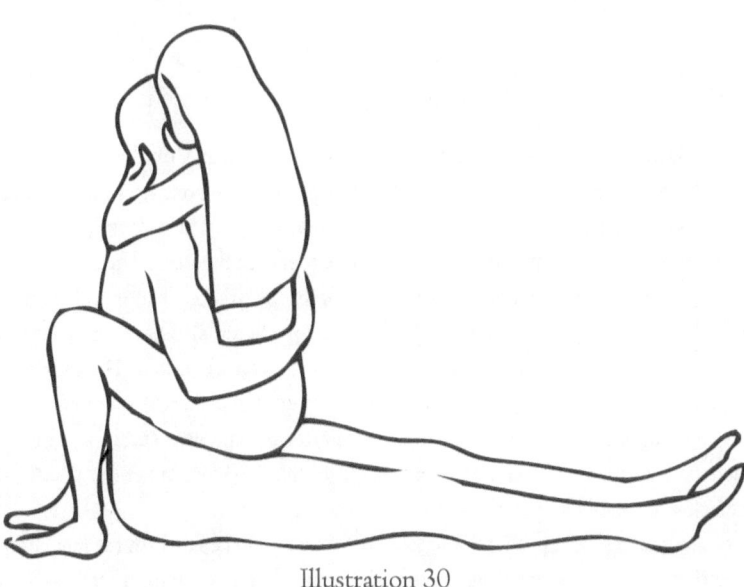

Illustration 30

In this position the woman controls the pace of the lovemaking, using her feet to provide leverage for her thrusts. The man remains fairly still and supports her body as she moves. Many couples find this position very romantic and intimate. Women enjoy this position greatly because they are in control of the thrusting.

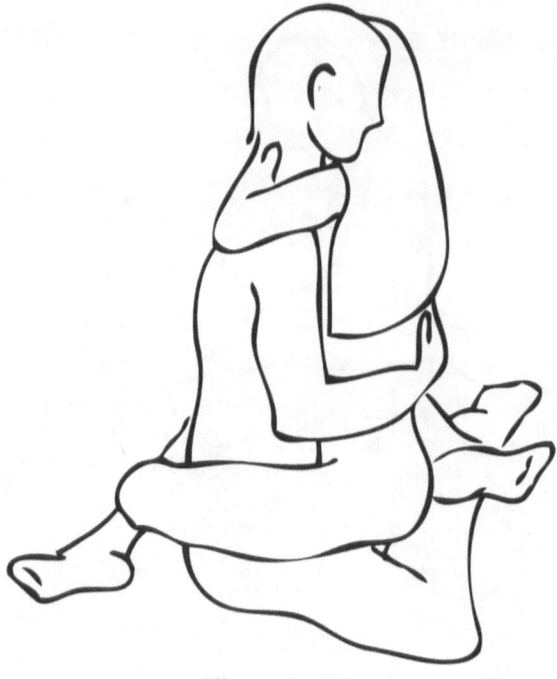

Illustration 31

A sitting position that many couples enjoy is to have the man sitting on the floor with both of his legs straight in front of him. Then the man can bend one leg so that the leg is bent close to his pelvis and its side is flat on the floor [above]. The outer thigh should be touching the floor. The inner thigh should not be touching the floor. Then he can bend the other leg so that the second leg is bent on top of the first one and its side is facing the floor and it is close to his pelvis. The second leg should also have the outer thigh touching the floor and the inner thigh should not be touching the floor. The woman can then sit on top of the man facing him with both legs around his waist. When she sits his penis should penetrate her vagina. The proximity of the couple's bodies and the face to face contact generate a feeling of intimacy. In this position, either the man or the woman can manually stimulate the clitoris during sex.

An alternative sitting position is to have the man sit on a chair with his feet straight on the floor. Then the woman sits on top of the man facing away from him, with each one of her legs on each one of his legs [see Illustration 32, opposite]. The man's penis should penetrate the woman's vagina. The woman takes control of the action. Her thighs' muscles enable her to rise and fall and set the tempo of the thrusts. The man benefits from seeing the woman's buttocks move rhythmically, which is a powerful primitive turn on. Just this visual experience for the man of seeing the woman's buttocks move up and down can be enough to drive the man wild with pleasure. The woman can use her free hands to stimulate her clitoris from the front. The man can use his free hands to massage the woman's breasts or clitoris or both. The man can kiss the woman's neck, face, and back of her head. The man can also whisper into her ear. In this position the woman's movements are not hindered, but the intimacy is decreased as the woman faces away from her partner. This position is used by couples who want a change. It is also used by couples who do not want to observe their partner's every facial movement during sex.

A sitting position that stimulates the woman's G-spot has the woman sit on the chair in a kneeling position with both of her knees on the chair supporting her weight facing away from the man. The man is in an upright position so he can rear entry her vagina and thrust away [see Illustration 33, below]. This position allows the man to stimulate the woman's G-spot. Many

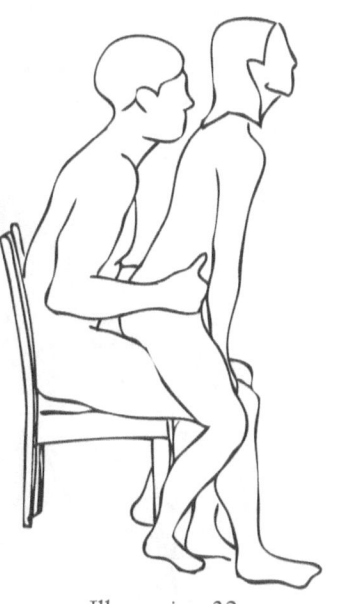

Illustration 32

women will orgasm from this position, provided that they have a sensitive G-spot. In this position the woman can manually stimulate her clitoris during sex for added pleasure.

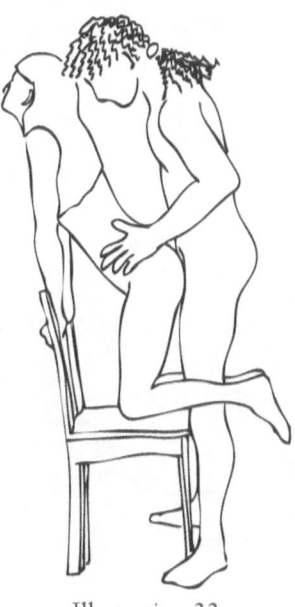

Illustration 33

A sitting position that is common has the man lie on the ground, flat on his back, with his legs straight. Then the woman should straddle his pelvis on her knees facing him [see Illustration 34 on next page]. After the penis is inserted into the vagina, the man should pull his body up to the sitting position, while keeping his legs straight. The woman can use her thigh muscles to control the thrusting. Both the man and the woman can hold each other in this position, and both can enjoy sensual caress. A variation of this position would be to have the man lie flat on the floor with both legs straight and have the woman straddle the man's pelvis on her knees facing away from him [see Illustration 35, next page]. After the penis is inserted into the vagina, the man should pull his body up to the sitting position, while keeping his legs straight. The woman can use her thigh muscles to control the thrusting. In this position the woman can stimulate her clitoris with her own hand. The man can stimulate the woman's clitoris or breasts with his own hands. He can also get an arousing view of her buttocks moving up and down. The man can easily kiss her back and face from this position. This variation is used by a couple for variety.

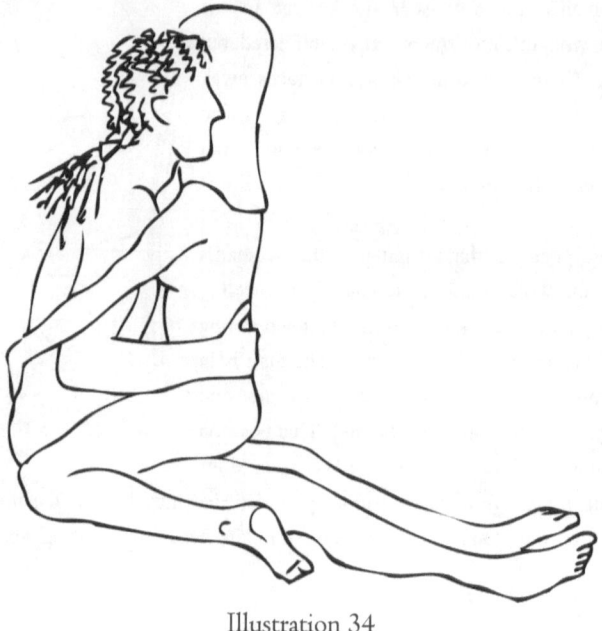

Illustration 34

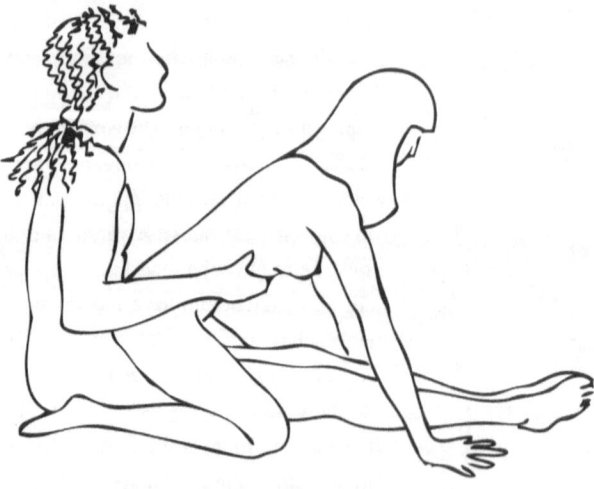

Illustration 35

An alternative sitting position is the kneeling position [right]. The woman kneels on the ground and the man kneels behind her. The man would press himself against his partner's back while caressing her with his hands. His penis would penetrate her vagina from behind. The man would use his thigh muscles for thrusting. Many women find it erotic to be kneeling and penetrated. Many men find it arousing to be kneeling and penetrating the woman. In this position, the man can stimulate the woman's breasts or clitoris. The woman can stimulate her own clitoris. Many couples enjoy the closeness and variety of having the woman's back close to the man's chest and both of their heads close to each other.

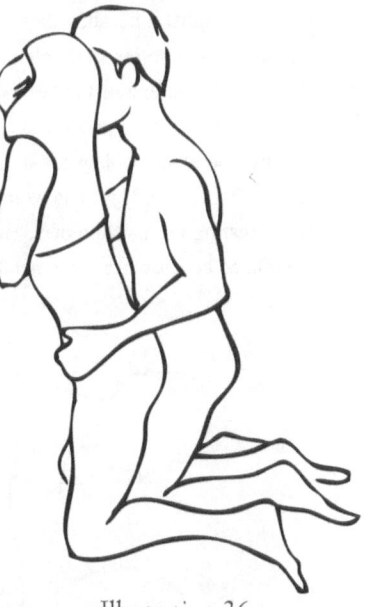

The next kneeling position is for the woman to lie on her chest with her legs straight and spread apart. Then the man is to kneel behind

Illustration 36

her, between her legs, and have her lift her legs and place them against his shoulders [below]. Then, while holding her legs, the man should move closer to the woman so that his penis penetrates her vagina. The man should make sure that the woman's legs

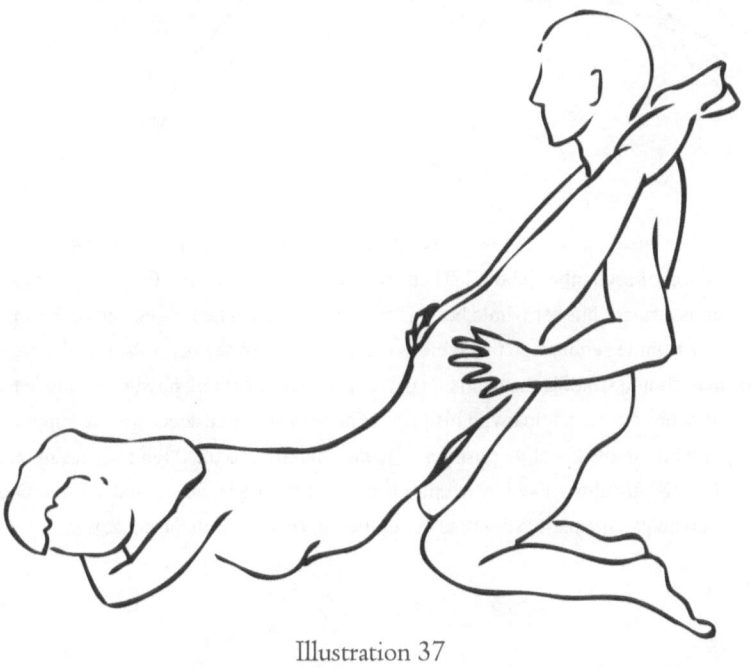

Illustration 37

remain straight on his shoulders. This position allows the man to thrust deep inside the woman so that he feels completely contained and she feels vulnerable and possessed. This position is one of the best ways to achieve deep penetration. Many women and men that enjoy deep penetration like this position. Many men like this position also because the woman's legs are in full view in this position, and men are usually greatly aroused by female legs. The woman's legs can also be clasped around the man's neck while resting on his shoulders. However, the woman may find that her clitoris is not stimulated because her movement is restricted.

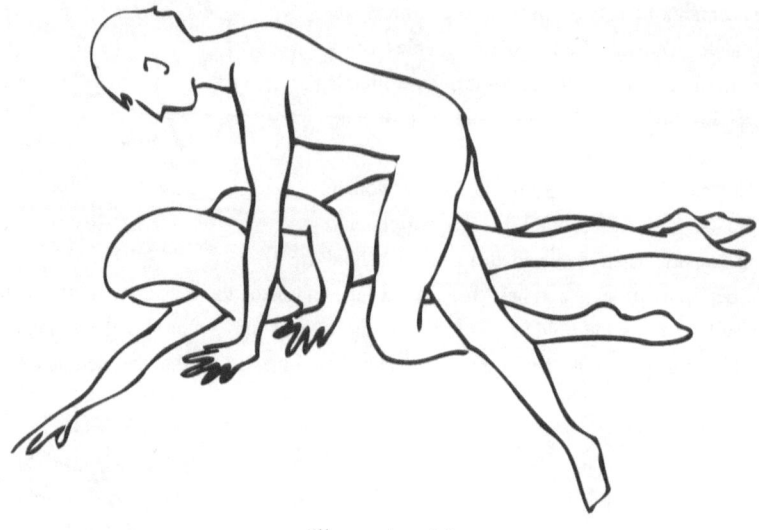

Illustration 38

Another kneeling position is to have the woman lie down on her right side with both legs on top of each other [above]. Then the woman should move her left leg so that her left leg is straight but her whole body is still on her side. The left leg should be spread from the right leg enough so that there is enough space for the penis to enter the vagina. The man should straddle the woman's pelvis while in a kneeling position facing her and should penetrate her vagina with his penis. The man should use his arms to support his weight while in the kneeling position. The man should use the thigh muscles to thrust. Usually this position is liked by couples because it is unique, novel, and not traditional. The woman can manually stimulate her clitoris in this position during sex.

Side-By-Side Positions

The side-by-side position is when the man and the woman lie down on their sides either facing each other [Illustration 39, below] or the man is facing the woman's back [Illustration 40]. The side-by-side position is a very relaxing way and a very pleasurable way for the couple to have sex. It is a good position to use when one or both partners are tired and want to have slow, relaxed intercourse. This position is liked by many couples because after orgasm, staying in this position is comfortable. It provides emotional closeness and relaxation during after sex play. The side-by-side position is a position that lends itself to falling asleep comfortably in each other's arms afterward. Many couples find this position romantic, since in this position, some couples doze off together and wake to find themselves tightly and sexily clasped. This is a very good starting point for making love.

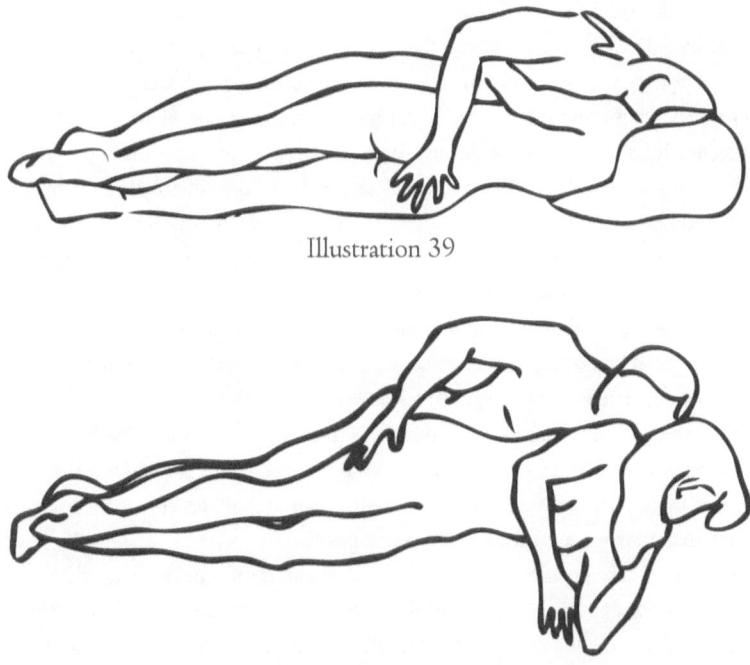

Illustration 39

Illustration 40

In this position penetration is not very deep. Therefore, women who have lovers with exceptionally large penises say the intercourse is more comfortable, in this position. This position allows for prolonged intercourse. In this position most men can thrust for a long time without climaxing, thus increasing the chances that the woman will orgasm during the sexual encounter. This position is also good for couples who want to have full body contact with their partner during sex. This position allows for manual stimulation of the clitoris to be achieved with ease by the man and the woman. The fact that this position allows for manual stimulation of the clitoris to be achieved with ease increases the chances that the woman will orgasm during intercourse.

This position is adored by many couples because it allows great emotional closeness. It allows great emotional closeness since the couple usually snuggles in this position and murmurs loving words to each other. This position is extremely restful, giving lovers a break if they find sex in other positions tiring. The side-by-side sex position is a very gentle position that can be used when one or both partners are physically frail or injured. It puts less strain on the body than other positions. It is also a position used by people recovering from surgery, or who are in old age. It is also a good position for pregnant women to use. It is a good position for men with premature ejaculation to use since it prolongs intercourse and slows down orgasm.

The side-by-side, face-to-face position is always more intimate and romantic than the side by side with the man's head facing the woman's back of her head. The reason is that in the face-to-face, side-by-side position, the couple can kiss and caress each other's face, chest, and other parts of the body. They can look at each other before, during, and after orgasm. They can also stare into each other's eyes during sex, which is very intimate, whereas in the face-to-back, side-by-side position, only the man can caress and kiss the woman. Also in the face-to-back position, the couple cannot look into each other's eyes, and cannot see each other's facial expressions before, during, and after orgasm. However, the face-to-back, side-by-side position has one advantage and that is that the woman's G-spot is easily reached by the man's penis during intercourse. A second advantage that the face-to-back, side-by-side position has is that the man gets great pleasure of seeing and feeling the woman's buttocks during intercourse. Third, the face-to-back, side-by-side position is the ideal sex position for the pregnant woman to have sex in because she will able to have sex with her abdomen comfortable. It is more comfortable for the pregnant woman in the face-to-back, side-by-side position than in the face-to-face, side-by-side position.

The side-by-side position is similar to the woman on top position or the man on top position, except that the partners lie on their sides. In the face-to-face, side by side position the couple embraces with both of them facing each other and both of their legs straight. The legs of both partners are straight and closed. The fact that the woman's legs are closed and straight will decrease the depth of penetration but will increase the stimulation of the clitoris. Both partners are limited in their movements but each have one hand free to stroke and massage each other as they gaze into each other's eyes.

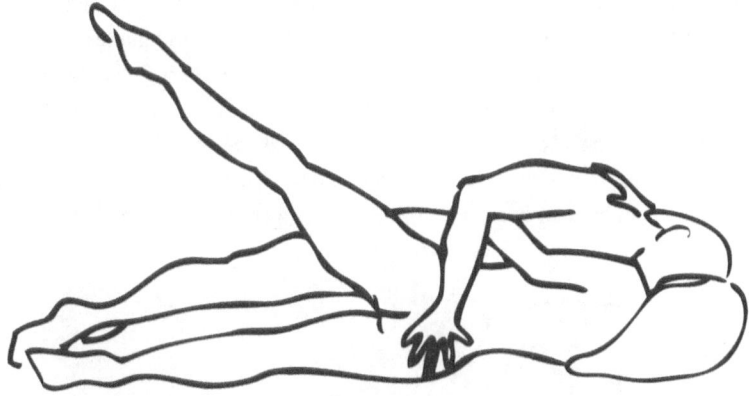

Illustration 41

Another variation of the face-to-face, side-by-side position is to have both partners lie facing each other with both of their legs straight [above]. Then the woman should lift her top leg so that the man can insert his penis into her vagina, while the man keeps both legs straight or he can spread them slightly apart by moving the top leg slightly forward. The higher the woman lifts her leg, the deeper the penetration can be and the more the man can stimulate the woman's clitoris with his hand. The woman can keep her leg raised throughout the intercourse, although that can get to be tiring, or the woman can lower her top leg resting it over the man's top leg. One favorite position of many couples is to have the woman's top leg over the man's top leg by bringing it forward slightly and then bringing the man's top leg forward slightly so it is resting on top of the woman's bottom leg.

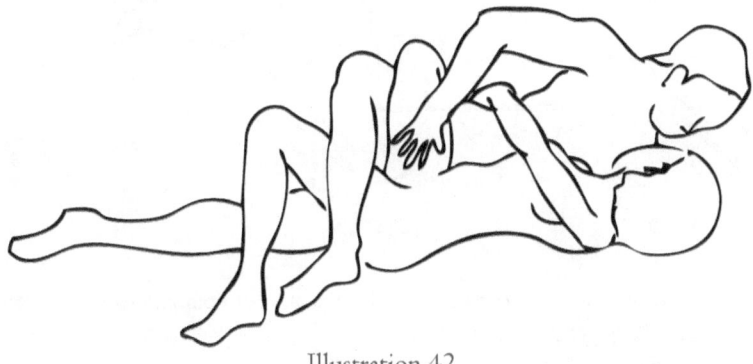

Illustration 42

A variation of the side-by-side position is called the scissors position [above]. In this position the woman lies on her back and the man lies beside her on his side. If the man is right-handed, he should lie on his left side. The woman raises her right leg and the man passes his right leg between both her legs making a kind of scissors with her legs; then the man enters the woman's vagina from the side and has his right leg rest on top of her left leg, which is bent on the floor. Her left leg should be bent with the sole of her foot flat on the floor. The man should have his right leg touch the floor while it is still on top of the woman's bent left leg. The woman's right leg should land on top of the man's right side towards his buttocks and it should be touching the floor. This is one of the best positions because it is not tiring and the weight of the man's thigh that is over the woman's bent leg gives extra clitoral pressure.

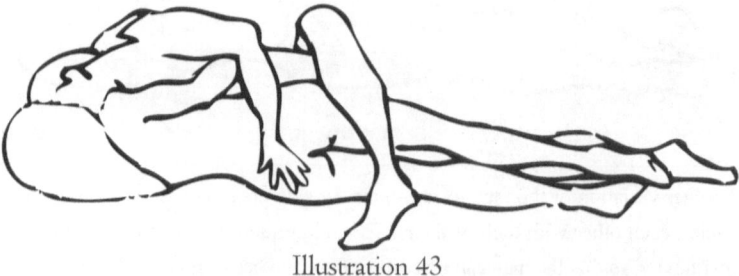

Illustration 43

A variation of the side-by-side, face-to-face position is for the woman to lie on her left side and the man to lie on his right side. When the man puts in his penis, he should lift up his left leg and lay it on the woman's right hip. His left leg should be dangling from the woman's right hip or it should be touching the floor with its sole [above]. If done right this allows for deep penetration with a direct connection to the G-spot. The man can also massage the woman's clitoris while having sex in this position.

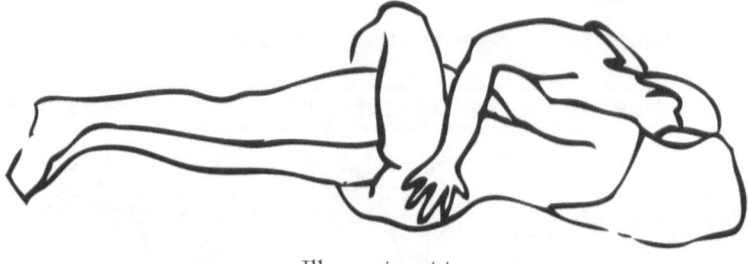

Illustration 44

An alternative side-by-side, face-to-face position is for both partners to lie down on their sides facing each other. Both partners should have both of their legs stretched out straight. Then the woman should wind her legs around the man's buttocks so that she can thrust against the weight of his body [above]. The woman should wrap her legs firmly around the man's buttocks and keep him in as closely as she likes during intercourse. The fact that the woman has her legs wrapped around the buttocks of the man assists the woman in her mobility. This is one of the sexiest and most pleasurable positions for a woman since the legs, particularly the inner thighs, are full of sensitive nerve endings and they are being stimulated in this position.

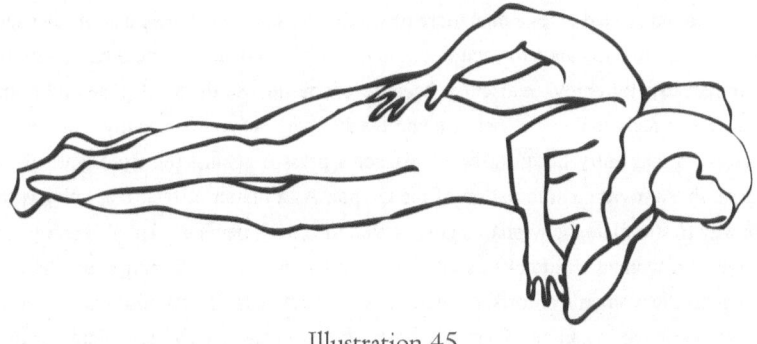

Illustration 45

Spooning is when the man and woman lie side by side with the man behind the woman, facing the back of her head [above]. It is the side-by-side, face-to-back position. This position allows the man easy access to the woman's entire body. This position is very sensual because there is total body contact between the man and the woman and the man's top hand is free to caress the woman's body or stroke her clitoris. Many women enjoy having their breasts fondled by the man's hand in this position. Alternatively, the woman is free to stroke her clitoris with her own hand in this position.

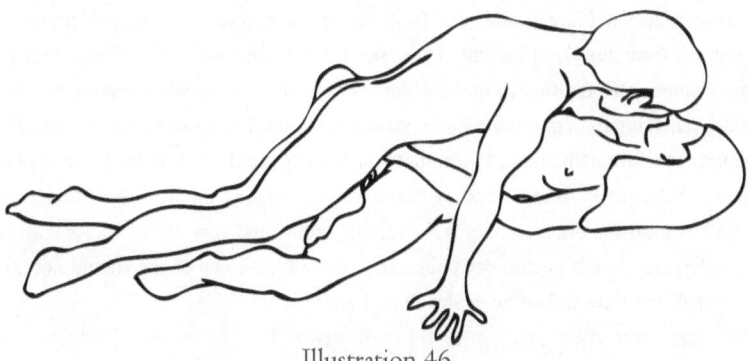

Illustration 46

Another modification to the spoon position is the modified spoon position [above]. In this position the woman lies on her back and the man is on top, but one of the woman's legs is drawn across the man's stomach and extended to the side, so that he is more or less lying on the woman's inner thigh. Then the man enters the woman at an angle that is halfway from the side, halfway from the rear. While the man is inside the woman the man or the woman can manually stimulate the clitoris during sex.

Rear Entry

Sex from behind is also called rear entry. It can be done in many different ways. Some couples love rear entry because it allows for deep penetration of the vagina by the penis. Rear entry also gives a man more pleasure than some other sex positions because the man has more distance to each thrust in this position than in some other positions. A woman usually enjoys rear entry because of the intense depth of penetration and because she feels that she is being taken by the man. A woman usually experiences pleasure in rear entry because the man's penis presses against the front wall of her vagina, thus providing stimulation of the G-spot. As a matter of fact, rear entry is the best way to stimulate the woman's G-spot with the man's penis. A man also enjoys the feeling of a woman's buttocks against his thighs in rear entry. In rear entry the man can caress the woman's clitoris, breasts, back, and buttocks. He can also kiss a woman all over her back, neck, and face. A woman in rear entry can also stimulate her own clitoris and bring herself to orgasm while the man is penetrating her. Some couples find rear entry enticing because it seems so primitive and animalistic because most animals copulate this way.

On the other hand, some couples do not like sex from behind at all. Some couples do not like it because they find it animalistic and primitive. Some do not like it because it is does not allow for face-to-face intimacy. Some women find rear entry painful when the man's penis penetrates very deeply and the woman feels pressure against her cervix. Rear entry is usually painful to the woman if the woman has a tilted uterus or a partner with a very large penis because he will likely hit the neck of her cervix. If the woman does not have a sensitive G-spot then the woman is unlikely to experience an orgasm from sex from behind. Thus, sex from behind would be disappointing to some women. The solution to this problem is to have the man while having sex from behind, reach his fingers around the woman's waist until he reaches the clitoris. Then the man, while thrusting, should stimulate the woman's clitoris with his hand until she orgasms. Having sex from behind, with the man stimulating the woman's clitoris with his fingers until she orgasms, can feel exciting, erotic, and very arousing. As with any way of having sex if a person does not like it this way, then he or she should not do it. But if he or she likes it then he or she should go for it.

The main rear entry position is called doggy style position [see Illustration 47, opposite]. It is when the woman is on her hands and knees with both open palms resting on the floor. Her hands can be straight, slightly bent, or greatly bent. The man kneels with his back remaining upright, behind the woman and then his penis penetrates her vagina from behind. The man can hold on to the woman's hips, thighs, waist, or shoulders in order to move her to meet his thrusts. The man does most of the thrusting in this position and the woman's movements are limited in this position. Some couples enjoy the speed that a man can create by holding on to the woman's hips and thrusting.

Sex Positions

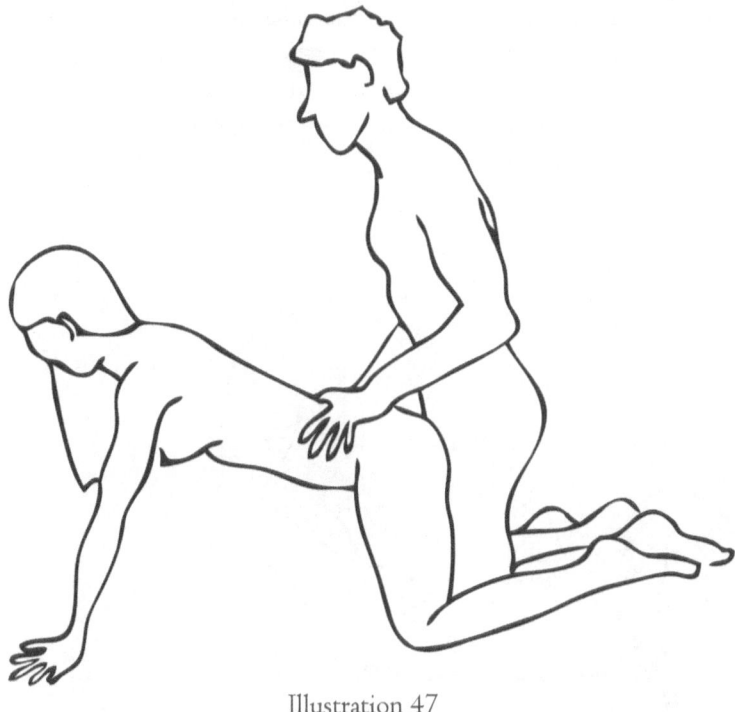

Illustration 47

Also in this position a man can control the speed of his thrusting, thus he can satisfy a woman whether she enjoys slow thrusting or a variation of speeds in thrusting. This position can be highly arousing, erotic, and charged for both man and woman. In this position the woman's vagina is especially tight. By the woman squeezing her thighs together the woman increases the tightness of her vagina and her ability to contract her pubococcygeal muscle group or PC muscles. The couple should try putting cushions underneath the woman's chest. This will improve the angle of penetration in the sex from behind position. The man can easily manually stimulate the clitoris in this position during sex, giving the woman a full body orgasm. For variety, in this position the woman can lift her leg by moving it slightly to the side, so that it is suspended in midair. Such an action causes the woman to stretch her vagina slightly, causing it to open more widely. This increases the chances of clitoral stimulation during intercourse in the rear entry position. This changes the sensations felt during sex by both the man and the woman. This can be done from time to time for variety.

Another variation of the rear entry position has the woman begin on her hands and knees with both open palms resting on the floor, then lower herself onto her elbows, so that she is resting on her elbows instead of the palms of her hands [see Illustration 48, next page]. The man then kneels with his back remaining upright behind the woman and then his penis penetrates the woman's vagina from behind. This position allows the woman to change the angle of her pelvis, the depth of the penetration and the sensation of sex for both her and the man. The woman's pelvis is pushed backward and upward. The man can easily manually stimulate the clitoris in this position during sex giving the woman a full body orgasm.

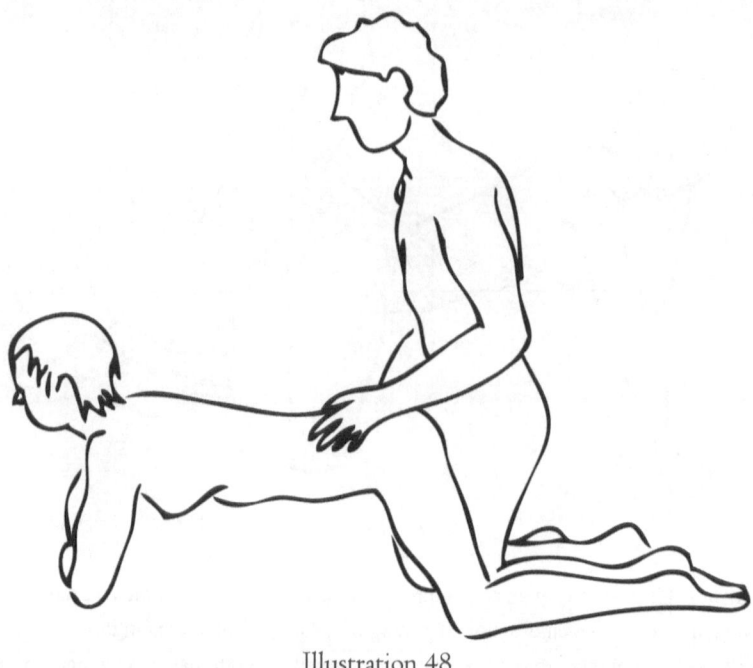

Illustration 48

Another variation of this position is for the woman to lie completely flat on her stomach, face down, with her legs open and her pelvis tilted up [below]. Then the man lies on top of her back, entering her from behind. This position allows the man and woman to experience a tight entry as the penis enters the vagina, which is very pleasurable for both. The penetration is shallow but can be increased by placing a pillow under the woman's pelvis. The woman can use her buttocks muscles to squeeze the man's penis as he thrusts. When lying flat, the woman is probably better off stimulating

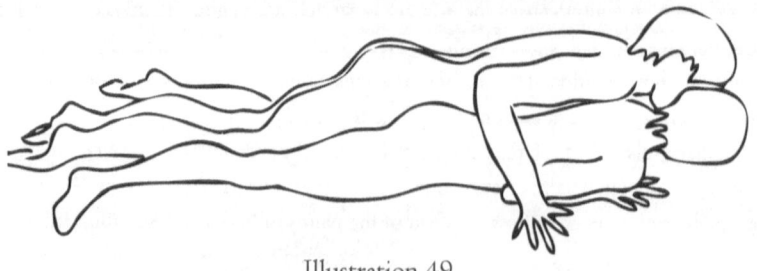

Illustration 49

her clitoris herself. A man lying down on his woman with her underneath him is an especially affectionate love position because the man's entire body is spread out along his partner's body. His head is next to hers and he can kiss and whisper to her during intercourse. In this position, the male pelvis rests at the rear of the woman's buttocks and pivots from that angle. This means this position is an easy and relaxing position for leisurely rhythmic and sensuous sex. However, this is not a position that is likely to greatly excite the woman, because the male is lying on top of her and she cannot really move that freely. This position is great for those times when the woman feels like taking a more passive role. It is also great for follow-up sex when she has already climaxed but wants to continue enjoying the intimacy of lovemaking. This position is also a good position to stimulate the woman's G-spot. However, in this position the woman's G-spot is stimulated through shallow thrusts.

Another variation of the rear entry position is for the woman to stand at the side of the bed and lean over, putting her weight on her elbows. The man stands behind her and enters her from the rear [right]. The man usually holds the woman from her hips or waist. Many couples like the novelty of the position.

Or, in an alternative position, the woman can kneel on the floor with her upper half resting on the bed and the man kneeling behind her [see Illustration 51 on next page]. Then he enters her with his penis. The fact that the woman's upper half is resting on the bed makes this position more relaxing than the regular rear entry position for the woman. However, many women still prefer the traditional rear entry position with the palms resting on the ground, because they enjoy the sexual sensation as they are resting on the palms of their hands and knees.

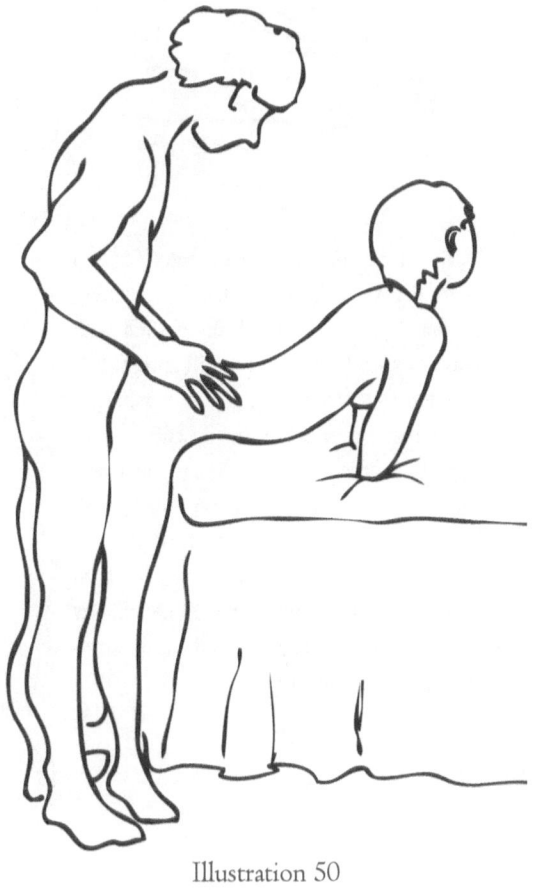

Illustration 50

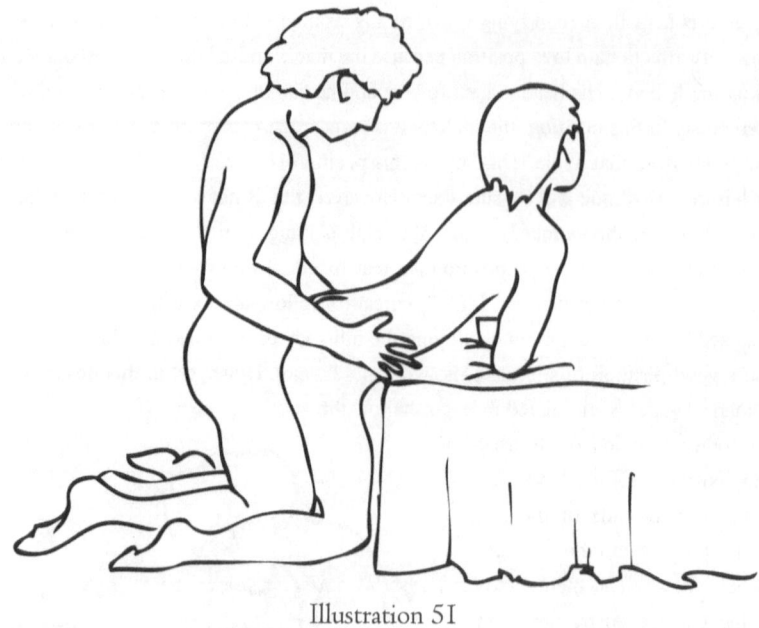

Illustration 51

Another variation of the rear entry position is for the woman, from a standing position, to stretch down and touch the ground with her hands while her legs are still upright, but slightly bent. Her partner stands, penetrates, and thrusts from behind while still upright [right]. In order for this technique to work, the man must hold his partner firmly with both hands around the hips. This position is likely to be an erotic adventure for both partners. Many women enjoy having sex with their head tilted towards the ground, so they enjoy this position.

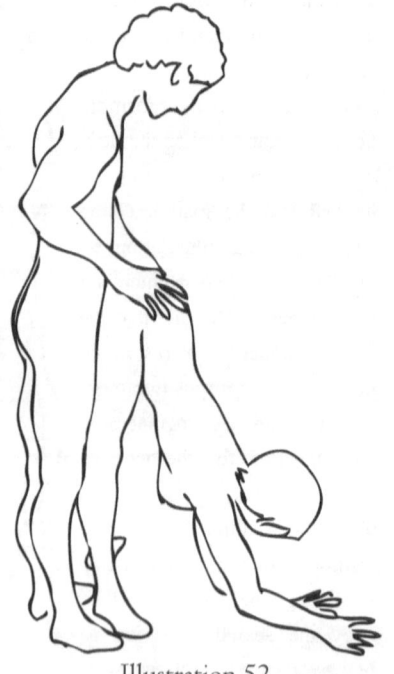

Illustration 52

Woman On Top Position—(Female superior position)

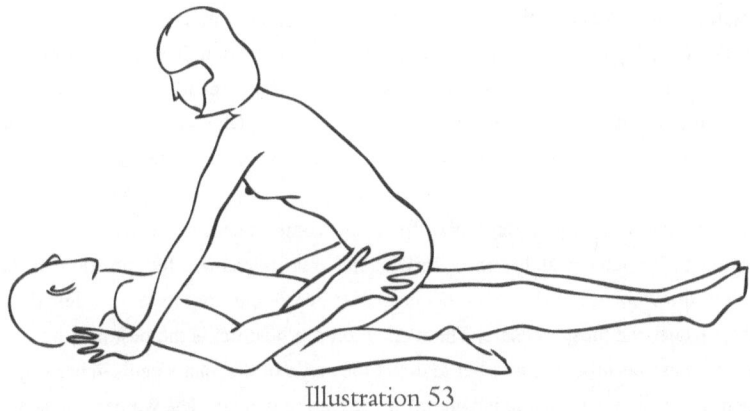

Illustration 53

To get into the woman on top position, have the man lie flat on his back, with both legs straight. Then the woman should straddle the man's pelvis with her knees. The woman should be facing the man's face and not his feet. The man then should place the penis at the opening of the vagina and then the woman should slowly lower her pelvis down onto the man's penis. The woman should start with shallow penetration. As she becomes more comfortable, she should lower her body further until she is in an upright sitting position. She should remain upright from the waist up as she moves up and down his penis during intercourse. A woman should try not to jerk up and down as she moves up and down the man's penis during intercourse. Rather, she should keep her movements fluid by keeping the pressure and speed the same as she switches the direction of her movement. Penetration is quite deep in this position. The man's most sensitive area on the penis is deeply buried within the woman's moist and warm vagina. In this position a woman can squeeze and massage a man's penis with her pubococcygeal muscles, or PC muscles, either while thrusting up and down on his penis or while sitting still with his penis inside of her. The woman can also direct the man's penis to her most sensitive vaginal spots as she thrusts and can use her pubococcygeal muscles, or PC muscles, to stimulate the shaft of his penis only as the head of the penis comes in contact with the sensitive vaginal spots. When the woman has her orgasm, the man can feel the contractions of her vaginal muscles much more intensely in this position than in any other position.

The woman on top position is also known as the female superior position. It is the second most popular of all sexual positions among people worldwide. Three-quarters of the couples use this sexual position at least occasionally. The woman on top position gives the woman the most control and freedom of movement during intercourse. The woman on top position is the easiest position for the woman to orgasm solely from penile and vaginal intercourse since the penetration is deep and because stimulation of the clitoris is achieved with greater ease than with any other position. As a matter of fact, the clitoris is usually stimulated more rapidly and with greater intensity in the woman on top position than in any other female sexual position. In some cases multiple orgasms are experienced by women in this position. The woman on top position is the best position that works well for the majority of women who want to have quick and easy orgasms. The woman on top position helps a woman speed her sexual response to climax.

The woman on top position works for most women because the female has great freedom of movement and is in control of her own orgasm in this position. In this position the woman can direct the penis against her G-spot, or any other vaginal area that gives her the most pleasure. The woman on top position is the best position for a woman to use because it allows her to direct the angle of the man's penis in her vagina, which results in great satisfaction and pleasure for the woman. The woman can control her degree of stimulation in this position. According to the level of sensation the woman is experiencing, she can speed up or slow down her thrusting in order to move toward an orgasm or hold off from climaxing until she is ready. In this position the woman can control the depth of penetration, the tempo and speed of thrusting. The female on top position works well for a woman that happens to be taller or smaller than the man.

The man finds it very erotic and arousing when the woman lowers herself onto his penis in this position. The man usually gets so excited as the woman lowers herself onto his penis in this position that he feels that he wants to be inside her. The woman should take advantage of her position in the woman on top sex position by displaying her body, because the man will love to watch her work by moving up and down his penis. The man usually gets great pleasure from seeing the woman's whole body displayed above him. He gets great pleasure from seeing the woman's vagina envelop his penis in this position. In the female superior position, the man experiences greater exposure of his penis to the woman's vagina than in any other position. The man is delighted to see the passion reflected in the woman's face as she moves up and down his penis. The man is gratified to see the woman's hair fall or hit her face or chest as she moves up and down on his penis. The woman on top position can be very gratifying to a man because he can look at and touch a woman's breasts during sex and enjoy seeing the breasts sway with the woman's every move. In this position the man can rub the woman's buttocks and belly which is thrilling to both partners. A man is delighted to be free from any responsibility in this sex position. The man is pleased to be lie on his back, relaxed and enjoying the sex. A man will find it highly erotic and exciting to see a woman masturbate herself and play with her nipples while in the woman on top position. She can be sitting still in this position or thrusting up and down in this position as she masturbates and plays with her nipples.

The woman on top position gives both partners easy access to the woman's clitoris. Either of the two partners can manually stimulate the woman's clitoris, with their own hand during intercourse in the woman on top position. In the woman on top position the woman can touch the man's chest and reach around to caress his scrotum and testicles, which many men find pleasurable. In this position both partners can see what they each look like during orgasm. In this position both partners make lots of eye contact, which contributes to intimacy.

Some women shy away from the woman on top position because they are afraid that their partner will view them as too assertive or aggressive. Some women do not enjoy this position because they feel self-conscious about having their bodies exposed and in full view. Some women are uncomfortable having freedom and control during sex so they do not like this position because it offers them both. Some women do not like this position because they are not comfortable pursuing their own pleasure, because they have adopted a double standard that it is acceptable for the man to be active in the pursuit of sexual pleasure but it is not appropriate for the woman to do so. They believe they should just lie there and let the man do all the work. Then they wonder why they do not have an orgasm. These women that shy away from the woman on top position need to adjust their attitudes so that they enjoy the woman on top position.

If a woman is inhibited about having sex in the woman on top position, she can do several things. First, she should understand that the man won't view her as too assertive or aggressive if she wants to have sex in the woman on top position. As a matter of fact, most men enjoy this position. Second, she should not be self-conscious about having her body exposed and in full view. She should not examine her body and worry about how her body looks. She should not try to analyze what the man is thinking throughout intercourse in the woman on top position. Third, she can ask her partner to reassure her that he loves her body and encourage her by telling her how beautiful her body looks and how erotic she looks moving up and down his penis. Fourth, the woman should feel comfortable to be in control and free during sex, because the clitoris is designed to encourage its bearer to take control of her sexuality. The clitoris operates at a peak performance when the woman takes control and is on top. The woman should feel comfortable pursuing her own pleasure because she needs more specific stimulation than the man. When the woman is in the woman on top position, she can be more active in going after the specific stimulation she needs.

Some men have trouble with the whole idea of a woman being in the superior position. They feel that their manhood and leadership are challenged when the woman is in the woman on top position. Sexual politics should not get in the way of good sex. Sexual politics should not be the couple's main concern. The couple's pleasure should be the couple's main concern. The couple should regard sex as a partnership that both can contribute to. If they have such an attitude they will have sensational sex. If they do not have such an attitude they will not enjoy sex to its fullest extent. Some men feel that the woman on top position is only for the take charge woman. That is not true. The woman on top position is for every woman. Despite the fact that the man has limited mobility in this position and has no control over the speed of thrusting that occurs in this position and has no control over the degree of penetration in this position, most men enjoy this position because they can rest and enjoy exquisite sexual sensations. Most men also enjoy this position because they enjoy seeing their woman experience pleasure in this position and because they enjoy seeing their woman take control in this position.

The woman's thrusts are powerful and erotic as she moves up and down the man's penis in the woman on top position. However, they can also become physically tiring for the woman and difficult to maintain. When the woman becomes tired in the woman on top position she can rest on top of her partner by laying her chest on top of his chest and enjoying the naked sensation of each other's bodies. In order to keep his erection going, the woman can rock gently from side to side. This way she is continuing love-making slowly and gently until she is ready to return back to sitting upright. While the woman is lying along the man's body face to face, both partners can kiss and whisper to each other, which creates intimacy and increases arousal.

A woman in the woman on top position, stimulates herself and her partner by moving up and down his penis. A woman in the woman on top position can also sit with the man's penis inside her and instead of moving up and down, she moves in a continuous circular motion stimulating both her vagina and the man's penis. The sexual sensations for both partners from a circular movement will be different than the sexual sensations from the up-and-down movement. Also, a woman in the woman on top position can sit with the man's penis inside her and she could move simultaneously up and down on the man's penis while moving in a circular motion at the same time. The sexual sensations for both partners from such movement will be different than sexual sensations from the woman moving only up and down or the woman moving only in a circular motion. The woman can vary the way she moves to add variety to the sex in the woman on top position. Also, while in the woman on top position facing the man's face, the woman can have her thighs around the man's waist and she could rhythmically squeeze her thighs and let go with her thighs. This pleasures the man's penis while stimulating the woman's clitoris.

In the woman on top position, the sex can last longer so that the woman can orgasm simultaneously with the man or even experience multiple orgasms. In order for that to happen, the man should communicate to the woman when he is close to ejaculating, and the woman should stop thrusting briefly, before the man reaches the point of no return. While this momentary interruption may seem irritating to the woman at first, it allows the man to control his ejaculation and to prolong lovemaking greatly, leading to far greater pleasure for her and for him.

For most men ejaculatory control is easier with the woman on top, versus the missionary position, for several reasons. First, the man in the woman superior position can just relax, which lets him gain ejaculatory control. On the other hand, in the missionary position the man cannot just relax since he has to do most of the work by thrusting. Second, in the woman on top position, the man is just lying down, so he does not get tired, while in the missionary position the man might get tired because has to do most of the work by thrusting. Third, many men find the stimulation in the woman on top position less intense than in the missionary position, so the sex can last longer in the woman on top position, because the man can delay ejaculation longer.

In the woman superior position, the man can ask the woman to hold off thrusting for a short while or to slow down thrusting. He can do so when he needs her to, so that he will have more control over his ejaculation. In the female superior position, a female can stop moving if she feels a premature ejaculation coming on. In the woman superior position, even if the man has climaxed before his female partner, the female can manually rub her clitoris or have the male manually rub it for her while his penis is softening inside her.

The couple can start off in the missionary position and then roll over, reversing their positions, so that they are in the woman superior position. But they should be careful that the man stays inside of the woman as they roll over together. In the woman on top position, the woman can move around and adjust the angle of the man's penis. She can get the penis into vaginal areas that the man would never have been able to if she were not on top. For some women, changing from the missionary to the female superior position may be all that is necessary to achieve orgasm. The fact that the woman is in control of the action and pacing of the thrusting in the woman superior position should enhance the woman's sexual response, but it may not be enough. Not all women can reach orgasm in the woman superior position, only through penile and vaginal contact. In order to orgasm, some women require direct stimulation to the clitoris that cannot be provided during sex in the woman on top position. That does not mean that there is something wrong with the woman if she needs direct clitoral stimulation in order to orgasm. Some women are different than others and require more stimulation of their clitoris.

When having sex many women feel the desire to orgasm. So even in the female superior position, if the woman cannot climax, she can usually have the male partner rub her clitoris while she goes up and down his penis to bring her to climax, or she can rub her clitoris herself. This can be done because the man and woman can easily access the woman's clitoris in the woman on top position. Many women are embarrassed to masturbate themselves when in the female superior position, because they feel awkward. Women should not be embarrassed to masturbate themselves while on top because the man usually never finds anything awkward about her pleasuring herself. As a matter of fact, the man is usually turned on by such an action. For some of the women that can reach orgasm in the woman superior position, only through penile and vaginal contact, it may not be fast enough. It may be faster than waiting for the man's penis to thrust her to orgasm, but it may still not be fast enough. This is another instance where the male partner can rub the woman's clitoris as she moves up and down his penis to bring her to climax faster. The woman can also rub her clitoris herself, while she goes up and down the man's penis to bring herself to orgasm faster.

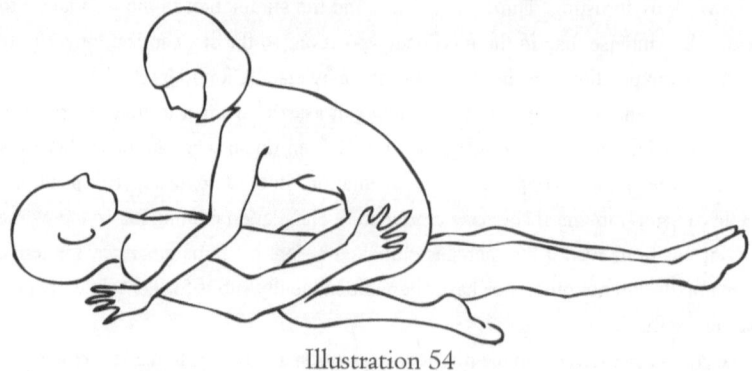

Illustration 54

If the woman is in the woman on top position, and she leans forward slightly [above], then her clitoris can come into contact with her partner's body. In order for the woman to be sure that she has an orgasm in the woman on top position, she can lean forward slightly to create friction between the man's pubic bone and her clitoris. Then the woman can rub her clitoris against the man's pelvis as she thrusts up and down the man's penis leaning forward. The slang term for this is called riding high because the woman is said to be riding the man while she controls the thrusts. The man can arch his back and raise his pelvis to help create more intense contact between the man's pelvis and the woman's clitoris. For a variation, the man could put a pillow under his hips. The fact that the pillow is under the hips of the man allows the woman to rub her clitoris against the man's pubic bone intensely as she moves up and down his penis. The woman should really feel the difference in pleasure as it intensifies. When the man sees the woman receiving great pleasure from this position, the man will reach new heights of pleasure as well.

For a variation, in the woman on top position, the woman can also thrust up and down the man's penis but keep the head of her partner's penis in the first two inches of her vagina. She can try to keep the head of the man's penis in the first two inches of her vagina because the first two inches of the vagina are the most sensitive part of the vagina and the head of the man's penis is the most sensitive part of the penis. Keeping the head of the penis within the first two inches of the vagina makes the sex produce different sexual sensations.

Another variation is when the woman is in the woman on top position, with the man's penis inside of her, she could part the vaginal lips and lean forward to the man's chest, bringing her clitoris directly into contact with the base of the man's penis. Then she should rub softly from side to side or in a circular motion the exposed shaft of the man's penis against her clitoris [below]. Usually this is all the direct stimulation of the clitoris the woman needs to reach orgasm. In this position also, the woman can move up and down her vagina on the man's penis while keeping her chest on the man's chest. The woman should not withdraw the penis completely from the vagina when thrusting up and down. This will stimulate the vagina, clitoris, and penis. This produces a different set of sexual sensations for both partners.

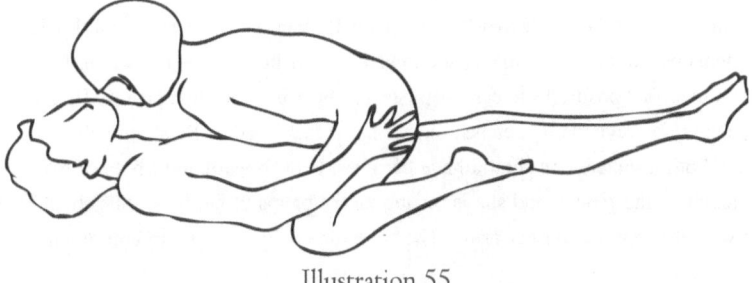

Illustration 55

For variety, in the woman on top position, the woman can lean back so that her palms are resting on the floor and her hands are supporting her weight [below]. She can move up and down on the man's penis while remaining in this posture. This is a good way to slow down her thrusting up and down the man's penis. This helps delay the time it takes the man to experience an orgasm. The anterior wall of the woman's vagina is stroked and massaged by the man's penis as a result of moving up and down the man's penis in this posture. Having sex in this posture is likely to result in stimulating the G-spot and in a G-spot orgasm for the woman if she has a sensitive G-spot. Some men, however, will find the backward pressure on their penis to be uncomfortable, especially if their erection tends to angle more toward their abdomen.

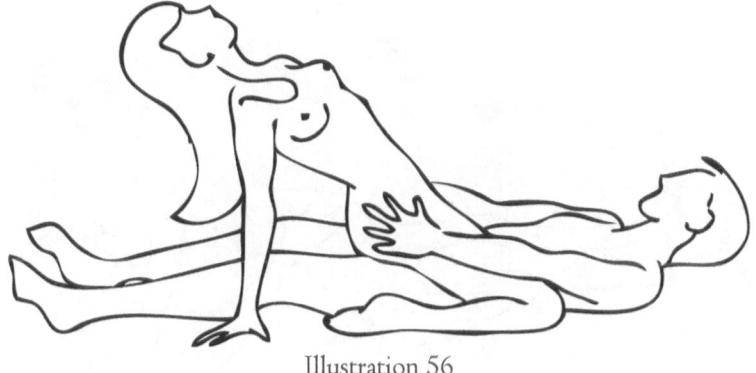

Illustration 56

The man can add to the woman's pleasure by manually stimulating her clitoris as she moves up and down on his penis in this posture. This greatly increases the likelihood that the woman will experience a full body orgasm. Another variation to this position is for the man to prop his back and head using some pillows. This makes the sexual sensations that both partners experience different than the sexual sensations that they experienced when the man did not have his back and head propped with some pillows.

Another variation to the woman on top position is to have the man lie flat on his back with both legs straight. Then the woman should straddle his pelvis with her knees. The woman should be facing the man's face and not his feet. The woman should slowly have the penis penetrate her vagina as she lowers herself into a sitting position. However, in this modified position she can keep her legs bent in a kneeling posture [Illustration 57, below], or have them stretched out along the man's sides [Illustration 58, bottom]. But in both instances she should have her chest bent forward, until both of her hands are touching the ground and she is resting on the palms of her hand. She should have her weight supported on her arms. Then she thrusts by moving up and down on the man's penis.

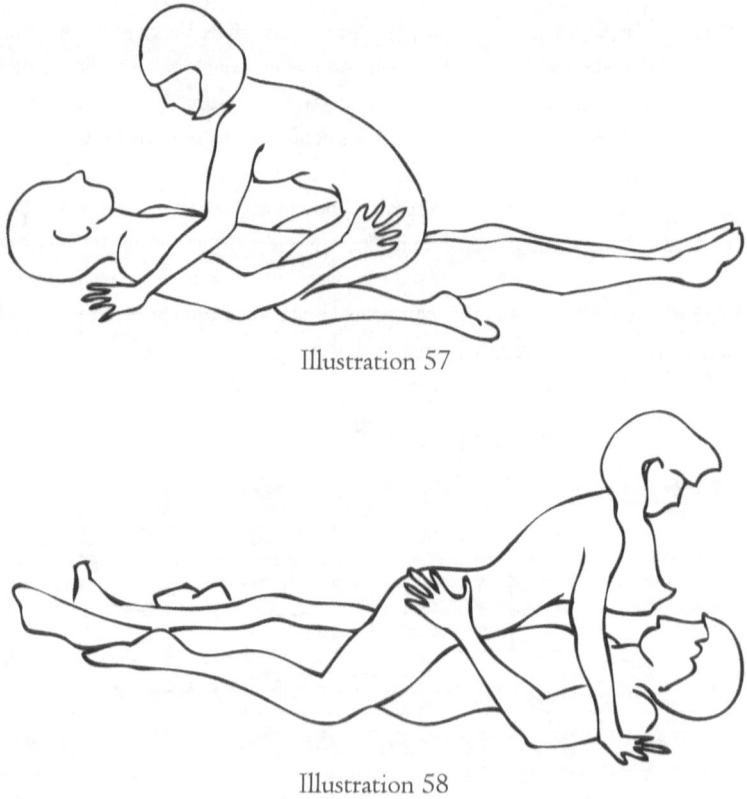

Illustration 57

Illustration 58

Another modified position to the woman on top position is for the man to lie flat on his back with both legs straight with the woman straddling his pelvis with her knees. The woman should be facing the man's face and not his feet. The woman should slowly have the penis penetrate her vagina as she lowers herself into a sitting position. However, in this modified position she lowers her chest until her breasts are touching the man's chest, but her chest is not touching the man's chest [below]. The woman has her weight supported by her hands that are touching the ground. Her palms should be resting on the ground supporting her weight. The woman should move forward and back with her breasts touching the man's chest. She should move forward and back to stimulate her vagina and the man's penis. The man enjoys having the woman's breasts caress his body as she moves forward and back. The man finds such a position very erotic and exciting. The woman finds it erotic and exciting that her breasts are caressing the man's body. The woman also can move from side to side to give a different sexual sensation to both partners.

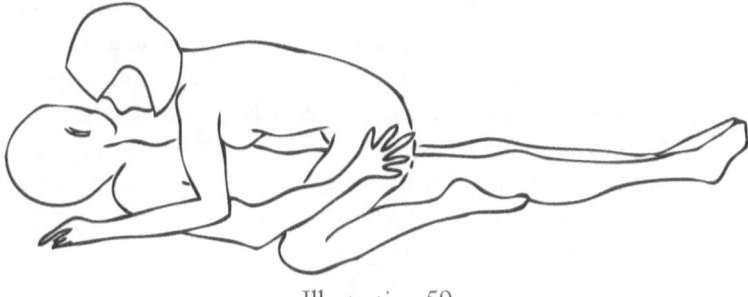

Illustration 59

An adjustment to the female superior position is to have the man lie on his back on the ground with both legs stretched straight. The woman is facing the man's face and not his feet. She straddles his pelvis with both of her knees. Then she lowers herself onto his penis until she is in an upright sitting position. While the man's penis is still inside her vagina, she leans forward and rests her elbows on the ground, on his shoulders, or on his chest [see Illustration 60 on next page]. This position allows the woman to thrust her hips freely. In this position, in addition to using her thigh muscles to thrust, a woman can use her shoulder muscles to help her thrust also. In this position, a woman can use her shoulder muscles to support her weight. The woman can nibble on the man's neck, ears, face, and lips in this position.

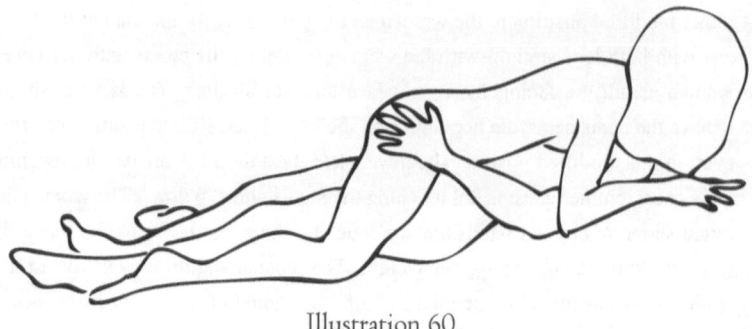

Illustration 60

A modification of the woman on top position is to have the man lie on his back with both legs stretched straight. The woman turns her back to the man so that she is facing his feet and straddles his pelvis with both of her knees [below]. She lowers herself onto his penis until she is in an upright sitting position with the penis inside her vagina. Then she moves up and down on his penis using her thighs to thrust. As she moves up and down, the man can support her with his hands. In this position, a woman can put one of her hands between the man's legs and cup and stroke his testicles from underneath. This will provide great pleasurable sensations. The woman can also massage the scrotum and testicles while thrusting or sitting still in this position. This brings great pleasure to the man. Some women like this position because it lets them fantasize and self-stimulate. Some people do not like this position because with the woman's back to her partner it decreases intimacy.

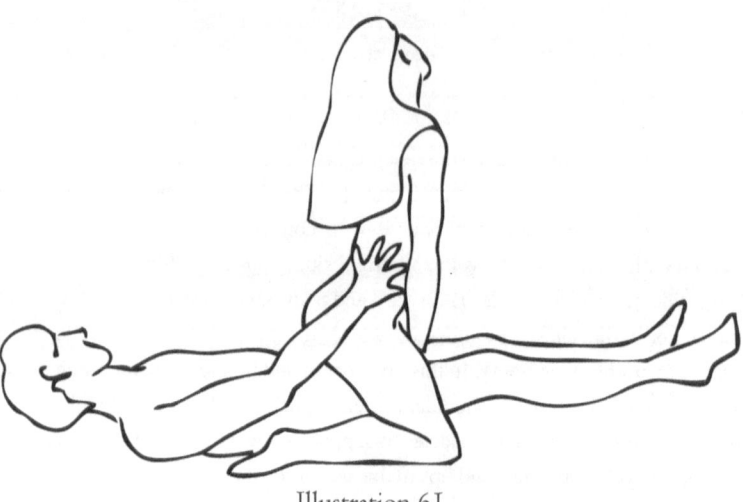

Illustration 61

A modification to this position is for the woman to lower her upper body backwards towards the man's chest until her upper body is supported by both of her hands [below]. The palms of both of her hands should be resting on the floor. The woman then thrusts up and down the man's penis using her thigh muscles to thrust. This position produces a different set of sexual sensations to both partners. In this position, the woman's G-spot is most likely to be stimulated. If the woman has a sensitive G-spot she is most likely to experience an orgasm as a result of the stimulation.

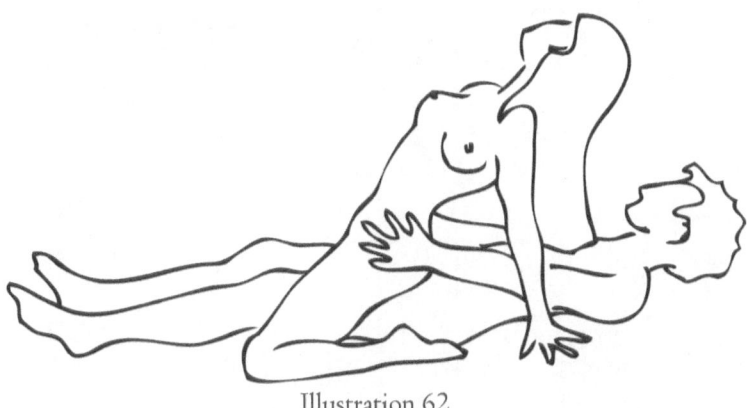

Illustration 62

Another variation of this position is to have the man lie flat on his back and the woman, while facing his feet, to straddle his pelvis with her knees. Then she should lower herself onto the man's penis until she is in an upright sitting position facing his feet. Then the woman should recline her upper body back until her back is on the man's chest with her legs straight together to keep the penis inside [below]. Then the woman can move forward and back stimulating the man's penis with her vagina. This position produces a variety of sensations that are pleasurable and erotic.

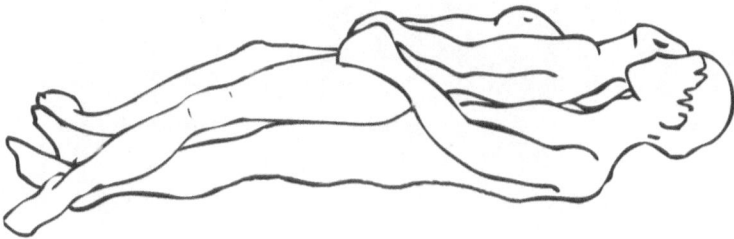

Illustration 63

Another modification to the woman on top facing the feet position would be for the man to lie flat on his back and the woman, while facing his feet, to straddle his pelvis with her knees. Then she should lower herself on to the man's penis until she is in an upright sitting position facing his feet. The penis should be inside the vagina. Then she should lie her chest and head on top of the man's feet [below]. Then she can move forward and back stimulating the man's penis with her vagina.

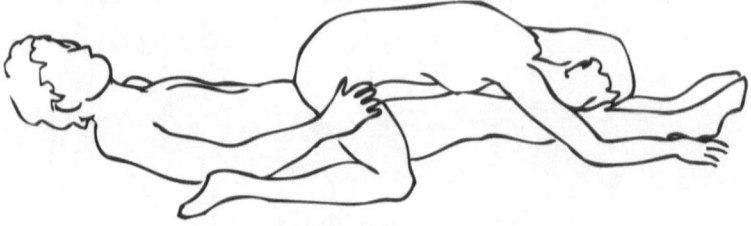

Illustration 64

Chapter 18

After Sex Play

To many people sex is considered over after the man ejaculates. Most women do not have orgasms every time during sex by the time the man ejaculates. So a couple should not consider sex to be over until the woman has had an orgasm also. There are many things that a couple can do for the woman to have an orgasm if the man has ejaculated and she has not had an orgasm. The man can masturbate the woman until she has an orgasm. She can masturbate herself until she has an orgasm. The man can perform oral sex on the woman until she has an orgasm. The man can use a vibrator on the woman until she has an orgasm. The woman can use a vibrator on herself until she has an orgasm. Depending on the man's age and physical condition, the man can get hard again quickly and then they can have intercourse again. Many women are multi-orgasmic, so if a multi-orgasmic woman experiences an orgasm during sex, that does not have to be the end of her sexual stimulation. The man can go on and have the woman experience more orgasms by masturbating her, using a vibrator, or through oral sex. Or the woman can go on and have herself experience more orgasms by masturbating herself or by using a vibrator. Before having sex, it is a good idea that the couple decides how many orgasms will be sufficient for the multi-orgasmic woman. If the woman is not multi-orgasmic and can experience only one orgasm, that is fine also. Once the woman has experienced an orgasm or a sufficient number of orgasms, then sex is considered over. Then after sex play begins.

Disappointing After Sex Behavior

Usually after sex, the man rolls over and goes to sleep, while the woman is left wide awake staring at the ceiling. The woman usually feels frustrated, cheated, and angry. It is a big disappointment and irritating for the woman to see the man sleeping peacefully and satisfied after an orgasm, while she is lying down in bed desiring more affection and attention from her man. The affection and attention that the woman desires after sex is known as after sex play. The man's behavior of falling asleep right after sex without giving his woman any after sex play is downright rude and inconsiderate. This behavior causes the woman to feel ignored.

The fact that many men usually after making love fall asleep immediately has led some people to wonder if a man's orgasm makes him fall asleep. In fact, having an orgasm does not need to make the man sleep. During the resolution phase of the sexual response cycle, a man may feel tired as his body recovers from orgasm. However, his body does not automatically fall asleep. A man chooses to sleep when he feels tired, that is all. If a man usually falls asleep after sex, he can change his way. He can make an effort to stay awake after sex, despite him feeling tired, and he should be able to stay awake.

Sometimes, immediately after sex, a man gets up, leaves and does not spend the night with his lover. By doing so, the man is not using the time after sex to get close to his partner. Sometimes after sex a man immediately jumps into the shower. This is also annoying to the woman, since she is still in need of affection and attention. Sometimes after sex immediately the man gets up to make a phone call, watch T.V., read a newspaper, or have a smoke. The woman hates that because she feels lonely and abandoned.

The Reason Women Want After Sex Play

Usually the woman enjoys foreplay and after sex play a lot, whereas the man does not care that much for them, but is concerned with the sexual intercourse only. The reason why a man does not care for after sex play, is not because he is an unfeeling brute. The man usually does that because there is a difference in the sexual response cycles of the man and woman. In the male resolution phase after ejaculation, the man's body returns to normal very quickly. The man loses his erection amazingly fast, within a minute. The huge amount of blood that was diverted to the man's penis and pelvic area during arousal rushes away. His muscles which tightened up so ferociously during sex relax. After losing his erection, the man's body goes into what is called the refractory period. A refractory period is a period of time before the man can have another erection. Usually after an orgasm, the man is tired.

A woman's resolution phase is quite different. In the resolution phase, the woman's body returns to normal steadily and not very quickly like the man's body. The swelling and florid coloration of the woman's genital that occurred during sex goes away. The woman's genital returns to normal much more slowly than the man's genital. The woman's body usually takes five to ten minutes to return to normal, while the man's body takes about a minute. Unlike men, women usually do not become sleepy after an orgasm, and their genitals do not become hypersensitive like the man's genital. The fact that the woman's body returns to normal steadily, over a time span of five to ten minutes, is the reason why the woman likes after sex play. The fact that the man's body returns to normal quickly, over a time span of one minute, is the reason why the man does not care for after sex play that much.

Proper After Sex Play Behavior

There are many things a person can do after sex to prolong the intimate experience. The things that the person does after sex are usually referred to as after sex play. Although after sex play is not as popular as foreplay, it should be. It should be popular because it is as important as foreplay. After sex play is all about doing things that are fun.

The first thing that a couple should do after sex is over with is to have the man lay next to the woman with the penis inside her for as long as he can, even though the penis is losing its erection. Men who maintain body contact with their lover after ejaculation retained their erections longer. The shrinkage of the erect penis after ejaculation actually occurs in two stages. In the first stage, it almost immediately shrinks to approximately 50 percent larger than its unaroused, flaccid state. But after that, its rate of shrinkage dramatically slows. If both people have sex play after orgasm, the penis will linger in this second, partially erect state for much longer than usual. If the man maintains his penis inside the woman after sex even though it is losing its erection, and both people cuddle, slowly caress, and kiss each other, then the man's need to sleep will usually quickly recede, and a new surge of growing arousal will start. Such an act will cause both people to feel an intense intimate connection to each other. It also brings both people great pleasure. While cuddling, kissing and caressing each other, both people should be sensitive to the needs of their partner in regards to cuddling, kissing, and caressing. Both people can whisper sweet compliments into each other's ears and talk together. Such acts promote closeness, and affection between both partners.

Both people should enjoy being close to each other while cuddling. They should relax their body and stop distracting, repetitive thoughts from entering their mind. By doing so, they will enjoy a relaxed state of mind and feel great pleasure throughout their body. Some people, while still cuddling, kissing and stroking, are already longing for another act of intercourse. Physiologically, men need time to recover before they can have intercourse again. Depending on the man's age and health, that time period might be short or long. For some men it is a matter of minutes, while for others it is a matter of hours. If both people like, they can continue to cuddle, kiss, and caress each other as they see fit until the man is ready for another sexual intercourse encounter. Then they could have sexual intercourse again. If both people do not want to have sex again, then after cuddling, kissing, and caressing each other, they could just lie down next to each other for a minute and just talk. Talking after all this helps prolong intimacy and keeps both partners connected.

After this there are a few possibilities that the couple could do as after sex play. One possibility is both people fall asleep in their lover's arms. Falling asleep in each other's arms can certainly be part of amazing sex. In fact, many people use sex to help them relax before bed and they enjoy the feeling of falling asleep right afterward. A second possibility is for the couple to shower together. Some people like to shower after sex because they get sweaty or sticky after sex. Showering together is a sexy way to have after sex play. Both people could shower each other, which makes it very pleasurable and erotic. A third possibility is for the couple to get some food from the kitchen and feed each other in bed. A fourth possibility is for the couple to get dressed in their clothes, with each partner dressing the other.

Sometimes after sex, either the man or the woman gets the urge to urinate. In fact, urinating immediately after sex clears the urethra of any bacteria that could have entered it and helps prevent urinary tract infections. So the person that gets the urge to urinate after sex should urinate, but then should come back to bed so that both partners resume the after sex play session. The way to resume the after sex play session is for the man to insert his penis inside the woman even though it is losing its erection, and both people should cuddle, caress, and kiss each other as they see fit.

Benefits of After Sex Play

Even if both partners experienced orgasms that felt great during sex, people can sometimes feel distant after sex if they do not stay close and enjoy after sex play. Sex is about intimacy, affection, pleasure, and love. That is why after sex play is an important part of amazing sex. The main important aspect of after sex play is for the man and woman to cuddle, kiss, and caress each other. They should also talk to each other. If this is not done then the woman will feel used, frustrated, and angry. The sex will not be fulfilling to the woman. She will feel sad and alienated from her partner. Women usually need to be loved after sex, while men do not care about being loved after sex. After sex play makes a woman feel very close to her partner and peaceful, in a way that sex itself does not. For many women, these moments of after sex play are very important. In some ways many women view them as better than orgasm itself.

Some of the most romantic and meaningful moments for a couple can happen during after sex play. People feel more vulnerable to each other after sex than at any other time. Therefore, after sex play makes a couple feel closer to each other, than they have ever felt. To some people after sex play can be as important, sensual, and erotic as the sex act itself. Even if one or both people want sex just for sex's sake, without deep intimacy or love, they should still do after sex play. They should do it because it is fun, and it makes the sexual experience more pleasurable and more amazing.

Talking During After Sex Play

The best conversations during after sex play are simply the ones the couple enjoys. They should be relaxing and keep up the high level of sexual intimacy that the couple experienced while having sex. The conversations during after sex play should be romantic and erotic. During after sex play, a person should talk about how close he or she felt to his or her partner during sex. Daydreams that a person had about romantic things he or she wants to do with his or her partner are another good topic to discuss during after sex play. Remembering the first time a person met his or her partner during after sex play conversations is exciting to both partners. During after sex play, talking about the little things that both people like about each other brings the couple closer together. Telling each other jokes and laughing during after sex play is very delightful. The most romantic thing that a person can do during after sex play is tell his or her partner that he or she loves him or her. It is important that the couple during after sex play only talk about things that make them feel good.

During after sex play, sharing what was good about the sex that the couple had is very informative and pleasurable. However, when the couple discusses that topic, they should talk about it in general and not be too specific. They should wait another time to be specific. After sex play is not about examining every aspect of the sexual experience. Rather, it is about enjoying the experience. If a person spends too much time describing every aspect of the sexual experience that the couple just had, it will take away from the excitement and pleasure of the after sex play experience. A person could tell his or her partner why he or she had an orgasm this time. A person could also inform his or her partner what he or she would like the partner to do in the next encounter. A person could also make known to his or her partner what he or she would have liked the partner to do in this encounter. It is important when talking about the sexual experience only to be positive and never be negative at all.

Conversations during after sex play should not include issues that a couple usually fights about. They should not also include talk about work or about family matters. In fact, if one partner brings up something that does not feel good to the second partner, the second partner can nicely tell the first partner not to discuss that topic anymore during after sex play. The second partner could let the first partner know that they will discuss that topic another time. Then both partners can resume talking about romantic and erotic things. A person should never criticize nor disrespect his or her partner during after sex play conversations. A person should always be respectful of his or her partner during after sex play conversations.

The conversations could be long or short. There is no predetermined length. Whatever length the couple sees fit for the conversation is the proper length. However, a person should observe his or her partner and make sure that he or she is not boring him or her during the conversations. The person should see that his or her partner is enjoying the conversations. The person should make sure that the conversations that he or she is discussing with his or her partner, are maintaining a level of intimacy that they had during sex. During after sex play conversations, both people should compliment each other so that they feel good about themselves and so that the experience would be pleasurable to both of them.

Chapter 19

Sex Techniques

A large number of people incorrectly think that sex is not complicated and that all it takes is to put a penis inside a vagina and just thrust. They believe that sex comes naturally and does not need to be learned. However, these incorrect beliefs cause a large number of people to lead unfulfilled and boring sex lives. They do not experience the utmost pleasure during sex as a result of these incorrect beliefs. However, the truth is that good sex does not just happen but it occurs by the couple being deliberate about it. Good sex is a learned skill that does not come naturally. Every person can have a passionate and deeply satisfying sex life. It is just a matter of the person learning how he or she could have a deeply pleasurable and satisfying sex life. The learning process can be a lot of fun.

In this chapter, numerous ways of making the sexual experience more pleasurable are discussed. More than one way of making the sexual experience more pleasurable is discussed because although the sexual response is the same in all men and it is the same in all women, the things that might be pleasing to a person during sex might be different from one person to another. Also, the things that might be pleasing to a person during sex might be different from one sexual encounter to another and from one minute to another during the same sexual encounter. A person should keep an open mind during sex towards all the techniques and possibilities. There is no right or wrong during sex; it is all about doing what feels wonderful for both the man and the woman. Sometimes the most unusual techniques will give the couple the most rewarding payoffs. A person should not dismiss a technique because it sounds weird. The main thing about applying these techniques during sex is for a person to always have a good time and do what feels right to both partners.

Even if a person already experiences pleasure and orgasms during sex, these techniques will help him or her to intensify the pleasure and orgasms he or she already enjoys. Also, a person reading this chapter not only will he or she bring more pleasure to his or her sexual encounters, but he or she will be a better lover bringing more pleasure to his or her partner. A person will be able to express his or her love to his or her partner through deep pleasure during sex in many different ways as a result of these techniques. Also, as a result of these techniques a person will have greater sexual confidence which will spill over into many other areas of his or her life. Finally, the shape and size of a person's body parts does not affect the quality of sex, it is the techniques that a person employs during sex that affect the quality of sex.

Making Sex a Priority—Timing, Frequency, and Duration of Sex

Making sex a priority is one technique that will make the sexual encounters of the couple more pleasurable. A couple needs to put sex as a top priority in their lives so that they have wonderful passionate sex lives. In the same way that they plan ahead for a Saturday night outing, they need to plan for intercourse. They need to think ahead and make a commitment for their intimacy. For most couples, the anticipation of planned times to have sex builds great excitement which leads to more pleasurable sex.

To have a healthy sex life, a couple should make sex a priority and exercise their passion regularly. The couple should have sex frequently, at least three times a week. Having sex three times a week seems to keep both partners satisfied sexually and feeling sexy and desirable. Sex is a crucial area of life that needs fulfillment, and a couple should strive never to have sex less than once a week in order to keep the passion alive.

Sex should be made a priority by the couple by them having sex any time during the twenty-four-hour day when they see fit. A significant number of people tend to think of sex as a nighttime activity, and have sex only the few moments before they go to sleep. The truth is sex is an activity that can be practiced any time during the day by the couple. The couple should schedule sex for the hours when they are both most energetic. Sex before bedtime can be very energizing and allow the couple to sleep more soundly and wake up more refreshed. However, sex in the morning is also energizing and allows the couple to greet the day with a lighthearted and joyous spirit. As a matter of fact, sex is energizing and fulfilling any time during the twenty-four-hour day. Some people think it is romantic and sexy if their lover wakes them up to make love in the middle of the night.

A couple can make sex a priority by devoting enough time to each encounter. Although the average length of time for the sex act itself is quite short, the amount of time that a couple could allocate for foreplay, sex play during the sex act, and after sex play can be incredibly varied. It can take a couple of minutes or a few hours. The average length of time that a healthy man can thrust non-stop is probably no more than 4 to 5 minutes. Most men experience a refractory period immediately after an orgasm during which they cannot have another erection for another twenty minutes. Therefore, the sex act itself usually takes only four to five minutes. With foreplay and after sex play, the average couple spends 10 minutes having a sexual encounter. However, the couple should spend at least 30 minutes on each sexual encounter. They should do so because it takes the average woman about 20 minutes during foreplay to become sufficiently aroused and sufficiently lubricated for penetrative intercourse. Then the sex act itself takes around 5 minutes and after sex play takes around 5 minutes, leaving the couple with a total of 30 minutes for sexual intercourse.

Also, the couple can make the sexual encounter longer than 30 minutes by increasing the duration of foreplay, after sex play, or both. The couple can also make the sexual encounter longer than 30 minutes by increasing the duration of the sex play during the sex act. The sex play during the sex act is when the man, before reaching orgasm, stops thrusting and withdraws his penis and the couple engage in kissing, hugging, and touching. Then the man resumes the sex act by continuing to thrust his penis into the vagina until orgasm. The sex play during the sex act can also occur when the man stops thrusting inside the vagina but keeps his penis inside the vagina so that it is not stimulated. As a general rule, the longer the sexual encounter the better. Some couples even spend hours in bed together having several sexual encounters. Pleasure during orgasm and sex decreases if the couple does not have enough time to take their time during sex. The best sex is when the duration of it is open-ended so that the couple can enjoy the leisure of lovemaking until they are satisfied. How long sex lasts usually changes from one sexual encounter to another.

Some people incorrectly believe that if a man can thrust his penis inside the vagina continuously for an hour then that will be very pleasurable. On the contrary, if the man thrusts continuously inside the vagina for longer than 12 to 15 minutes, then that will not be very pleasurable to the woman and the woman might become sore. Usually, the man should take a break from thrusting before 12 to 15 minutes have elapsed. Also, having sex all night long does not mean having penetrative intercourse all night long. A couple may spend hours in bed together, but usually sex play happens and there are breaks. The idea that the couple is engaging in one behavior (oral sex, penetration, or kissing) for hours without a break is not likely. Taking breaks during a sexual encounter and in between several encounters makes the sex less vigorous and more enjoyable.

Making Circumstances Right for Sex

The second technique that will make the sexual encounters for the couple more pleasurable is to make circumstances right for sex. The couple can make circumstances right for sex several ways. The first way is by making sure there are no distractions in the environment by taking the phone off the hook, making sure no one is in the home but them, and putting a do not disturb sign on the door of the home so that no one rings the doorbell. If they have kids, they could send the kids to a babysitter or a family friend. Having distractions will only decrease the pleasure during sex. The second way is by making sure that where they have sex is a warm and comfortable place. Having sex in a place that is uncomfortable or cold will make the sexual encounter very unpleasant. The third way is by making sure that the man and the woman's state of mind is good for the sexual encounter. If there are some persistent things that are on either person's mind, it is best to clear those out of his or her mind by having a brief conversation before sex so that the person leaves the concerns of his or her day aside and can be totally involved in the sexual encounter. If a person does not have the proper state of mind during sex because of his or her concerns of the day, the sex will not be pleasurable to its greatest extent. The fourth way is by making sure that the man and the woman are physically ready for sex. If either the man or the woman is tired or sleepy, that person should postpone the sexual encounter until he or she has gotten the proper rest. If a person has sex when he or she is sleepy or tired, the sexual encounter will not be very pleasurable to the couple.

The fifth way the couple could make the circumstances right for sex is by both of them having good hygiene. A person is repulsed from his or her partner if his or her partner emits body odor or has bad breath. In order for both people to be clean and smelling nice before the sexual encounter, they should take a shower before approaching their partner for sex. Both people should make sure that they do not have bad breath by brushing their teeth or using mouthwash before approaching their partner for sex. The couple should make sure that the sheets are clean before having sex because dirty sheets will make the sexual encounter very unpleasant. Beginning a lovemaking session with a freshly made bed contributes to having a more pleasurable sexual encounter. The sixth way the couple could make circumstances right for sex is by both of them urinating before sex to make sure that their urinary bladder is empty. By doing so both people can have sex and not worry about expelling urine during sex. Plus both people can relax and let their muscles go during sex, not having to tense up their muscles because of fear that urine will be excreted. The fact that a person is not worried about urinating during sex and his muscles are not tense during sex makes the sexual encounter more pleasurable to him or her and his or her partner.

The seventh way the couple could make circumstances right for sex is by both of them using lubrication. Even if lubrication is not needed because the woman produces sufficient lubrication, both the man and the woman using lubrication will make the sex more enjoyable. Also, thrusting is made more enjoyable with lubrication. Adding lubrication during sex will add new pleasurable sensations to the couple's lovemaking. Lubrication can be applied on both the vagina and penis for better sex. The skin covering the penis is elastic. It stretches and becomes thin as the penis enlarges during an erection. This tender skin may become scraped during prolonged vigorous sex, resulting in friction burns. This might cause discomfort to the man during sex. Also, a woman's vagina might become dry during sex, resulting in discomfort to the woman during sex. Adding lubrication to the penis and the vagina will prevent the penis from becoming scraped and will prevent the vagina from drying during sex, thus keeping the sex pleasurable and preventing it from becoming uncomfortable.

If a woman does not lubricate sufficiently, that does not mean that there is something wrong with her. Also, if a woman does not lubricate sufficiently, that does not mean that she is not sufficiently aroused for sex. Each woman lubricates to a varying degree. Also, each woman's lubrication varies from one encounter to the next. The degree that the woman lubricates depends on where she is in her menstrual cycle, whether she is taking certain medications, whether she is under stress, and other factors. It is best to use water-based lubricants because they do not damage a condom and do not irritate the genital areas of the man and the woman. Oil-based lubricants will destroy a latex condom and sometimes will cause irritation to the vagina.

The eighth way a person could make circumstances right for sex is for him or her to have sex with the right partner. A person should not have sex with a partner he or she does not like. Sometimes a person gets stuck with his or her partner because he or she cannot find anyone else to date. So he or she continues to date his or her partner even though he or she does not like his or her partner. If a person does not like his or her partner, the sexual experience will not be pleasurable at all. On the other hand, a person who is in love with his or her partner and has sex with his or her partner will have a sexual encounter that is pleasurable to the greatest extent. Sex is meant to be an expression of love between two people. Therefore sex with love is far more rewarding and enjoyable than sex with no love.

Initiating and Rejecting Sex

The third technique that will make the couple's sex life more pleasurable is the way sex is initiated and how it is turned down. A large number of people think that only the man should initiate sex. They think only the man can openly start the sexual encounter and they think the woman can start the sexual encounter only by giving subtle signals. They think the man can openly start the sexual encounter by talking about it openly or by physically starting the sexual encounter. They think the woman can give subtle signals that she wants sex by either wearing special lingerie to bed, by mentioning that she wants to go to bed early, or by walking in the nude in front of the man. Unfortunately, many men do not pick up on those subtle signals and do not understand that the woman wants to have sex. As a matter of fact, it is not uncommon for some women to be frustrated, crying and complaining that nothing is happening sexually between them and their male partner. The reason why these women suffer is because they were not open about their desire to have sex and never let the man know the real meaning of their subtle signals.

Women should be open about their desire to have sex. Women should be willing to initiate sex when they feel like having sex. As a matter of fact, men find it arousing when the woman takes the initiative in starting the sexual encounter. Also, women find it exciting when they take the initiative in starting the sexual encounter. Great sex exists in a relationship when both the man and the woman are free to express their sexual desires and initiate sex when they feel like it. Whether the man or the woman initiates the sexual encounter, it should be done in a romantic and loving way and not in a demanding way. If a person initiates sex by demanding it, it will cause the sexual partner's sexual arousal to drop to zero. It will also cause the sexual partner to feel resentment and annoyed. However, if a person initiates the sexual encounter in a romantic and loving way, then the sexual partner will most likely welcome the sexual encounter and will be very excited about it. Openly initiating sex can be done either by the person talking about it or by physically starting the act. Physically starting the act can occur by kissing, hugging, touching, or undressing the sexual partner. The sexual act can be initiated spontaneously without it being prearranged. It can also be initiated at a prearranged time.

Sometimes people are different in their sexual appetites. Some people might like a lot of sex, while others might like a little sex. When one person in a couple has a high sex drive and the other person in the couple has a low sex drive, this condition is known as the couple having a mismatched libido. When the couple has a mismatched libido, one person is initiating sex more than his or her sexual partner wants. This is normal since every individual is different and has different preferences. However, if a couple experiences such a situation both of them should compromise so that both are satisfied sexually. If both compromise and are satisfied sexually then the relationship most likely will be maintained. For example, if the man wants sex three times a week and the woman wants it once a week, they could compromise and have sex twice a week so that both of them are satisfied sexually.

Sometimes, when a person comes to initiate sex, he or she might find that his or her sexual partner's sexual appetite changed. For example, a woman might have wanted to have sex frequently, but all of a sudden she does not want it often. This change might be temporary because of stress, health issues, medications, relationship issues, or self-esteem issues. This change might be permanent because the person changed and his sexual desires changed. If the partner's sexual appetite changed, the person should not be alarmed. He or she should communicate with his or her sexual partner and find out the cause of the change. If the change is temporary because of relationship issues, stress, health issues, or medications, the person should help his or her sexual partner deal with the situation so that his or her sexual appetite is restored. If the change is permanent because the sexual partner's preferences changed, then the person should accept that. If the person cannot adapt to the change then he or she and his or her sexual partner can come to a compromise that is satisfying to both of them. It is unfortunate that sometimes when the person finds out that his or her partner's sexual appetite changed, he or she incorrectly assumes that the sexual partner no longer finds him or her attractive or no longer loves him or her. This causes the person to withdraw from his or her sexual partner, causing the relationship to end. Had the person and his or her sexual partner communicated, then he or she would have found out that his or her fears were unfounded and the relationship would not have ended.

As a general rule, sex increases a person's sex hormones and his or her sex drive. The more a person has sex the more he or she will want sex. The opposite is also true that if a person goes for a long period of time without sex, he or she will have less desire for it. For this reason, a couple should try to be sexually active as often as possible, ideally at least once a week. The right amount of sex that a couple has is whatever amount that makes both of them happy. Both the man and the woman having equal freedom to initiate a sexual encounter when they desire contributes to the couple having the amount of sex that makes both of them happy.

Whenever a person initiates sex and his or her sexual partner rejects it, the person should just back off calmly without showing any sign of being upset. The person should accept his or her partner's rejection politely, while still showing affection and kindness. The person should show that he or she understands that his or her partner is not in the mood. If the person does that the next time he or she tries to initiate sex, the sexual partner will most likely accept it. But if the person, when rejected, shows he or she is upset or criticizes his or her partner, then the partner will most likely be resentful and hurt. This will cause the sexual partner to avoid sex with the person the next time the person tries to initiate it. The sexual partner should turn down the person politely while showing affection. It is a good idea that he or she touches the person with his or her hand or lips after turning him or her down to convey love and affection. By the sexual partner touching the person this will increase the affection and bonding of both people, even though the person initiating sex was turned down. Also the sexual partner should encourage the person to choose an alternative time for sex after turning him or her down. The sexual partner should do that so the person does not get discouraged from initiating a sexual encounter, and does not avoid having sex with his or her sexual partner. Furthermore, if the sexual partner is not interested in having sexual intercourse, but is willing to be sexual, then he or she could participate in oral or manual sex to satisfy the person. If the sexual partner participates in oral or manual sex to satisfy the person sexually, the person will not feel hurt that he or she got turned down for initiating sex.

Sexual Arousal and Entering the Woman When Ready

The fourth technique that will make the couple's sex life more pleasurable is both partners becoming sufficiently sexually aroused before sex and the man penetrating the woman's vagina with his penis when the woman is ready for penetration. Both the man and the woman becoming sufficiently sexually aroused before sex will make the sex more exciting, satisfying, and fulfilling for both of them. Getting a person sufficiently sexually aroused before sex will cause the smallest touch by the person's partner to cause the person great pleasure. Also, if a person is sufficiently sexually aroused before sex, he or she will be yearning for sexual fulfillment. This yearning, when satisfied, brings great pleasure to the person satisfied. The more sexually aroused a person is, the more sexual energy he or she has and the more intense the orgasm will be. Also, the more sexually aroused a person is the more he or she is open to receive sexual pleasure and passion. In addition, the more sexually aroused a person is the more he or she is willing to give sexual pleasure and passion. Although foreplay was discussed in great detail in another chapter, sexual arousal is very important to an extremely pleasurable sexual encounter and certain aspects of it are emphasized in this section.

There are several ways for a person to arouse his or her sexual partner before sex. Touching, kissing, and talking seductively are the three main ways for a person to arouse his or her sexual partner before sex. A person touching his or her sexual partner before sex is greatly arousing to both people. Touching is an expression of loving care between both people that is very sensuous to both the giver and the receiver. It lets both people feel emotionally and physically close to each other. A person can touch using not only his or her hand, but by using any part of his or her body. A person can rub any part of his or her body against any part of his or her partner's body to give himself or herself pleasure and to give his or her partner pleasure. Any part of the body can do the touching, including the chest, back, stomach, neck, ears, breasts, face, tongue, and mouth. Touching is a great way for a person to relax the stiff muscles and ease the tension of his or her sexual partner.

Kissing is the second way a person can arouse his or her sexual partner before sex. When a person kisses his or her sexual partner before sex, both of them become sexually aroused as a result of the kissing. Kissing lets both people feel emotionally and physically close to each other. A person can kiss his or her partner anywhere on his or her body. As a matter of fact a person smothering his or her partner with kisses all over his or her body is very sexually exciting to both people because it builds a great anticipation of the sexual act to come.

Kissing and touching should be done by a person all over his or her partner's body so that his or her partner is sexually aroused to the greatest extent. Both the man and the woman should kiss and touch each other so that both of them are sexually aroused to the greatest extent. It is important that both partners are turned on by each other's bodies before sex for the most pleasurable sexual encounter. The man usually has the tendency not to touch and kiss the woman all over her body and be concerned only with her genital area. This usually happens because a man can enjoy sex to a greater extent than a woman even if his body is not touched and kissed all over. Also, this usually happens because a man can orgasm during sex if his body is not touched and kissed all over. It is important that the woman is touched and kissed all over her body because usually, if she is not she won't get aroused sufficiently to enjoy sex to the maximum extent. Also, usually she won't get aroused sufficiently to orgasm during sex.

Kissing and touching before sex is sexually arousing because it builds anticipation to the sexual encounter. Kissing and touching, as well as hugging and cuddling, make a couple feel secure, safe, loved, and relaxed. These feelings are important for pleasurable sex. When kissing, touching, hugging, or cuddling a couple should be flexible and spontaneous. There are numerous ways to touch and kiss before sex for a person to get his or her sexual partner sexually aroused. However, there are several methods of touching and kissing that are worth mentioning. One way for a person to touch and kiss his or her partner to arouse him or her sexually is for a person to kiss his or her partner's ear softly and then using the tip of his or her tongue to encircle his or her partner's ear. A person would do so while talking seductively to his or her partner. This will drive the sexual partner wild with sexual arousal. A second way to touch and kiss before sex is for the woman to fondle gently the man's testicles, and to gently kiss and suck on them. The woman can also touch and kiss the man's penis before sex since both the man and the woman find it very erotic. The woman can touch different areas of the man's penis to generate different sexual sensations in the man. The entire length of the penis is sensitive to touch, pressure, and temperature. However, the glans or head is more responsive than the shaft. The rim of the penis head is called the corona and it is more sensitive than the head of the penis. The frenulum is the skin just below the head of the penis on the underside of the penis. It is above the shaft of the penis. It is where the head and shaft meet. If the woman stimulates the frenulum it will drive the man wild with pleasure and sexual arousal because the frenulum is the most sensitive area on the penis.

A third way to touch and kiss before sex is for the man to gently touch and kiss the vagina, the clitoris, and the area surrounding it. Both the man and the woman find it very erotic. A fourth way to touch and kiss before sex is for a person to touch and kiss the eyelids of his or her partner, since they are very sensitive to touch. A fifth way to touch and kiss before sex is for the man to kiss and touch the woman's breasts and nipples. If the man does so, it will quickly result in the woman becoming aroused and the vagina getting very excited. The man also finds it arousing that he is touching the woman's breasts. A sixth way to touch and kiss before sex is for the man to use his thumb to pressure the bottom of the vagina entry within the first two inches and kiss the area surrounding the vagina. This causes both the woman and the man to become very aroused. A seventh way to touch and kiss before sex is for a person to kiss and touch his or her partner's legs and inner thighs. The inner thighs are very sensitive and almost all people find that having them touched and kissed by their sexual partner is very sexually exciting. It is exciting because it creates a sense of anticipation of the sexual act to come.

An eighth way to touch and kiss before sex is for the man to stimulate the woman's labia minora and labia majora by kissing and touching them. This will drive the woman wild with pleasure and the man will have great pleasure seeing that happen. The ninth way to touch and kiss before sex is for a person to stimulate the perineum of his or her partner by touching and kissing it. This will get the partner very sexually aroused. The tenth way to touch before sex is for the person to grope, rub, and squeeze the buttocks of his or her sexual partner. This gets the blood flowing in the genital area of the man and the woman, which leads to an intense orgasm during sex. A person can also use his or her fingertip to gently rub the outer rim of the anus. Because this area contains a large number of nerve endings, this type of stimulation will send shivers up a person's spine.

Talking seductively is the third way a person can arouse his or her sexual partner before sex. When a person talks seductively to his or her sexual partner, both of them become sexually aroused. A person can talk seductively by telling his or her sexual partner what he or she is going to do with him or her sexually. A person can talk seductively by describing his or her partner's body parts in a seductive way. A person can talk seductively by talking dirty. Talking dirty is when the person tells his or her partner what he or she is going to do to him or her sexually using obscene language. A fourth way a person can arouse his or her sexual partner before sex is by both of them bathing or showering together. A bath or shower before sex can make both people feel relaxed and in the proper mood for sex. A fifth way a person can arouse his or her sexual partner before sex is by sucking his or her toes. A person sucking his or her sexual partner's toes before sex produces a very pleasurable sexually arousing feeling in his or her sexual partner.

A sixth way a person can arouse his or her sexual partner before sex is by sucking his or her fingers. This will cause the blood to rush to the partner's genital area in preparation for sex. It is extremely sexually arousing. A seventh way a person can arouse his or her sexual partner is by the woman using her breasts to touch and massage part of the man's skin, including his nipples. If a woman does that it is very sexually exciting to both her and the man. A lot of men like their nipples to be stimulated, not just women. An eighth way a person can arouse his or her sexual partner before sex is for the man to play with the woman's breasts, devoting generous attention to everywhere except the nipples. The teasing will drive the woman wild. Eventually, the man can touch the nipples gently and slowly driving the woman wild with pleasure and satisfaction. The ninth way a person can arouse his or her sexual partner before sex is for the woman to grab the guy's head and press his face into her breasts. He will love her for it. The man can also press his face into her breasts. She will love him for it. The tenth way a person can arouse his or her sexual partner before sex is to tie his or her sexual partner to the bed with handcuffs, rope, or some type of cloth. The sexual partner could be stimulated by the person while he or she is restrained. This will drive him or her absolutely wild because he or she can see but cannot touch.

The eleventh way a person can arouse his or her sexual partner before sex is for the person to blindfold his or her sexual partner and then touch and kiss him or her all over. This will drive the sexual partner wild with sexual arousal because he or she cannot see, so his or her sense of feeling is enhanced, making the experience much more pleasurable. The twelfth way that arousal before sex could occur is for the man to tease the woman's clitoris and vulva with his penis by rubbing it all around the clitoris and vulva. The man can tease the woman by occasionally inserting the tip of his penis inside the vagina and taking it out again. The man should not penetrate the woman's vagina with his penis, even when the woman is ready, so that she becomes greatly aroused. The man should wait until the woman is practically begging for him to penetrate her. A variation of this technique is for the woman to take the penis, fondle it, and use it to massage and play with her vulva and clitoris before she puts it inside her vagina. She could tease the head of the penis by sliding it inside and outside the vagina occasionally. If this occurs, it is a great visual for the man to see the woman enjoying his penis and using it for her satisfaction.

The thirteenth way that a person could arouse his or her sexual partner before sex is for the woman to roll the man's penis between her hands like she is trying to start a fire with a stick. As a variation she could also sway the man's penis from side to side until it becomes fully erect. Both ways would cause the man to become sexually excited. Both ways also cause the woman to become sexually aroused because she sees the man become sexually aroused. The fourteenth way that a person can arouse his or her sexual partner before sex is for the man to lie down on his back with his legs straight and the woman to get on top of him and place his penis head inside her vagina and hold it tight with her vaginal muscles. As she does that she can caress the soft shaft with her hand and use her other hand on his groin and testicles until he gets an erection. This method excites both the man and the woman sexually, but it particularly drives the man wild.

Both the man and the woman should know that their sexual arousal builds in a way that might be best described as waves. That means that there is a peak in arousal and then an ebb, or diminishing of the intensity of feelings, and then a new wave of sexual arousal. The new wave of arousal is usually more intense than the preceding one. If the man and the woman know that their sexual arousal builds in waves, then when their arousal decreases, they won't worry and their arousal will continue without being hindered. However, if the man and the woman worry that their arousal is decreasing, then their arousal won't continue and they will be hindered from experiencing sexual pleasure to the greatest extent.

When a person is trying to arouse his or her sexual partner, he or she should be flexible and spontaneous. The key to arousal is to be unpredictable. When the sexual partner cannot guess the person's next move the sexual partner's arousal will intensify. A person should make his or her sexual partner feel comfortable, desirable, attractive, and safe in order to arouse him or her to the greatest extent. It is very important that a person make his or her sexual partner feel wanted before sex in order to arouse him or her. A person could do that by letting him or her know how much he or she wants him or her and how sexy and desirable he or she finds him or her. A person should show that he or she is paying attention to his or her partner during the arousal stage because this lets the sexual partner relax, get rid of his or her anxiety, and enjoy the physical pleasure to the greatest degree.

A couple arousing each other should be fun and never a chore. It should remain fun by a person not criticizing his or her partner. It should remain fun by a person not demanding his or her partner get aroused. A person should give his or her sexual partner good feedback when they are trying to arouse each other because that makes both people get sexually aroused. As a matter of fact, by a person telling his or her sexual partner how much he or she is enjoying the experience and is enjoying being with him or her, the sexual partner will get sexually aroused greatly. A couple arousing each other should remain fun by a person not worrying that he or she is not getting sexually aroused. A person should not force himself to get aroused sexually because the more he or she tries, the harder it becomes. As a matter of fact, the man should not force himself to get an erection because the more he tries the harder it is for him to get an erection. If a person criticizes his or her partner or demands his or her partner get aroused then the person will most likely cause his or her partner not to get sexually aroused. If a person worries that he or she is not getting sexually aroused, then he or she will most likely not get sexually aroused.

Both people should participate equally in the arousal stage. When both people participate equally in the arousal stage there is a buildup of sexual tension that works well for both of them. Also, by both people participating equally in the arousal stage, the burden of performance is removed. Both people should participate equally in the arousal stage because most people want a sexual partner who is responsive so that the sex is fun and makes them feel good. Furthermore, the key ingredient for sexual arousal is for a person to be enthusiastic so that his or her sexual partner gets sexually aroused. Also, a person's enthusiasm is contagious and will cause his or her sexual partner to become enthusiastic about the sexual encounter.

The couple, when trying to arouse each other before sex, should go slow and gently. They should even make the act of removing clothing sensual and erotic. The slower and gentler they go the more sensation is provoked, and the quicker they become aroused. If the couple goes fast in their motions when trying to arouse each other, a lot of pleasure will be lost and it will take them a much longer time to get aroused. Also, when a person goes slow and gentle in the arousal stage it is evidence to the sexual partner that the person cares about him or her as a person. This is very important for the woman. It is very important to the woman because the woman usually cannot get aroused if she does not feel the man cares about her, whereas the man can get aroused even though he feels that the woman does not care about him. It is also very important to the woman to go slow and gentle in arousing each other before sex because a woman usually cannot get aroused if they do not go slow and gentle in arousing each other before sex, whereas the man can get aroused even though they are going fast and not gently in arousing each other before sex. Another way for the couple to get each other aroused is for them to go slow and gently and then build in speed and intensity as long as it keeps feeling amazing. A person prefers different forms of stimulation at different places, from one encounter to another, so a couple should remember that when trying to arouse each other before sex, and they should do things that both of them find sexually arousing at that particular encounter.

It is important to remember that both the man and the woman becoming sexually aroused before sex is very important in order for the couple to have sexual pleasure during sex to the greatest extent. Both the man and the woman becoming sexually aroused before sex not only makes the man and the woman experience sexual pleasure during sex to the greatest extent, but it also lets them experience orgasms that are much more intense and satisfying than if they were not sexually aroused before sex. Also, a longer time period of foreplay contributes to a man having a strong hard erection. Usually the man is sexually aroused at a moment's notice before sex, while a woman usually needs a lot more time to get sexually aroused before sex. Usually the woman needs 15 to 20 minutes to get sexually aroused, while the man needs minute to two to get aroused sexually. Men usually have the tendency to rush to start the sexual act and start the sexual act before the woman is ready for it. So it is important for a man to make sure that he provides his woman with sufficient stimulation before sex to get her sexually aroused and ready for intercourse. As a matter of fact, most women cannot have an orgasm during sex unless they are sufficiently sexually aroused. Also, most women have their sexual pleasure decrease during sex greatly if they are not sufficiently sexually aroused prior to the sex act.

A couple should wait to have the physical sexual act until the woman is yearning for sex and is ready for it. Entering the woman too early does not allow time for the woman's genital area to become fully engorged with blood and results in her genital area being less sensitive and less stimulated by penetration. The act of the penis penetrating the vagina is what changes the experience from sexual play to sexual intercourse. Penetration should occur only when both partners feel ready and desirous of having the penis inside the vagina. The physical signs that the man and woman are ready for sex are that the woman has natural vaginal lubrication and the man has an erect penis. When the woman is ready for sex she may also open up her vagina by spreading her legs while relaxed. She may arch her back and raise her genital area toward the man's penis. In addition, her labia majora (outer lips) are folded back out of the way of the vaginal opening and the labia minora (inner lips) are swollen and gape widely to create a funnel into the vagina when she is ready for sex. When the woman is not ready for sex, it would be demonstrated by stiff legs tightening close to each other or by the woman withdrawing from being penetrated. When the man is not ready for sex, it would be demonstrated by the man not having an erection. Both the man and the woman would be more comfortable with penetration and will have more pleasurable sex if they both were ready for penetration when it occurs. A man feels best about penetrating the woman when he senses her warm and desirous wish for entry.

When penetration occurs, it should occur slowly and gently. If it occurs slowly and gently, the woman will be much more receptive and desirous of the man's penis stroking her vagina. Also, the man will be much more desirous of stroking the woman's vagina with his penis if the penetration occurs slowly and gently. Slow and gentle penetration will bring both the man and the woman's sexual desire to a rapid and eager boil. It will cause the vagina and clitoris to be much more sensitive and will cause the woman to experience a lot more pleasure during penetration and during sex. Also, slow and gentle penetration will make the man's penis more sensitive to pleasure and will cause the man to experience a lot more pleasure during penetration and during sex. If penetration occurs quickly and intensely, it will be a lot less pleasurable to both the man and the woman. Also, the sexual act will be a lot less pleasurable to both the man and the woman if penetration occurs quickly and intensely.

Be Deliberate About Making the Sexual Act More Pleasurable

Sex is a means for a couple to express their love and commitment to each other through deep pleasure. Unfortunately, for many couples after a while, sex becomes a mechanical act where the woman lies on her back while the man thrusts his penis back and forth until he reaches orgasm. Sex to them is no longer pleasurable, but is a boring chore that has to be done out of duty. Good sex in a relationship does not just happen, but the couple can make it happen by being deliberate about it. There are numerous things that a couple could do to make the sexual experience exciting, passionate, and extremely pleasurable. The man or the woman's capability as a lover depends on the sexual techniques that he or she puts to use, not on the size or shape of his or her sexual organ. Although there are numerous sex techniques for a couple to use during sex, every couple is unique sexually and will use only certain techniques for their own sexual expression. Also, although physically, the sexual response is the same in all men and it is the same in all women, the things that might be pleasing to a person during sex might be different from one person to another, from one sexual encounter to another, and from one minute to another.

A Person Should Be Comfortable with His or Her Body

During the sexual act itself, a person should be comfortable with his or her body. It is important for a person to have a feeling of being at ease with his or her own body, since this lets a person be relaxed during sex and enjoy the sexual encounter to the greatest degree. If a person does not feel comfortable with his or her own body, then he or she won't feel comfortable during the sexual encounter and the sexual pleasure during sex will decrease. If a person feels comfortable about his or her body, then he or she will feel closer to his or her partner during sex because he or she can reveal all of himself or herself to his or her partner. If a person is uncomfortable with his or her own body, then his or her partner will sense that, and that will make the partner himself or herself uncomfortable during sex and decreasing the partner's pleasure, too. In order for a person to be comfortable with his or her own body, he or she needs to love, respect it, and not be self-conscious about it. A person can become comfortable with his or her body by acting like he or she is comfortable with his or her own body, although he or she is not.

Confidence and Enthusiasm

Another technique for a person to employ during the sexual act itself is for him or her to be confident. The sexiest thing is a confident person during the sexual act. If a person is not confident in himself or herself during sex, he or she will turn his or her lover off and the sex will be less enjoyable. Confidence is the quality that distinguishes a poor lover from a good lover. Confidence during sex is an attitude of control, self-assurance, and coolness. Confidence during sex means that a person believes in the correctness and appropriateness of his or her actions. Also, a person has to be confident and believe that he or she can experience pleasure during sex. A person should do so because pleasure does not just happen during sex; a person has to believe that it will happen. Another technique for a person to employ during the sexual act itself is for him or her to be enthusiastic. A key ingredient to good sex is to have an enthusiastic sexual partner. One of the biggest turnons during sex is for a person to have a partner that is enthusiastic.

A Person Should Not Focus on Having an Orgasm

During the sexual act itself, a person should not focus on having an orgasm. A person cannot be concerned about whether he or she will orgasm during the sexual encounter because this will reduce his or her pleasure during sex. Also, this might decrease a person's chances that he or she will orgasm during sex. If a person focuses only on having an orgasm, he or she will run the risk of rushing past or denying oneself and his or her partner the pleasures to be enjoyed along the way to an orgasm. There are a lot of emotions, sensations, and pleasures to be experienced on the way toward orgasm and returning from orgasm. For the sexual experience to be delightful, satisfying, and complete, a person needs emotional abandonment during sex. That means a person cannot be focusing his or her attention on how his or her body is responding during the sexual encounter and whether he or she is getting closer to orgasm. Rather, a person must focus on the joy and delight of the physical sensations produced during the sexual encounter and the experience of loving and being loved. A person must enjoy his or her body and his or her partner's body during sex by losing himself or herself in the experience and not being self-conscious. A person must relax and enjoy each moment as it comes during sex rather than worrying whether he or she will orgasm. Sex is not simply about orgasming; each minute of it should be a pleasure in itself.

The best orgasms tend to happen when the person is not thinking of having one. This is because when a person tries to will an orgasm or focuses on orgasming, he or she interferes with his or her involuntary sexual response. The goal of sex should not be orgasming. Rather, the goal of sex should be for both people to have emotional closeness, share a leisurely, understanding atmosphere, and enjoy the fun of each other all night. In other words, the main goal of sex is to become intimate with another person. Also, how both people make each other feel during sex through touching, kissing, and talking brings greater satisfaction to a couple than orgasms do. There are many couples that experience a pleasurable sexual encounter without orgasming. The intimacy, physical closeness, caring, and love that these couples share with each other is fulfilling in its own right.

A Person Should Not Worry During Sex

A person should not worry during sex. A person should not worry about how his or her body parts look during sex because that will decrease his or her sexual pleasure. A person should feel good about his or her body so that he or she can reveal all of himself or herself to his or her partner and feel closer to his or her partner. A person should feel good about his or her body parts so that he or she feels at ease with his or her body during sex and enjoys the sexual pleasure each moment during the sexual encounter. A person should not worry about his or her sexual performance in bed or what his or her partner thinks of his or her sexual performance in bed. When a person worries about his or her sexual performance he or she will be inhibited, anxious, and unable to enjoy the sexual encounter. Some people, because of worrying, might not be able to climax during the sexual encounter. A person should not worry about his or her sexual performance, but should feel free to perform sexually the way he or she wants.

If a person feels free to perform the way he or she wants during sex, then he or she will have no anxiety and no inhibition during sex, which will make the sexual encounter delightful to the greatest extent. Also, a person will be able to climax more readily. It is important that a person does not worry about anything during the sexual encounter, not even daily chores that have to be done. Instead, a person should focus all his or her attention on the pleasurable sensations occurring during the sexual encounter, so that he or she experiences sexual pleasure to the greatest extent during the sexual encounter. Also, a person's partner will enjoy the sexual encounter more if the person does not worry during sex because the person is uninhibited and enjoying the sexual encounter greatly.

A Person Should Not Pressure His or Her Partner During Sex

An additional technique for a person to employ during the sexual act itself is not to pressure his or her partner to enjoy the sexual encounter or to orgasm. A person could pressure his or her partner by telling him or her that he or she has to orgasm or enjoy the sexual encounter. A person could also pressure his or her partner by continuously asking him or her before sex, during sex, or after sex whether he or she enjoyed the sexual encounter. If a person pressures his or her partner to enjoy the sexual encounter, that will stress the partner out and cause his or her pleasure during sex to decrease. The chances that the partner will orgasm will also decrease. Instead of pressuring the partner, a person should reassure the partner that it is okay for him or her to enjoy sex to the extent that he or she does and that it is okay for him or her not to climax during sex. If a person does that, the partner's pleasure during sex will be greater and the partner's chances of orgasming during sex will be greater.

Letting Go

Letting go is another technique for a person to employ during the sexual act itself. A person should let go during sex, experiencing the sexual act with no inhibitions and without being self-conscious. A person should let the natural noises and behaviors typical of the sexual response occur freely without any inhibitions. As the man or the woman gets aroused during sex, he or she has his or her heart rate increase, breathes faster and louder, experiences slight muscular contractions, moves in certain ways, and makes noises. Also, the man or the woman's face sometimes contorts in ugly ways during sex and during an orgasm. Some people are embarrassed to let their natural noises and behaviors during sex occur, so they cut off the body movements, facial grimaces, intense breathing, and groans that occur naturally during sex because they seem silly. The body movements, facial grimaces, intense breathing, and groans should never be cut off because they are necessary for the person's sexual pleasure and his or her ability to orgasm. Also, they are arousing to the person's sexual partner during sex. As a matter of fact, there is no greater aphrodisiac for a person than the sight and sounds of his or her lover in ecstasy. If a person cuts the natural behavior off during sex, he or she will decrease his or her pleasure during sex and will decrease his or her chances of orgasming during sex. It is important for a person to understand normal physical responses and let himself or herself fully experience them without any inhibitions.

A person should also let go during sex by relaxing and not tensing up. Sometimes during sex, a person tends to tense up, especially when he or she comes to orgasm. Tensing up during sex will decrease a person's pleasure during sex and orgasm and will decrease the person's chances of orgasming. A person should relax during sex by focusing on the pleasurable physical sensations and letting them take up his or her full attention. A person should enjoy the feeling of his or her body touching his or her lover's body during sex. A person should also enjoy the feeling of his or her sex organ being stimulated.

Another way for a person to let go during sex is by being spontaneous and flexible. A person should be spontaneous and flexible by letting his or her body move as it wishes. He or she should follow his or her inner urges and desires during sex. A person can do anything during sex as long as it feels good to himself or herself and his or her partner. If anything does not feel good to a person or his or her partner during sex, he or she should not do it. Even though a couple may have prepared a list before sex of what they like during sex and what they do not like, that is okay as long as each person does the things on the list that the couple approves spontaneously and flexibly. In other words, the person can do some of the things that the couple approves, in any order he or she likes, and can add some stuff that they did not talk about. However, under no circumstance should a person do anything that the couple put on the "do not do" list. By a person being spontaneous and flexible during sex, he becomes more accepting of himself or herself and his or her partner. By a person being spontaneous and flexible during sex, he or she can turn a mildly interesting sexual encounter into a deeply exciting one. Being spontaneous and flexible during sex makes the sexual encounter exciting because it makes the sexual encounter unpredictable. The key to arousal, excitement, and pleasurable sex is being unpredictable. If the sexual encounter is predictable and routine, it will be very dull and uninteresting to the couple, reducing their pleasure and excitement during sex.

An orgasm is triggered when there is enough buildup of sexual tension from effective stimulation. A person cannot will an orgasm, since it is a reflex that is under the involuntary nervous system, but he or she can stop it from happening by interfering with the involuntary nervous system by not letting go. A person cannot give his or her partner an orgasm. All he or she can do is create the right conditions and provide sufficient stimulation for the orgasm to occur. Therefore, a person should let go, relax, and enjoy the sexual encounter, providing the right conditions for his or her partner to orgasm. He or she should let go and know that providing the right conditions for his or her partner to orgasm is all he or she can do for his or her partner to orgasm.

Fantasizing

During the sexual act itself a person could fantasize, which is a delightful technique. Fantasies do not detract from a person's concentration during sex and they do not hinder a person's ability to enjoy the pleasurable sensations during sex or to have an orgasm. If, while having sex, a person fantasizes, that is okay as long as a person concentrates on the sexual feelings produced during the sexual encounter. Fantasizing will serve to intensify the pleasurable sexual feelings produced during the sexual encounter. It will also make a person's climax more intense and pleasurable.

Taking the Lead During Sex

Both partners alternating in taking the lead during the sexual act is a thrilling technique. The best sex comes when a person and his or her partner spontaneously pick up on each other's emotions and desires during sex and create a cycle of increasing arousal. Good sex becomes like a wonderful dance with one partner following where the other leads. Both partners should alternate the lead role, each contributing to the final masterpiece. Sex is a partnership and each partner should participate in and enjoy sex on an equal basis. They should do so to make the sex encounter truly sensational. By a couple alternating taking the lead during sex, they allow new ways of sharing themselves in the actual sexual experience to emerge.

It is important that a couple alternate in taking the lead in the sexual act because both the man and the woman should give and receive during sex. It is important that both the man and the woman give and receive during sex so that they both have a mutually exciting, pleasurable, and satisfying sexual encounter. If only one partner gives and the other only receives during sex, then the sexual encounter will not be pleasurable to the greatest extent. However, if both partners give and receive during sex, then the sexual encounter will be pleasurable to both of them to the greatest extent.

It is important that both people give and receive during sex so that both people are responsive during sex. If only one partner gives during sex, then the receiver will only be passive during sex. He or she would not be responsive during sex. Most people want someone during sex who is responsive. Both people should be responsive during sex so that they both enjoy each other's body and experience mutual sexual satisfaction. If both the man and the woman are responsive during sex, that makes both of them feel connected to each other in a most intimate way.

Most people find the least pleasant element of a sexual encounter is an unresponsive partner or a cold fish. If a partner is not responsive during sex, then the sexual encounter will become a chore. It is important that a partner be responsive and return the kisses, touches, and sweet talk of the person during sex. It is important because the person does these things not just because of wanting to do these things, but because he or she wants the partner to reciprocate and do these things to him or her. It is important that a partner reciprocate these things because these things create the mood to make the couple feel aroused during sex. Sex is emotional, requiring the proper mood, not a cold race to orgasm. Also, by both people being responsive during sex, the burden of sexual performance is removed from the man, since both are working towards the same end: a mutually satisfying sexual relationship. Being responsive also means giving feedback. By giving feedback, a partner signals that he or she is appreciating the person's efforts during sex and enjoying them. A partner can give the person feedback during sex by providing him or her with hot sighs and sensuous gestures in response to getting aroused. Giving hot sighs and sensuous gestures in response to getting aroused during sex are the hottest things that a partner can do to arouse the person he or she is with.

Some people incorrectly believe that only the man can take the lead during sex. They incorrectly believe that the woman should remain passive during sex. It is important that both the man and the woman take the lead during sex at an equal basis. They should do so, so that they both have a mutually satisfying sexual encounter. However, from time to time, only the woman can take the lead during a sexual encounter, or only the man can take the lead during a sexual encounter. This could be done because it is exciting for a couple to have the woman be in control throughout the sexual encounter from time to time and it is exciting for a couple to have the man be in control throughout the sexual encounter from time to time. When a woman is in control, she knows the positions and angles that work best for her. A woman should not be afraid of taking the lead during sex for fear that she will be labeled pushy or a slut. Rather a woman should know that there is nothing slutty or pushy about her taking the lead during the sexual encounter.

Intimacy

A very important technique for a person to employ during the sexual act is to be intimate with his or her sexual partner. A person being intimate with his or her sexual partner means that he or she is close and affectionate to his or her partner. A person can become intimate with his or her partner by being romantic, loving, and affectionate during sex. This intimacy results in a person having a strong passion for sex with his or her partner.

A large number of couples do not enjoy their sexual encounters because their sexual encounters lack intimacy and tenderness. The reason for the lack of intimacy during sex is because the sexual act lacks the necessary level of holding, touching, caressing, romancing, cuddling, and hugging. When intimacy is lacking during sex, a person may not feel loved, appreciated, desired, and secure enough to relax and enjoy sex. This causes a person's sexual pleasure during sex to decrease. Lack of intimacy between a couple during sex usually happens because for many men the man penetrating the woman's vagina with his penis and thrusting is enough for intimacy, while women usually want more than that during sex to feel intimate. They want more touching, holding, caressing, hugging, kissing, and romancing during sex to feel intimate with their partner.

Therefore, in order for a person to cultivate intimacy during the sexual act to make the sexual act more pleasurable he or she should caress, hug, romance, kiss, and hold his or her partner during the sexual act. A second way for a person to cultivate more intimacy during the sexual act with his or her partner is for him or her to look his or her partner in the eyes during sex. Both the man and the woman looking into each other's eyes during sex is a powerful way for them to connect, feel intimate, and to feel love for each other. A third way for a couple to cultivate more intimacy during sex is for the couple to remain still for a while, hold each other, and then resume sexual intercourse. A fourth way for a couple to cultivate more intimacy during sex is for the couple to try having their breathing coincide with each other. A fifth way for a couple to be more intimate during sex is for them to talk to each other. Talking to each other during sex and being honest and open cultivates intimacy because it leads to emotional closeness. It leads to emotional closeness because both people are sharing their feelings during sex. A sixth way for a couple to be more intimate during sex is for them to be sensitive to each other's feelings. A couple should show that they care for each other. It is important for a person in any sexual encounter to feel loved and cared for, because without that feeling he or she is not going to feel intimate with his or her partner. As a result, the sexual encounter will lack pleasure.

A seventh way for a couple to be more intimate during sex is for them to spend more time together. If the couple does not spend enough time together during sex, then the sexual act will lack intimacy. A couple should allocate at least thirty minutes to each sexual encounter in order to give sufficient time to cultivate intimacy. An eighth way for a person to become more intimate with his or her partner during sex is for the person to make his or her partner feel as if he or she is very important to the person. A person should not let his or her partner feel like a piece of meat during sex by not showing him or her importance. A person can make his or her partner feel important during sex by telling him or her how much he or she enjoys having sex with him or her. A person can also make his or her partner feel important by treating him or her as very special during sex. A ninth way for a person to become more intimate with his or her partner during sex is for him or her to focus his or her full attention on his or her partner making his or her partner feel special. This releases the partner's sexual inhibitions and turns him or her on. The partner completely lets go during sex as a result of this attention and experiences his or her body and its reactions on a completely different level of pleasure than usual.

A tenth way for a person to become more intimate with his or her partner during sex is for him or her to play, tease, and laugh with his or her partner. It is easy for a couple to get in the habit of rushing through all the fun and playfulness that they used to go through during a sexual encounter and just concentrate on the penis thrusting inside the vagina. As a result, the intimacy between them fades away and they drift far apart emotionally. This usually results because the man is more concerned with the physical sexual release, while the woman wants more playfulness and fun during sex to satisfy her emotional intimacy. Shared experiences in bed that are fun breed intimacy between the couple and can shine up a lackluster love life. An eleventh way for a person to become more intimate with his or her partner during sex is for him or her to smile. People who smile during sex look friendly, warm, and open which leads to intimacy. They also have a more pleasurable experience.

Having a nubile body and doing acrobatics during sex is not the secret to great sex. Thrusting in and out until the woman orgasms is not the secret to great sex. Orgasming during sex is not the secret to great sex. The secret to great sex is sharing love, affection, and romance with one's partner. In other words, the secret to great sex is for the couple to have intimacy between them. The intimacy, emotional closeness, caring, and love that the couple shares during sex can be fulfilling in its own right, more fulfilling than an orgasm. Sex with intimacy, emotional closeness, caring, and love without an orgasm is more fulfilling than sex without intimacy, emotional closeness, caring, and love, but with an orgasm. Sex should be enjoyed and shared by a couple as a beautiful act that gives great pleasure and brings two people closer together. The deeper the level of intimacy, the greater the pleasure during sex for both the man and the woman. When the couple have a deep connection with each other as a result of intimacy that is created from previous sexual encounters and daily hugs, and kisses, then they will experience great sex.

When the couple becomes truly intimate with each other, each of them will feel free to do anything during the sexual encounter and will know that it will be okay with his or her partner. Intimacy lets a person be himself or herself during sex without any inhibitions. Intimacy lets a person be himself or herself during sex without being criticized or put down by his or her partner. Intimacy lets a person be himself or herself during sex and be received with understanding and warmth by his or her partner. The couples who are most satisfied are those who have the greatest levels of bodily freedom with one another. Intimacy during sex will make a person feel loved, appreciated, desired, and secure enough to relax and enjoy sex. Intimacy during sex will make a couple feel that an empty void has been filled. Intimacy can keep the couple's sex life exciting and alive. It can make a dull sex life exciting. It can help a couple with a non-existent sex life rediscover the exciting and pleasurable sex life that they once had. It can save a loveless relationship and restore it to a happy and fulfilling relationship.

Talking During Sex

A very effective technique for a person to employ during sex is for him or her to talk with his or her partner. Talking during sex is sometimes referred to as pillow talk. A large number of couples do not enjoy sex because they do not communicate during sex. In a large number of couples, one partner does not let the other partner know what he or she likes and dislikes sexually. One partner is afraid to let the other partner know how to please him or her sexually. He or she thinks the sex will get better over time, but unfortunately it does not. When both partners communicate with each other during sex and let each other know the right way to satisfy each other sexually, then both of them will be satisfied sexually. Another advantage of talking during sex is that it is effective in making both partners more sexually aroused. This leads to a more pleasurable experience and more intense orgasm for both partners. Talking during sex uses the mind of both people to amplify the sensations they are feeling.

There are several ways to talk during sex. One way is for a person to tell his or her partner in great detail exactly what he or she is going to do to him or her sexually. That should get the partner sexually excited. Another way to talk during sex is for a person to compliment his or her partner. During sex, a person can tell his or her partner how physically attractive he or she is or what a good lover he or she is. A third way to communicate during sex is for a person to utter sounds and words of pleasure to let his or her partner know what he or she finds pleasurable during sex. Most sexual partners appreciate feedback during sex so that they know how they are doing. It can be frustrating for a sexual partner to try to pleasure a person during sex if he or she does not receive feedback. A fourth way to communicate during sex is for a person to express his or her intimate sexual feelings using vulgar terms. This is known as dirty talk. Many people find it exciting and arousing during sex to hear and talk dirty talk.

A fifth way to communicate during sex is using non-verbal communication. During sex, a person can guide his or her partner using his or her hands to show him or her what feels good. The bedroom is a vulnerable place where both people are naked physically and emotionally. Therefore, it is important that a person does not criticize his or her partner during sex since this will result in the partner feeling hurt and resentful, which will make the sexual encounter less pleasurable to both people. The criticized partner's desire to have sex and to please the person during sex will decrease as a result of the criticism. During sex, a person should not discuss anything not having to do with the sexual encounter since it decreases the pleasure during sex.

Sex is about exciting a person's mind and body, not just the body. Communication during sex is very important in exciting a person's mind. Sexual openness and honesty about all sexual matters is very important for a good sexual relationship. Effective verbal and non-verbal communication during sex can enhance the sexual experience. As a matter of fact, talking during sex is an aphrodisiac.

Touching

A person touching his or her partner's whole body during sex is a technique that should not be overlooked. Both people should touch each other's whole body during the sexual encounter for amazing sex. Both people should enjoy the pleasure of being touched by his or her partner during sex; it is an amazing feeling. If both partners go through sex with just thrusting occurring and no touching occurring, then the sex will not be pleasurable to the greatest extent. Touch during sex is a great way to relax stiff muscles and ease tension. Touch is the strongest of all senses during sex. In fact, the nerve endings in the skin are more sensitive to touch when a person is aroused during sex. Touching during sex is a way of expressing love and affection during sex. It brings both people closer emotionally and physically. Touching during sex makes a person more aroused sexually, makes the pleasure during sex more pleasurable, and makes the orgasm during sex more intense.

A person can use any part of his or her body to touch any part of his or her partner's body during sex. A person rubbing another person's skin anywhere can be exciting during sex. The touching should usually be done slowly and gently, because slow and gentle touching by a person during sex produces the greatest pleasure during sex to the sexual partner. Also, slow and gentle touching during sex shows that a person cares about his or her partner, which causes the partner great pleasure during sex. Another way to touch during sex is to start the touching slowly and gently and then increase the speed and intensity of the touch to a level that both people find amazing. The way to touch during sex is not to use one stroke in a spot for too long, because the area may become less sensitive to pleasure. The key to good touching during sex is for a person to use variety and be unpredictable. A person touching his or her partner predictably during sex takes away from the pleasure of the encounter. However, if a person touches his or her partner unpredictably during sex, that makes the sexual encounter pleasurable to the greatest extent.

Kissing

Kissing during sex is a very passionate technique. Both partners should kiss each other all over their bodies during sex. Kissing is erotic when it is done on its own, but it is more erotic when done during the sexual act. If a person kisses his or her partner during sex then the partner will get more sexually aroused during sex, will experience more pleasure during sex, and will have a more intense orgasm. Kissing is a way for a person to express love and affection during sex. It lets both people become closer physically and emotionally. As a matter of fact, most prostitutes will not kiss their customers because they find it too personal and intimate. So kissing during sex will make the sexual act extremely personal and intimate.

A partner will find that any part of his or her body, when kissed, is sexually arousing and pleasurable. As a matter of fact, if a person smothers his or her partner's body with kisses all over, then the partner will find that extremely delightful. When a person kisses his or her partner's body, the partner should enjoy being kissed and feel the pleasure all over his or her body. It is important that when a person kisses his or her partner's body during sex, that he she does not kiss one area for too long since that will decrease the pleasure during sex. A person should change the spots where he or she kisses during sex so that the kissing remains pleasurable to the greatest extent. Plus, the kissing should be unpredictable, not following a predictable pattern. If the kissing pattern is predictable, that will decrease the pleasure derived from the kissing. If the kissing is unpredictable, the kissing will be pleasurable to the greatest extent during sex.

Most couples slack off on the kissing during sex after being in a relationship for a while. It is important for both partners not to slack off on the kissing during sex. Kissing during sex will add new sensations to the sexual act and makes both people feel amazingly turned on. A slightly open-mouth kiss on the partner's mouth during sex is more sexually arousing to both people than a closed-mouth kiss. Kissing using full mouth kissing (French Kissing) during sex is the most passionate form of kissing. When French kissing during sex, a person can insert his or her tongue into his or her partner's mouth. That is very erotic. However, if a person inserts his or her tongue into his or her partner's mouth gradually, this will drive his or her partner wild with pleasure. Then the person can move his or her tongue around the partner's mouth which will even add more pleasure to the experience. While French kissing during sex, if a person flicks his or her tongue against the roof of his or her partner's mouth, that will cause great pleasure to both people. While kissing during sex a person should kiss slowly and gradually. He should also kiss passionately with deep intense feelings. Such kissing will cause the partner sexual pleasure during sex to the greatest extent. A person should not kiss quickly without any feelings since that will not produce a great amount of pleasure during sex. French kissing during an orgasm creates one of the most amazing passionate moments during sex.

Stimulating the Whole Body

A delightful technique for a person to employ during the sex act is for him or her to stimulate his or her partner's whole body during sex. The genital area is not the only area that is sensitive to stimulation during sex. It is not the only area that gives pleasure during sex. A person can stimulate his or her partner's whole body during sex to give him or her pleasure to the greatest degree. The skin is the largest sexual organ, so during sex a person should take advantage of that fact. If, during sex, a person thrusts only without stimulating other parts of his or her partner's body, then the result of such a sexual encounter is that the sex will not be very pleasurable. As a matter of fact, it might be very boring. The partner's body will be in need of attention. The skin is highly sensitive and is full of nerve endings waiting to be aroused, so a person letting his or her hands, lips, or tongue wander over the partner's body during sex is very arousing, loving, and intimate.

The best sex does not come just from the penis stimulating the vagina. The best sex is when both people stimulate each other's whole body, including their genital area. Stimulating the whole body during sex takes the pressure off the man's penis, helping him last longer. It also takes the pressure off the woman, making her more likely to orgasm. Both people stimulating each other's whole body during sex will release tension in their bodies, and will make them relax greatly.

Men can usually get a climax during sex just from stimulating their penis, whereas women usually need whole body stimulation in addition to having their genital area stimulated to orgasm. Usually, during sex, the man just concentrates on thrusting his penis inside the vagina and does not stimulate the woman's whole body. If the man does that the woman may not orgasm, and the sex will not be pleasurable to the greatest degree to both the man and the woman. The man should stimulate the woman's whole body during sex in order for her to most likely orgasm and in order for her to have a very pleasurable sexual encounter. A woman should also stimulate the man's whole body during sex even though he can have an orgasm without his whole body being stimulated. The woman should do so, so that the sexual encounter is pleasurable to the man to the greatest extent.

Sexual Positions

Choosing the positions to have sex in is a sexual technique that is very effective. There is no set number of positions for a couple to use during one sexual encounter. The couple can use one position during a sexual encounter or they can use more. Usually, a couple uses two or three positions during one sexual encounter, moving from one position to another. It is better to use two or three positions during one sexual encounter because the couple finds the sex pleasurable and exciting if they change from one position to another during the same sexual encounter. Using more than three sex positions during one sexual encounter tends to reduce the pleasure during sex because changing positions too frequently during sex can be distracting and disruptive to the flow of lovemaking. However, the major determining factor in the number of positions to use is for the couple to do what works best for both of them in terms of pleasure.

A sexual encounter is a time when the couple is in harmony, moving, enjoying each other's bodies, and pleasing each other. In that process a couple is likely to change from one position to another. The positions should flow naturally out of the couple's enjoyment of being together so that the sex is pleasurable to the greatest degree. If the positions do not flow naturally, the sex will be less pleasurable. The choice of position that the couple uses should grow out of the feelings of both people at the moment. The positions in sequence should not involve a lot of climbing over legs or turning the partner around. There is no right or wrong position to use during sex. A couple should just do what feels natural and pleasurable. The couple should choose positions that are pleasurable for both of them. Usually, the simpler the position, the better it is for the couple to enjoy the sex. However, an exotic position from time to time is exciting because it adds variety to the sex. Different positions produce different sensations during sex to both the man and the woman, so the couple should alternate positions to alternate the sensations felt during sex to keep the sex exciting. The couple should move into each position with a great deal of gentleness, patience, ease, and relaxation. Doing so will lead to great sex. It is important to remember that sex can be loving in any position. To make the sex more exciting, from time to time a couple can change positions during sex without withdrawing the penis from the vagina.

Moving During Sex

Moving during sex is a technique that could be employed to make the sexual encounter more pleasurable. Sometimes a couple does not move at all during sex except for a little thrusting movement, enough to stimulate the penis to orgasm. Sometimes that thrusting is enough to stimulate the woman to orgasm and sometimes it is not. When a couple moves a little during sex, the sexual encounter is not pleasurable to the greatest degree. However, during sex a couple should move to make the sexual act pleasurable to the greatest extent. The movement during sex should be a lot more than just a little thrusting movement enough to stimulate the penis. Both the man and the woman during sex should relax and let their body move the way it wants to. This will make the sex intensely as pleasurable as possible. Also, during an orgasm some people tend to stiffen and not move. This reduces the pleasure of an orgasm. During an orgasm a person should relax and move the way his or her body wants to make the orgasm as intensely pleasurable as possible.

Breathing

Breathing correctly during sex is a technique of great significance. Usually during sex, a person's breathing is excited, erratic, fast, and shallow. This is true especially at the point of orgasm. Such breathing is practically instinctual. However, such breathing increases stress and anxiety during sex, causing tension in the body. Such breathing decreases the pleasure during the sexual encounter and decreases the pleasure of an orgasm making an orgasm less intense.

The proper way for a person to breathe during sex is to breathe slowly and deeply, rhythmically. He or she should breathe in from his or her nostrils and not from his or her mouth, and he or she should exhale from his or her nostrils and not from his or her mouth. He or she should breathe deep from the belly and not from the chest. When a person breathes that way during sex, he or she should relax throughout his or her body. He or she should feel every part of his or her body relaxing, from his or her toes to his or her fingers, to the top of his or her head. When a person breathes that way during sex he or she should relax his or her mind, quieting distracting thoughts that distract him or her from sexual pleasure.

Such breathing makes a person focus only on the pleasurable sexual feelings felt during the sexual encounter. Such breathing makes the pleasurable sexual sensations felt during the sex act felt not only in the genital area, but throughout a person's body. Such breathing makes the pleasurable sexual sensations felt during an orgasm felt not only in the genital area but throughout a person's body. Such breathing will increase the blood flow to the genital area, making the sexual pleasure felt during the sexual encounter pleasurable to the greatest extent. It will also make the orgasm intense, making the pleasure felt during an orgasm pleasurable to the greatest extent. Such breathing helps a man have a stronger longer lasting erection and makes him last longer before ejaculating. Such breathing helps a woman relax and attain an orgasm more readily and more quickly. Such breathing lets both the man and the woman have greater sexual stamina during sex. The slower and the deeper the breathing, the more relaxed a person is during sex, and the more pleasurable and intense the sexual encounter is.

It is important that a person breathes from the nose during sex and not the mouth. If a person breathes from the mouth during sex, he or she is keeping the pleasurable feelings of sexual pleasure from going to the head. If a person breathes from the mouth during sex, it is like breathing from the mouth during an allergy or a cold. He or she does not feel completely satisfied from his or her breathing. However, if a person breathes from the nostrils during sex, he or she lets the pleasurable feelings of sexual pleasure go to the head completely. Also, he or she feels completely satisfied and fulfilled from his breathing. In addition, a person being able to breathe effectively through the nose during sex will make kissing possible for a long period of time, and will make doing things with the mouth a lot more possible without gasping for air.

During sex, a person usually holds his or her breath and tightens his or her muscles from time to time. Unfortunately, breath holding happens unconsciously and a person is usually not aware of it. Breath holding during sex can result in increased muscle tension and decreases the pleasure during sex. It also results in a decrease of sexual arousal during sex. In addition, a person usually holds his or her breath just before an orgasm, which is quite normal, however that decreases the pleasure of an orgasm and makes it less intense. A person should be aware of his or her breathing during sex and make sure that he or she continuously breathes during sex without holding his or her breath. By a person continuously breathing during sex without holding his or her breath, he or she will release the tension in his or her body, causing his or her body to relax. By a person continuously breathing during sex without holding his or her breath, the sexual act will be pleasurable to the greatest degree. Also, by a person continuously breathing during sex, he or she will make his or her sexual arousal go to the greatest extent. By a person continuously breathing before an orgasm and during an orgasm, he or she will experience the pleasure of the orgasm to the greatest degree. Also, the orgasm will be intense to the greatest degree.

Once the couple have mastered the proper way of breathing during sex, if they like, they could try to synchronize their breathing at the same time. Both of them would inhale at the same time and then exhale at the same time. This creates an amazing connection between both partners which can translate into great pleasure during sex. This will lead to a feeling of total oneness between the couple which can lead to incredible orgasms.

Thrusting

Proper thrusting during sex is a very useful technique for a person to use. Thrusting during sex usually is the act of the penis penetrating the vagina by backward and forward movement. The movement can be by the man or the woman. Some people incorrectly assume that only the man does the thrusting during sex. This is not true. Women sometimes do the thrusting during sex. Who does the thrusting during sex is determined by the position that the couple is in. For example, if the couple is in the missionary position, the man usually does the thrusting. However, if the couple is in the woman on top position, the woman does the thrusting. Most couples find the sex extremely pleasurable when the man does the thrusting. However, most couples also find the sex extremely pleasurable when the woman does the thrusting. The woman enjoys it when she does the thrusting because she is in control of the situation for a change. She also enjoys it because she can manipulate the angles of the thrusts to stimulate the areas of the vagina that she finds sensitive. The man enjoys it when the woman thrusts because she is in control of the sexual encounter for a change. He finds it erotic that the woman is taking charge of the sexual act. Also the man enjoys it because he can relax, enjoy the encounter, and let the woman do all the work.

Whether the man or the woman is doing the thrusting, there are several types of thrusts that could be done during sex. The first type of thrust is the shallow thrust. Shallow thrusts stimulate the highly sensitive first one, two, or three inches of a woman's vagina and, depending on her position, her G-spot. The shallow thrust is deeply satisfying to the woman while not being overly stimulating to the man. They do not overstimulate the man's penis so that he climaxes before the woman climaxes. The shorter thrusts place less friction on the man's penis, which makes him last longer during sex, while they still provide sufficient stimulation to the woman's vagina since the first two inches of the vagina have the most nerve endings and are very sensitive. Shallow thrusts bring excitement to the sexual encounter because they tease the person on the receiving end of the thrusting. They tease a person because they cause a deep desire for deeper thrusts in the person on the receiving end of the thrusting. When the man is thrusting shallow thrusts, the woman's desire for deeper thrusts heightens. When the woman is thrusting shallow thrusts, the man's desire for deeper thrusts heightens. The man could thrust only shallow thrusts without taking the penis out completely from the vagina. This will greatly satisfy the woman and has a great possibility of having the woman climax during sex. This will also satisfy the man.

The second type of thrust is the deep thrust. Deep thrusting is when the penis penetrates the vagina from the entrance of the vagina to the back end of the vagina. These are the thrusts that are depicted in the media and in pornography. They are highly stimulating for both partners because the head of the penis pulls along the whole length of the woman's vagina. If the man is having difficulty getting or keeping an erection the long deep thrusts are extremely good for resolving this problem. However, the long deep thrusts are highly pleasurable to the man and can make it hard for him to control his ejaculation. They might bring him to orgasm very rapidly, so that he orgasms before the woman orgasms.

Whether the man or the woman is doing the deep or shallow thrusting, the movement is usually in and out. However, a person can produce different sensations while thrusting by thrusting in and out while moving in a circular motion. Also, while thrusting in and out a person can move from side to side. That will also produce different sensations. In addition, while thrusting in and out a person can move from top to bottom or in a diagonal direction. However, the easiest way to do deep or shallow thrusts is to simply move in and out.

A person should try thrusting at different angles. A person could thrust towards one side of the vagina, creating different pleasurable sensations. A person thrusting at different angles allows the couple to find the angles that are pleasurable during thrusting. The couple finding the right angles during thrusting that produce pleasure during sex is one of the easiest and satisfying ways to improve their sex life. The secret to great sex can be as small as a light change of angle during thrusting. The key to good thrusting is variety. A person should not use one type of thrust in one spot for too long or the area may become less sensitive to the stimulation. A person should change the areas that are being stimulated by thrusting. While thrusting, the person doing the thrusting should not jerk up and down but should keep his or her movement fluid as he or she thrusts in and out. The pressure and speed should not lessen as the person thrusting switches direction. When thrusting, the penis should not be pulled out completely from the vagina. This should be done to maintain a suction feeling.

Both types of thrusts could be used together. When the deep thrusts are used with the shallow thrusts, the deep thrusts push the air out of the woman's vagina and create a vacuum that can be intensified by using the shallow thrusts. As long as the penis does not come out completely, the vacuum effect is maintained. The vacuum effect makes the sexual encounter more pleasurable to both the man and the woman. The shorter thrusts should be more than the deep thrusts. A person can try nine shallow thrusts to one deep thrust. He or she can try 6 shallow thrusts to one deep thrust. He or she can try 3 shallow thrusts to one deep thrust. Varying the depth of the thrusts is one of the most important ways for a couple to spice up their sex life. By using both types of thrusts, a couple can stimulate different parts of the penis and vagina. Also, varying between shallow thrusting and deep thrusting is a way for a man to control his ejaculation so he can help the woman reach orgasm. The long deep thrusts are often very stimulating to the man, while shallow thrusts are often less intense for the man but still quite stimulating to the woman.

While having sex and thrusting deeply, shallowly, or both, a person can suddenly stop thrusting without any prior warning and have the penis out of the vagina. He or she can wait briefly and then slowly and gradually have the penis penetrate the vagina. Then he or she can resume thrusting but gradually build up speed. This makes both partners hotter than ever. This works because stopping and restarting thrusting builds on the previous sensation and it lets both partners skip up a few rungs on the pleasure ladder.

Another way of thrusting that could be done is to stimulate only the shaft of the man's penis. Whether the man or the woman is doing the thrusting, the woman can squeeze her PC (pubococcygeus) muscle around the shaft of the man's penis when the penis is inside her vagina without stimulating the head. The woman should keep her PC muscle squeezed during this thrusting technique. Then the thrusting is done to stimulate only the shaft of penis while it is inside the woman's vagina by the PC muscle only squeezing around the shaft of the man's penis during thrusting. The thrusting should not pull so far that the woman's PC muscle squeezes around the head of the penis or that the penis comes out of the vagina. Such thrusting prolongs sexual intercourse because only the shaft of the penis is stimulated during sex and the head of the penis is not. The shaft of the penis is not as sensitive to stimulation as the head of the penis is. Such thrusting makes it more probable that the man will orgasm the same time that the woman does. For a variation, the woman can squeeze her PC muscle around the head of the man's penis or frenulum and the thrusting motion can stimulate only the head of the man's penis or frenulum which will be very exciting to the man. It will be very exciting to the man since the head of the man's penis is very sensitive to stimulation and the frenulum is the most sensitive to stimulation. Such stimulation will drive the man wild with pleasure but will make him last longer because the whole penis is not stimulated, causing less friction to the penis. This will make it more likely that the man will orgasm the same time as the woman. The woman will enjoy such stimulation because she sees the man in ecstasy, and she might orgasm from such stimulation at the same time the man orgasms.

The third type of thrusting during sex is grinding. Grinding does not involve the usual thrusting in and out. Grinding involves keeping the penis inside the vagina at the same depth, but having the man or the woman thrusting in a circular motion. The circular motion can be done in any direction. The person doing the circular thrusting is the person that is in control in that particular position. The clitoris will be stimulated through such action, by the man's pelvis stimulating it. The stimulation of the clitoris by the man's pelvis usually causes the woman to orgasm the same time as the man. This sexual technique offers close, intense contact and provides deep, prolonged pressure that is sometimes preferable to rhythmic thrusting, particularly for G-spot and clitoral stimulation. This sexual technique will stimulate more areas of the penis, making the encounter more pleasurable for the man. Even though it stimulates more areas of the penis, it makes the man's erection last longer during intercourse because of its movement. This technique is good if a man is prone to quick ejaculation. This sexual technique will stimulate more areas of the vagina making the sex more pleasurable to the woman. When many women masturbate, they often rub their clitoris using circular movements. During grinding, the clitoris is stimulated using circular movements similar to those when the woman masturbates. That is why many women like the grinding technique. As a variation, while laying on top of each other the couple could have the penis remain in the vagina at the same depth while the person thrusting moves up and down. The person is moving up towards the face of his or her partner and then down towards the feet of his or her partner. He or she is not moving in and out like regular thrusting. This is usually a rocking motion. This will also cause the man's pelvis to stimulate the clitoris, leading to orgasm. Since there is not a lot of moving in and out in this technique whether the man or the woman is lying on top, the man does not get overstimulated, but the woman is deeply pleasured. This technique allows the man to orgasm at the same time as the woman.

A person should thrust slowly and gently during sex in order to enjoy the pleasurable sensations during sex to the greatest degree. Also, a person can start thrusting slowly and increase the speed gradually as long as it keeps feeling amazing to both people. Once the person finds the maximum speed that is amazing to both people, he or she can maintain that speed while thrusting. This technique of thrusting is also pleasurable. One bad habit is for a person to thrust rapidly in and out. In real life, such a move reduces the pleasure for both the man and the woman and may even cause irritation. But such a move is portrayed in movies because it looks good on video and sells more copies. However, a person could try it from time to time, since the fact that it is not usually done will make it very exciting. A person could go fast, but not extremely fast, so that he or she does not irritate his or her partner. Most people need a consistent, repetitive motion during thrusting in order to feel satisfied. While thrusting, a person should maintain a rhythm that is pleasurable to both people. The right rhythm will make sex pleasurable to the greatest degree and will make an orgasm intense to the greatest degree.

What type of thrusts to use during a sexual encounter differs from one couple to another, and differs from one sexual encounter to another. It also differs during the same sexual encounter from one moment to another. This is so because a person's tastes during sex differ from moment to moment. The type of thrust to use during a sexual encounter depends on the couple's feelings at the moment. For example, sometimes a couple would want a sexual encounter only with shallow thrusts. Other times, the couple might want an encounter only with deep thrusts. At other times, the couple might want an encounter with a combination of shallow thrusts and deep thrusts. A person could gauge from his or her partner's body language what thrusts his or her partner likes.

When thrusting, a person should be unpredictable because being unpredictable is the key to sexual arousal. If a person thrusts routinely, the thrusting will not be very pleasurable. However, if a person thrusts in an unpredictable fashion, the sexual encounter will be pleasurable to the greatest extent. Also, the further apart the sensations are on a spectrum of feeling, the more intense they will feel when done in succession. In other words, if a person thrusts shallow thrusts and right away he or she changes to deep thrusts, then the feeling that he or she feels during thrusting will be more intensely pleasurable because the thrusting are further apart on a spectrum of feeling.

Most men can thrust for four to five minutes before orgasming. After orgasming, they have a refractory period of around 20 minutes where they cannot thrust any longer. Some people incorrectly believe that a man should be able to last longer than four to five minutes thrusting. If a man can last only 4 to 5 minutes thrusting during sex, that is normal and sufficient time to provide the woman with sexual pleasure and satisfaction.

Speed During Sex

Utilizing the speed during sex is a technique that can be used to enhance the sexual experience. During sex, a person should do everything slowly and gently. That includes thrusting, kissing, hugging, cuddling, touching, and moving. The slower and gentler a person goes during sex, the more pleasurable sensations are provoked from the sexual encounter in both people. The slower and gentler a person goes during sex, the more intense and pleasurable the sensations are during an orgasm from both people. By a person going slowly and gently during sex, it is evident to his or her partner that he or she cares about him or her as a person. This is very important to a woman because, usually, a woman cannot become fully aroused and experience an orgasm unless she feels that the man cares about her as a person. However, this is not very important to the man because the man can experience an orgasm whether or not he feels the woman cares for him. However, if the man feels the woman cares for him then the pleasure during sex and the orgasm will be a lot more intense.

If a person goes fast or is rough during sex, the sexual experience won't be pleasurable to the greatest extent to both people. It will even make the orgasm less intense for both the man and the woman. As a matter of fact, moving extremely fast during sex sometimes may be irritable and sometimes it may cause a sensation of numbness during sex in the areas of the body stimulated. For example, if the man thrusts into the vagina in and out extremely fast, this sometimes may irritate the woman and sometimes may cause a sensation of numbness in her vagina. Also, if the man rubs the clitoris extremely fast during sex, this sometimes may irritate the woman and sometimes may cause a sensation of numbness in the clitoris.

If a person goes slowly during sex, his or her partner is more receptive and desirous of his or her stimulation. The woman would be more desirous of the man stroking her if he goes slowly during sex. The man would be more desirous of the woman stroking him if she goes slowly during sex. If a person goes slowly during sex he or she will bring his or her sexual arousal and his or her partner's sexual arousal to a rapid and eager boil. This is because a person's body becomes much more sensitive to stimulation if he or she goes slowly during sex.

A person could slow down the sexual arousal process of both people, especially the man's, by changing positions, varying speed, and changing the pattern of the thrusts during the sexual encounter. Doing such things lets a couple slowly build up to orgasm and lets them both enjoy the sexual experience fully. Also, in order to slow things down, the couple should make sure that there is sufficient time for the sexual encounter and that they are not rushed. The best sex is when it is open-ended and there is no deadline to finish the encounter by. This is because a person can enjoy leisurely lovemaking because he or she is not in a rush to finish the sexual encounter. It is important that a couple is not in a rush during sex since that causes both of them to be stressed and tensed during sex, which will greatly reduce their pleasure during sex.

Although going slow during sex is extremely pleasurable, there is another way to have sex. That way is to start slow and then increase the speed as long as it feels amazing to both people. The couple should stop increasing the speed at the maximum speed that is amazing to both people. They should maintain that speed throughout the intercourse. This way of having sex is also pleasurable, but not as pleasurable as going slow throughout the encounter. Also, although going fast during sex is not very pleasurable because the sensations produced are not pleasurable to the greatest degree, it could be done once in a while to make the encounter exciting. It will make the encounter exciting since that is something different than usual. The excitement during the encounter makes going fast during sex very pleasurable, although the sexual sensations are not very pleasurable. However, it is important that when the couple goes fast during sex, they go fast but not extremely fast, because going extremely fast can sometimes be irritable and cause numbness in the areas of the body being stimulated.

In conclusion, a couple rarely enjoys the sex to the greatest degree when it is fast and furious. A couple usually enjoys sex to the greatest degree when it is gentle and slow. This is because the sexual encounter is sensuous, full of feeling, and longer. This type of sex lets both people feel the pleasurable sexual sensations fully to the greatest degree. This type of sex is very loving and caring that leads to a more intimate relationship. Slower sex makes a man's erection firmer and longer lasting. The woman has a greater chance of climaxing when the sex is slow than when it is fast. The couple have a greater chance of experiencing a simultaneous orgasm when the sex is slow than when it is fast.

Rhythm

Maintaining a consistent and steady rhythm during sex is a very effective technique to make sex more satisfying and fulfilling. A person could maintain that rhythm during all aspects of the sexual encounter. He or she could maintain the rhythm while thrusting, touching, kissing, licking, or moving during sex. Each couple has a different rhythm that they like to have sex to. A couple should have sex using a rhythm that is satisfying to both of them. A couple can find their proper rhythm during sex very easily.

If the rhythm is broken during sex the sexual encounter won't be very pleasurable. A consistent rhythm should be maintained during sex because a person's body naturally wants a consistent rhythm of stimulation during sex. The vagina and the penis especially want a consistent rhythm of stimulation during sex. As a matter of fact, a large number of women cannot orgasm during sex unless there is a consistent rhythm of stimulation. If the man breaks the rhythm of stimulation during sex, the woman's sexual arousal will usually drop and she won't be able to climax unless he again maintains a consistent rhythm. The man can orgasm even if there is not a constant rhythm of stimulation. However, if there is a constant rhythm of stimulation, the man's sexual pleasure during sex will be more intense and his orgasm will be more pleasurable and intense. During sex, a person must maintain a consistent steady rhythm to make the sexual encounter pleasurable to the greatest extent for both the man and the woman. Maintaining a steady and consistent rhythm will make an orgasm more pleasurable and more intense for the man and the woman.

It is important as the partner is about to orgasm that the person keeps on doing whatever he or she is doing and maintain a steady rhythm. A person should not vary the pace, pressure, or activity. This is very important for the woman because most likely she won't be able to orgasm if the man varies the pace, pressure, or activity as she is about to orgasm. So if a woman moans with delight during sex it does not mean to speed up or do it harder, it means that the man should keep doing what he is doing. Although the man can still orgasm even though his partner does not keep doing whatever she was doing as he is about to orgasm, it is important that the woman keep doing whatever she was doing as the man is about to orgasm because if it is not done, a man's sexual pleasure during sex and orgasm will be less.

More Tips on Making the Sexual Encounter More Pleasurable

This section discusses more tips on intensifying pleasure during sex. Whether the man or the woman is doing the thrusting during sex, to intensify the pleasure during sex, combine acts of affection with slow and steady penetration of the vagina by the penis. These acts of affection include kissing, hugging, and caressing. These acts of affection combined with penetration of the vagina by the penis are more satisfying than anything seen in pornographic flicks. As a result of this technique, almost all people would be perfectly content at the end of the lovemaking session even if they do not orgasm. Women especially, as a result of this technique, would be perfectly content at the end of the lovemaking session even if they do not orgasm. An orgasm is merely a peak in sexual pleasure. It is not the sole source of sexual pleasure. Sex is not something a person does to someone or for someone. Sex is an experience a person does with someone. The main purpose of sex is for it to be an expression of love and closeness between two people. This technique satisfies that, while orgasming does not satisfy that. That is why this technique is more pleasurable than orgasming. The loving exchange and joy of sex is much more important than whether a person orgasms during sex. Using this technique, a person should feel refreshed invigorated, happy, satisfied, and fulfilled, even though he or she did not orgasm.

A person should spend time talking, hugging, kissing, and touching during sex because it lets his or her partner feel safe, secure, loved, and relaxed during sex. This is important so that his or her partner becomes sexually aroused enough to reach orgasm. A woman usually cannot orgasm during sex unless she feels safe, secure, loved, and relaxed. A man can orgasm during sex even though he does not feel safe, secure, loved, and relaxed. However, the experience is not very pleasurable. During the sexual encounter, moving through several sex positions, kissing, touching, and hugging creates more sexual arousal and brings feelings of exquisite sensuality in both people. A person should focus on the stimulation that he or she and his or her partner find most arousing. A person should be himself or herself during sex and not try to imitate movies. This make the sexual encounter more comfortable for both people. This will make the sex more exciting and extremely passionate to both people. During sex, a person might seem silly and awkward. He or she may stumble, laugh, or fall. No one should care. Sex should be fun and playful in order for it to be pleasurable to the greatest extent.

A person should relish the feeling of his or her skin against the skin of his or her partner during sex. He or she should concentrate on that pleasurable feeling and let his or her sexual arousal increase during sex. This lowers inhibitions and increases the emotional comfort level between both partners. When a person's body gets very aroused, then the smallest touch could send him or her into ecstasy, which makes the sex extremely pleasurable to the greatest degree. When the body is aroused, the vagina and the penis especially become very engorged with blood, which makes them extremely sensitive.

During sex, a person should be guided by his or her own internal desires and urges. A person should go with what is comfortable to him or her and his or her partner. Sex should not be an acrobatic ordeal or an act requiring great strength and agility. During sex, a person should keep moving towards stimulation that produces feelings of pleasure. He or she should back away from any form of stimulation that does not produce any good feelings to him or her or his or her partner. In sex, if a person pleases his or her partner, the partner's sexual satisfaction increases the person's pleasure.

A person should be unpredictable during sex. He or she should not make sex a routine or mechanical. Being predictable during sex or making the sexual act routine takes away from the pleasure during sex. By a person being unpredictable during the sexual encounter, he or she makes the sexual encounter very exciting and pleasurable. The fact that the sexual partner does not know what is going to happen next during the sexual encounter makes the sexual encounter extremely thrilling and delightful. Also, the orgasms during sex are a lot more intense and pleasurable if the sexual encounter is unpredictable. Even good sex becomes boring when it is predictable. It is very important to remember this point. One way to make the sex unpredictable is to sometimes do delayed stimulation. Delayed stimulation is when a person stops thrusting, touching, kissing, or licking suddenly, waits briefly and then starts again with the same form of stimulation. For maximum effect, when the person restarts the stimulation he or she should restart the stimulation in slow motion and then build back up to speed gradually. Stopping and then restarting a form of stimulation builds on the previous sensation and lets a person skip up a few rungs on the pleasure ladder. It makes the sex more thrilling and pleasurable.

Furthermore, a person should not stimulate the same area for too long during sex, because stimulating the same area for too long only tends to reduce the pleasure level that the sexual partner feels. Sometimes stimulating the same area for too long during sex may cause the area to become numb. Even though a person should not stimulate the same area for too long during sex, a person should keep stimulating the same area in the same way when his or her partner is very close to orgasming. Changing the area that is being stimulated or the way it is stimulated when a woman is close to orgasming will usually cause a woman not to orgasm. Changing the area that is being stimulated or the way it is stimulated when a man is close to orgasm will decrease a man's sexual pleasure even though he still orgasms. Variety is very important in a sexual encounter to keep it from being boring and routine.

The couple could keep the lights on during sex so that they have visual stimulation during sex. Both the man and the woman, if they see sex, will enjoy the sex a lot more because they will be stimulated visually in addition to being stimulated physically. The visual stimulation intensifies the pleasurable sensations during sex and orgasm. The couple could make the sex more pleasurable and intense by being romantic during sex. They could be romantic during sex by talking affectionately to each other during sex. They can also be romantic during sex by touching and kissing each other gently and affectionately during sex. They could be romantic during sex by being sensitive to each other's needs during sex.

One thing that a person can do during sex to make the sex more pleasurable is to squeeze his or her thighs together several times. During sex, as a person's sexual arousal and pleasure begin to build, he or she can start squeezing his or her thighs together to intensify the feelings. He or she could continue doing so while he or she climaxes. Even though a person's legs are next to each other, a person squeezing his or her thighs together several times during sex it intensifies the pleasurable sexual feelings. This will also make the pleasure during an orgasm more intense.

A woman can touch the man's testicles during sex to make the sex more pleasurable. Usually men feel that their testicles do not get enough attention during sex. While the man is thrusting gently during sex, a woman can squeeze his testicles to the rhythm of his motion. Also, if the woman is thrusting, she can touch the man's testicles gently during sex to the rhythm of her motion. A man's testicles are highly sensitive and love to be gently stroked. If a woman does so she will make the man's pleasure during sex more intense and she will make his orgasm more intense.

The man can squeeze the shaft of his penis tightly at the base of his penis before sex or during breaks that occur during sex. This temporarily prevents the blood of the penis from flowing back, causing the penis to swell. This increases the sensitivity of the penis shaft and head. This makes the sex a lot more pleasurable to the man and makes the man's orgasms a lot more intense and pleasurable.

Where Thrusting Should Be Done During Sex

During sex, when the man or the woman is thrusting, the thrusting could be concentrated near the opening of the vagina. This could be done because the nerve endings in the vagina appear to be concentrated near the opening of the vagina. As a matter of fact, the outer third of the vagina, close to the opening of the vagina, contains nearly 90 percent of the vaginal nerve endings and is more sensitive to touch than the inner two thirds of the vagina. The nerve endings in the outer third of the vagina provide significant sexual pleasure when stimulated. The number of the vaginal nerve endings in the middle third of the vagina is more than the number of vaginal nerve endings in the deep inner third of the vagina close to the cervix. There are few nerves at the back of the vagina, so there is little sensation in that area. Therefore, when the man or the woman is thrusting during sex the stimulation of the deep part of the vagina should not be a major concern.

However, when the man or the woman is thrusting deep into the vagina during sex, the stimulation of the cervix might be of concern. Stimulation of the cervix might be of concern because stimulation of certain parts of the cervix produces an intense orgasm for the woman. However, stimulating certain parts of the woman's cervix during sex can be painful to the woman and result in a sensation similar to being kicked in the stomach. It is up to the woman to find out which parts of the cervix are pleasurable for her when stimulated and which parts of the cervix are painful for her when stimulated. The woman should do so because every woman is different when it comes to which parts of the cervix produce pleasure when stimulated. However, one area of the cervix in particular that produces pleasure to every woman is a ring-like structure that encircles the cervix. This ring-like structure is highly erogenous. This ring-like structure, when stimulated during sex, produces intense orgasms for the woman. The ring-like structure in a sexual context is referred to as the deep spot sometimes. The best way to stimulate the cervix is during deep sexual penetration such as when the man enters the woman from behind. During sex, if the woman finds it painful when the man's penis hits the cervix she can simply adjust the angle of penetration.

During sex, whether the man or the woman is thrusting, the G-spot or the area where the G-spot is supposed to be could be stimulated to make the sex more pleasurable to the woman. The G-spot is located about one and a half to two inches from the opening of the vagina. It is located on the front wall of the vagina. It is not responsive to gentle touching. It responds best to firm, deep, continuous pressure. The reason many women do not think they have a G-spot is that the G-spot responds only to firm pressure and that may not occur during sex. However, during sex, the man or the woman can press on the woman's G-spot or the area where the G-spot is supposed to be located from the outside. This can bring her G-spot or the area where the G-spot is supposed to be into fuller contact with the penis and trigger mind-blowing orgasms or intense pleasure. Since the exact position of the G-spot or the area where the G-spot is supposed to be varies between women, a person needs to go by the feel. A person should start by pressing the ball of his or her hand against the woman's navel. If the woman squeals with delight he or she will know that he or she has come to the right place. If the woman does not squeal with the delight a person should gradually move down until the woman does squeal with delight. However, the G-spot does not appear to be present in all women. In many women the G-spot is present and when it is stimulated it produces an orgasm. However, in some women the G-spot does not appear to be present and when that area is stimulated it does not produce an orgasm. Rather, it only produces a great deal of pleasure and that place becomes their favorite place. So it is a good idea to stimulate the G-spot or the area where the G-spot is supposed to be during sex so that the woman experiences intense pleasure.

Stimulating the Clitoris, the Labia Minora, and the Labia Majora

During sex, whether the man or the woman is thrusting, sometimes the thrusting of the penis into the vagina alone does not bring a woman to climax. This is because sometimes the clitoris does not get enough direct stimulation during the thrusting. Therefore, the man or the woman could stimulate the woman's clitoris by hand during sex, so that the woman orgasms consistently during sex. This makes the sexual experience more pleasurable to both the man and the woman. The stimulation of the clitoris during sex should be done slowly and gently, because the clitoris is highly sensitive. The man or the woman can stimulate the clitoris directly or indirectly. He or she could stimulate the clitoris indirectly by stimulating the area around it.

During sex, the man or the woman could stimulate the labia minora and labia majora by touching and stroking them gently with his or her hand. This will send a pleasant sensation rushing through the woman's body during sex, making the sex a lot more pleasurable. This will also make the orgasm a lot more pleasurable. The delicate inner lips that surround the clitoris the labia minora are highly sensitive. As sources of erotic arousal, the labia minora seem to be fully as important as the clitoris. The labia majora pair of outer lips tends to be much less erotically sensitive than the inner lips. However, both the labia majora and labia minora could be stimulated during sex because a large number of women stroke them along with the clitoris when they masturbate.

Breaks During Sex

A couple can make a sexual encounter longer than it takes both the man and the woman to orgasm. A couple can even make the sexual encounter take hours, even though the man and the woman can climax in only 4 or 5 minutes. The woman can climax in 4 or 5 minutes if her clitoris is stimulated sufficiently. A couple can make the sexual encounter take hours by taking several breaks during the sexual encounter. Every time the man or the woman feels getting close to an orgasm the couple could stop the sex and take a break. The couple could do this process as many times as they feel like it. The break should be at least one minute or until the urge of the man or the woman to orgasm subsides. During the break, the couple could kiss, touch each other, hug, cuddle, talk affectionately, and laugh together. All this stuff that leads up to an orgasm is really the main part of having sex. Taking breaks during a sexual encounter makes the sexual encounter more exciting and more pleasurable for both the man and the woman. It makes the orgasms more intense for both the man and the woman. As a matter of fact, the longer the sexual encounter is, the more intense the pleasure during sex and the more intense the orgasm.

Also, if the sexual encounter is over with because the man orgasmed or because both the man and the woman orgasmed, the couple can still make the sex longer by taking breaks. Even though the sexual encounter is over, the couple could continue showing acts of affection to each other like kissing, touching each other, hugging, cuddling, talking affectionately, and laughing together. The couple could continue to do so until the man and the woman are ready to have sex again. Then the couple could have sex again. The couple could repeat this process several times. By the couple doing so, the sexual encounter becomes longer. The separate sexual encounters become one long pleasurable and intense encounter as a result of the breaks in between. The pleasure during sex becomes more intense, and also the orgasm becomes more intense.

There is a third way to make the sexual encounter longer by taking a break. A man can have the woman orgasm through manual or oral sex. Then the couple could take a break, showing acts of affection to each other during the break. Then when both the man and the woman are ready, the couple could resume having vaginal sex. The two separate encounters become one long encounter as a result of the break. This will make the sex a lot more exciting, pleasurable, and fulfilling to both the man and the woman. It will also make the orgasm more intense to both the man and the woman.

Intensifying an Orgasm

It is possible to intensify the pleasure of an orgasm. The intensity of an orgasm depends on the level of sexual arousal or stimulation a person gets during sex. If a person gets a lot of stimulation during sex, the orgasm will be intense. If a person does not get a lot of stimulation during sex, the orgasm will be mild. Stimulation during sex includes kissing, hugging, talking, touching, and licking. A second way a person can intensify an orgasm during sex is for him or her to maintain the same rhythm, continue stimulating the same areas, and maintain the same pressure as his or her partner is getting close to an orgasm. This will make an orgasm intensely pleasurable to the sexual partner.

A third way a person can intensify an orgasm during sex is for him or her to hold off his or her sexual partner's orgasm for a short while. When the sexual partner is about to climax during sex, the person can stop the genital stimulation for 30 to 60 seconds and then restart again. When he or she restarts again he or she cannot zero on the genital spot that his or her sexual partner wants to be touched the most. He or she should stimulate other genital spots until the sexual partner cannot stand it anymore and is very close to orgasming. Then the person can stimulate that spot that the sexual partner wants touched the most. When the person zeros on the spot that his or her sexual partner wants to be touched the most, the person should continue the stimulation until his or her sexual partner orgasms. This will make the orgasm extremely intense for the sexual partner. A person can tell when his or her sexual partner is about to climax from his or her body language and breathing. A person can tell which genital spot the sexual partner wants touched the most by him or her looking at the genital spot he or she is touching when he or she feels his or her sexual partner getting extremely excited and close to an orgasm. If the man is doing this technique, he would look at the vaginal spot that the woman wants touched the most with his penis during sex. If the woman is doing this technique she would look at the penile spot that the man wants touched the most with her vagina during sex.

A fourth way a person can intensify an orgasm during sex is for him or her, right before reaching climax, to squeeze his or her legs tightly together and contract the thigh muscles continuously several times. Each contraction of the thigh muscles should send sexual pleasure through the person's pelvic region. This will give the woman or the man such an intense orgasm that he or she is going to cry out with joy. A fifth way a person can intensify an orgasm during sex is for the person right before his or her partner climaxes to grab his or her partner's buttocks and pull his or her partner deeply into him or her. The thrusting should continue while the partner is pulled deeply into the person. This will not only make the sexual partner's orgasm intense but it will also make the person's orgasm intense. The sixth way a person can intensify an orgasm during sex is for the person to take breaks during sex making the sex longer and delaying the orgasm. The longer the sexual encounter, the more sexual tension there is to release at the time of orgasm, leading to a deeper and more pleasurable climax for both the man and the woman.

A seventh way a person can intensify an orgasm during sex is for the person doing the thrusting to stop the thrusting when his or her sexual partner is feeling intense pleasure before reaching orgasm. He or she would stop the thrusting and watch his or her partner beg for more. This will tease his or her sexual partner greatly making the sexual encounter a lot more pleasurable and exciting. Then the person can resume the thrusting making the pleasure from the thrusting a lot more pleasurable than before. An eighth way to make an orgasm more intense during sex is by the man and the woman climaxing when the penis is still inside the vagina. When the woman climaxes with the penis inside the vagina the climax is a lot more satisfying and fulfilling than if she climaxes with nothing inside her vagina. When the man climaxes with the penis inside the vagina the climax is a lot more satisfying and fulfilling than if he climaxes with the penis not being in the vagina. Both the man and the woman find the fact that the penis is inside the vagina during climax to be very arousing.

A ninth way to make an orgasm more intense during sex is for the man and the woman to know what an orgasm actually is and not have unrealistic expectations about it. An orgasm is a reflex response that is triggered when there is enough buildup of sexual tension from effective stimulation. Sometimes an orgasm is very powerful and intense. Other times, an orgasm is just a gentle wave of release. Sometimes it may be long in duration and other times it may be short in duration. All orgasms are good.

One type of orgasm should not be held up as superior to another type of orgasm. There is no bad orgasm. If a person knows that all orgasms are good and that it is okay to experience mild and short orgasms, then the person will enjoy his or her orgasm more intensely than if he or she did not know that.

Some people, when they orgasm they do so noisily, by panting, moaning, and yelling. Other people, when they orgasm, do so virtually silently. Some people thrash around during climax; others barely move at all. Some people have unrealistic expectations about an orgasm and expect their partner to moan nosily and thrash around during a climax. If a person has unrealistic expectations about how his or her partner should act when he or she orgasms, and if his or her partner does not move around during climax and orgasms silently then the person will not have an intense orgasm. The person will not have an intense orgasm because he or she incorrectly believes that his or her partner is not climaxing. However, if a person has a realistic expectation how his or her partner should act during an orgasm, then he or she will experience an orgasm intensely.

It is important for a person to know that an orgasm is just a peak in sexual pleasure. He or she should know that an orgasm is not a necessity during sex. If a person knows that then the orgasms during sex will be a lot more pleasurable and intense because the person is not worried about having an orgasm.

Full Body Orgasm

An exciting sexual technique is for a person to experience a full body orgasm. An orgasm is a reflex response that is triggered when there is enough buildup of sexual tension from effective stimulation. During an orgasm, involuntary muscle contractions and spasms may occur in various parts of the person's body including the legs, stomach, arms, pelvis, neck, and back. The involuntary muscular contractions and spasms may be felt in the genital area of a person. As a matter of fact, the male experiences rapid, rhythmic contractions of the anal sphincter, the prostate, and the muscles of the penis, while the woman has the muscles of the vagina and uterus relax and contract rhythmically and rapidly. All people find the involuntary muscular contractions pleasurable.

During an orgasm, involuntary muscular contractions occur in various parts of the body, but not in the whole body. The orgasm is usually felt in the genital area and in some parts of the body. However, during a full body orgasm the whole body is involved in muscle contractions. The orgasm is intense and every part of the body is vibrating in orgasm. The orgasm is felt in every part of the body. The full body orgasm is an intense, earth-shattering, romance novel type of orgasm.

Both the man and the woman can experience full body orgasms. In order for a person to experience a full body orgasm, he or she should relax and let go during sex and while orgasming. He or she should focus on the pleasurable sexual sensations throughout his or her body. A person should stay in the moment and aware of himself or herself and his or her partner. He or she should not block out the world when climaxing as people often do. During sex, he or she should breathe deep, slow breaths from the belly and not the chest. Slow, deep breathing will move the pleasurable sensations throughout the whole body. It also tends to make the orgasm longer. The breathing should be in and out from the nostrils. While breathing, a person should make sure that every part of his or her body is relaxed. If any part of his or her body has muscular tension, he or she could relax it during sex by breathing into that area. This will help a person to attain a full body orgasm by integrating his or her whole body into the sexual and orgasmic experience. A person should breathe continuously during sex and during an orgasm and not hold his or her breath, which is typically what most people do. If a person holds his or her breath, the orgasm will be less intense and he or she will not experience a full body orgasm. A person should let his or her body ease into orgasm and let it move any way that feels natural. Also, a person can keep his or her eyes open during sex and look at his or her partner during sex and while orgasming, in order to help him or her experience a full body orgasm.

However, the most important thing that could be done to a woman during sex for her to experience a full body orgasm is the simultaneous stimulation of the G-spot and the clitoris. Usually, the woman can have sex in a position where her G-spot is stimulated by the man's penis. Then she can manually stimulate her clitoris or have her partner stimulate her clitoris manually during sex. The clitoris can be stimulated either directly or indirectly. It can be stimulated indirectly by stimulating the area around it. This simultaneous stimulation of the G-spot and clitoris during sex will cause the woman to experience a full body orgasm. Also, the man should keep his penis inside the vagina when the woman has her full body orgasm since the vaginal muscles contracting around the man's penis increases the orgasmic sensation making a full body orgasm much more intense. For a variation, the man or the woman can manually stimulate the G-spot while the man or the woman manually stimulates the clitoris. This will also produce a full body orgasm.

Furthermore, the most important thing that could be done to a man during sex for him to experience a full body orgasm is the simultaneous stimulation of the penis and the prostate. There are two ways to stimulate the prostate during sex. The first way is for the man to get in a sex position where the woman can easily access his prostate externally during sexual intercourse. The woman should place her index and middle finger on the perineum during sex and apply external pressure to the perineum. The external pressure is applied to the perineum by the woman running her fingers up and down the perineum softly and gently. When the woman moves her fingers up and down the perineum she will find where exactly on the perineum the prostate could be stimulated. She will find that point by seeing the man becoming extremely ecstatic when she touches that point. The perineum is a hairless patch of skin located between the scrotum

Sex Techniques

and the anus. When the perineum is massaged externally, the prostate is indirectly stimulated because the prostate is located just behind the perineum.

The second way to stimulate the prostate during sex is for the man to get in a sex position where the woman can easily access his prostate internally during sexual intercourse. The woman should insert a well lubricated finger into the anus. The prostate gland is reachable with the smallest lady index finger because it can be reached two or three inches inside the anus. The woman should insert her finger while it hooks toward the man's stomach. She should stimulate the prostate by moving the finger in gentle circular or up-and-down strokes against the front wall of the rectum. She should move it slowly and gently in a sustained regular rhythm to give maximum pleasure to the man. Stimulating the front wall of the rectum should stimulate the prostate because the prostate gland is near the front wall of the rectum even though it is not inside the rectum. As a matter of fact, it is located at the base of the penis. The woman can know which area of the front wall of the rectum, when stimulated, stimulates the prostate by feeling for a small bulge at the front wall of the rectum. The small bulge at the front wall of the rectum is the prostate. It feels firm and is the size of a walnut. Stimulating the prostate during sex not only gives the man a full body orgasm, but it makes the man's erection stronger and longer.

There are numerous positions for the couple to use during sex that will give only the woman a fully body orgasm. However, two positions that are worth mentioning are the doggy style position and the face-to-back, side-by-side position. In the doggy style position, the woman is on her hands and knees and the man penetrates her vagina from the rear. This position allows for deep penetration of the vagina by the penis. In this position, the man's penis presses against the front wall of the woman's vagina, thus providing stimulation of the G-spot. The woman can stimulate the clitoris with her hand when the man stimulates her G-spot with the penis, thus providing simultaneous stimulation of the clitoris and the G-spot. This results in a fully body orgasm for the woman. In the second position, the face-to-back, side-by-side position, the woman lies on her side and the man lies on his side behind her. His face is facing the back of her head. He penetrates her vagina with his penis from behind. In this position, the woman's G-spot is stimulated by the man's penis during sex. The man or the woman can stimulate the clitoris manually during sex, thus providing simultaneous stimulation of the clitoris and the G-spot. This results in a fully body orgasm for the woman.

There are numerous positions for the couple to use during sex that will give only the man a fully body orgasm. However, two positions that are worth mentioning are the missionary position and the face-to-face, side-by-side position. In the missionary position, the woman lies flat on her back and the man lies on top of her. He penetrates her vagina with his penis while keeping his legs straight. In this position, the man's penis is stimulated during sex and the woman can stimulate his prostate gland during sex. She can stimulate the prostate gland by stimulating the perineum or by stimulating the front wall of the rectum. The simultaneous stimulation of the prostate and the penis in this position results in a full body orgasm for the man. In the face-to-face, side-by-side position, the man lies on his side and the woman lies on her side facing him. The man penetrates the woman's vagina with his penis. The woman can stimulate the man's prostate in this position by stimulating the perineum or by stimulating the front wall of the rectum. In this position, the penis and the prostate of the man can be stimulated simultaneously during sex, resulting in a full body orgasm for the man.

There are numerous positions for the couple to use during sex that will give the man and the woman a fully body orgasm simultaneously. However, one position that is worth mentioning is the woman on top position. In this position, the man lies flat on his back with his legs straight and the woman straddles his hips with her knees. She sits on top of him with her knees bent. She can be either facing the man's face or facing his feet. In this position, the woman is in control and she can guide the man's penis to stimulate her G-spot as she thrusts up and down on the man's penis. The man can stimulate the woman's clitoris in this position with his hand as she thrusts on his penis. As all this is going on, the woman can stimulate the man's prostate either by stimulating the perineum or the front wall of the rectum. In this position the stimulation of the man's penis and prostate occurs simultaneously with the stimulation of the woman's clitoris and G-spot. This results in a full body orgasm for both the man and the woman simultaneously. This results in an intense explosive moment of happiness and pleasure for both the man and the woman simultaneously.

When is Sex Over With?

Some people incorrectly assume that sex is over with when the man orgasms, whether the woman orgasms or not. They assume so because usually the man orgasms either at the same time that the woman orgasms or earlier. This is the case because the penis is stimulated sufficiently during intercourse, while the clitoris does not always receive sufficient stimulation during intercourse. When the man ejaculates there is usually a refractory period of at least 20 minutes where he cannot get another erection, thus he cannot resume sex. The fact that the man usually cannot resume sex after ejaculation for 20 minutes makes people incorrectly assume that sex is over with when the man orgasms, whether the woman orgasmed or not. Sex is not penetration of the vagina by the penis until the male orgasms only. Sex should continue until both the man and the woman orgasm.

Blue Balls

Although an orgasm is not necessary for a man's sexual fulfillment, sometimes a condition called blue balls occurs in some men. Blue balls is a slang term referring to testicular aching that may occur in some men sometimes when they do not orgasm after getting aroused sexually. This may occur when the blood that fills the vessels in a male's genital area during sexual arousal is not dissipated by orgasm. During blue balls, the testicular aching can range from a mild ache to pain worse than getting kicked in the crotch. During blue balls, the testicles also might feel heavy. The man might also experience pelvic heaviness and aching as a result of blue balls. The term blue balls came to be because of the bluish tint that the balls take on when blood engorges the vessels in the testicles. Technically, it is not the testicles themselves that take on the bluish tinge but the skin of the scrotum that turns blue. The blue occurs because the blood that fills the vessels in a male's genital area becomes stagnant and de-oxygenated. Blood lacking in oxygen becomes darker, hence the skin of the scrotum appears blue. The blood in the man's genital area becomes stagnant and de-oxygenated because the man did not orgasm.

Blue balls can hurt enough to ruin an otherwise pleasant evening. It is not dangerous. The condition blue balls does not usually last long. It usually takes thirty minutes to an hour for the condition blue balls to disappear since that is the time it takes the blood in the genital area to normalize. A man can deal with blue balls by just waiting for the blood in the genital area to normalize or by masturbating himself to orgasm.

Discomfort in a Woman if She Does Not Orgasm

Although an orgasm is not necessary for a woman's sexual fulfillment, sometimes some women experience discomfort if they get sexually aroused and do not orgasm. They will feel nervousness, edginess, or even aching discomfort in their pelvis area. They will also experience discomfort in the clitoris and the area around it. This happens because when a woman gets sexually aroused, her clitoris and genital area usually become engorged with blood that, if not released via orgasm, might cause discomfort in some women sometimes. It usually takes 2 to 3 hours for the blood in the genital area to normalize and for the discomfort to go away. The woman can deal with this discomfort either by waiting for the blood in the genital area to normalize or by masturbating herself to orgasm.

If the Man Ejaculates Before the Woman Climaxes

If the man ejaculates before the woman climaxes, it is not a disaster. Although many people think a fully erect penis is necessary for a woman's sexual satisfaction, this is not true at all. A soft penis can provide a multitude of wonderful sensations for a woman. Also, a fully erect penis is not necessary for a man's sexual satisfaction. Even when the penis is soft, a man, including an impotent man, can experience pleasurable sensations and get sexual satisfaction. Some penises remain erect after an ejaculation while others go limp very quickly. If a man ejaculates before the woman climaxes, it is possible to make the sexual experience pleasurable and satisfying to both. One way is to get into a position where the man inserts his penis into the vagina and he or the woman can stimulate the clitoris with his or her hand. A good position to try is the woman on top position. Then the woman or the man can rub the woman's clitoris and the area surrounding it with his or her hand. A woman will feel great pleasure and will feel satisfied and fulfilled to climax with a limp penis inside her. She may find herself having a strong orgasm around his penis.

A second way the woman can get satisfied sexually with a limp penis is for the couple to get into the woman on top position. The man lies on the floor with his legs straight and the woman straddles his hips with her knees and sits on top of him facing towards his face. The limp penis should be inside the vagina. The woman should get her clitoris to press against the man's pelvis. Then she should slowly rotate her pelvis in small circles without lifting up. The intense stimulation of the woman's clitoris by the man's pelvis will give the woman an orgasm. This stimulation of the limp penis will give the man sexual pleasure even though he does not orgasm. The woman may find herself having a strong orgasm around the man's penis.

A third way the woman can get satisfied sexually with a limp penis is for the couple to get into the woman on top position facing the man. The woman should have her knees straddling the man's hips. She should place the penis up against the man's pubic bone or lower abdomen. Then she should lower her vulva, spread her labia, and then place her clitoris on top of the soft penis. Then she should rub her clitoris continuously back and forth against the soft penis. The woman can lean forward to give the man kisses and massage his chest and arms while doing this technique. The friction of the clitoris against the penis will give both the man and the woman great pleasure. The woman should be able to orgasm from this technique as a result of the clitoris being stimulated.

It is important that the woman gets a chance to orgasm if the man orgasmed before her. This is important so that she gets a chance to get sexual fulfillment and satisfaction, too. Using any of the three techniques described in this section will allow the woman to orgasm with a limp penis. These three techniques are not the same as sex with a man with a great erection. However, in many ways they are more pleasant to the woman. They are more pleasant to the woman because there is more concentration on the clitoral area and on the woman's pleasure. However, the first two techniques are more fulfilling than the third technique to the woman because orgasms are more fulfilling to a woman when the penis is inside the vagina, even if the penis is limp. Orgasms are more fulfilling when the vagina contracts around the limp penis than if it contracts around nothing. The woman should keep the attitude that this is something pleasant in itself when she does either of the three techniques. She should never have the attitude that this is second best. She should do so because in reality this experience is pleasurable and fulfilling to a woman to the greatest degree.

If the Woman Climaxes Before the Man

If the woman climaxes before the man, most of the time the couple could continue having sex because most women are multi-orgasmic. That means that most women can experience several orgasms within one sexual encounter without a refractory period. Therefore, if the man continues having sex after the woman orgasmed, if the woman is multi-orgasmic, the woman will able to continue the sexual intercourse and experience several orgasms during the intercourse. However, some women are not multi-orgasmic. If a woman is not multi-orgasmic, that means that she can experience only one orgasm per sexual encounter and needs to have a refractory period after the orgasm. During the refractory period, the woman usually cannot have sex. Therefore, if a woman orgasmed before the man and she is not multi-orgasmic, she can bring the man to orgasm either manually or orally. If the woman orgasms before the man during sex, she should bring him to orgasm to satisfy and fulfill him sexually.

Multiple Orgasms

If the woman and the man climax during sex, the man's climax is usually sufficient for him. However, sometimes the woman's climax is not sufficient for her. Sometimes the woman might want to climax more because she is multi-orgasmic. A multi-orgasmic woman can experience at least two successive orgasms without a refractory period during a sexual encounter. Therefore, if a woman climaxes during sex and she is multi-orgasmic, she might not be satisfied from one orgasm and might want another one or more. Therefore, if the man sees the woman orgasm during sex he could try stimulating her clitoris manually or orally after she orgasms. If the woman is multi-orgasmic, she will enjoy the continued stimulation of the clitoris and will experience several orgasms from the stimulation.

However, if the woman is not multi-orgasmic, then she will not enjoy the continued stimulation of the clitoris and will find it uncomfortable. The man should not continue stimulating the woman's clitoris or having sex with the woman if he senses that she is not comfortable with the continued stimulation. The man should remember that a large number of women are multi-orgasmic, but not all are multi-orgasmic. A woman that is not multi-orgasmic will find that she can no longer tolerate any more contact with her clitoris and genital area after an orgasm because they are extremely sensitive.

On the other hand, if the man does not continue stimulating the clitoris after the woman orgasms during sex, if the woman still feels she wants more stimulation to orgasm more, she should tell the man that she is with. She should do so, so that the man she is with provides her with the needed stimulation. The woman could also provide her clitoris with continued manual stimulation after an orgasm during sex so that she experiences multiple orgasms if she desires so.

When the man or the woman continues stimulating the clitoris after the woman orgasms, he or she should not wait too long to restart stimulation of the clitoris after the woman orgasms. This is because if he or she waits too long the woman's body may move into a refractory period, making a second orgasm less likely. When the man or the woman continues stimulating the clitoris after the woman orgasms, he or she should do so gently and slowly. It should be done gently and slowly since the clitoris is most likely to be very sensitive after an orgasm.

Do Not Worry about an Erection and Arousal During Sex

During sex, the intensity of the man's erection tends to fluctuate several times. It may rise to the maximum then decrease then rise again to the maximum. This may happen several times. Neither the man nor the woman should be alarmed if this happens during sex. This is perfectly normal. If either the man or the woman worries about it then the person worrying about it will have his or her pleasure during sex reduced. Also, the woman may not be able to have an orgasm if she worries about the man's erection decreasing during sex. The man also may not be able to regain his erection and have an orgasm if he worries about his erection decreasing during sex. Both the man and the woman should ignore the fact that the erection decreased during sex and they should continue the sexual encounter. It is important that the thrusting continue. If this happens then the erection will return and the pleasure during sex will be the maximum for the man and the woman. Also, the orgasm will be intense and pleasurable to both the man and the woman.

It is important to note that if the man lies on his back during sex sometimes he will lose an erection during sex because by him being on his back gravity will draw blood away from his penis. However, if the man were to turn on his stomach during the sexual encounter and thrust he will regain his erection. Also, when a man is totally receptive during sex and not giving any form of stimulation to the woman, sometimes he will lose his erection. When the man becomes active again, taking the initiative and pleasuring his partner, he will usually become erect very quickly.

From time to time, a man cannot get an erection. This is normal and happens to all males. The man might be tired or under stress and not in the mood to have sex. The man can use manual or oral sex techniques to satisfy his partner sexually if this happens. After a while, the man can try having sexual intercourse if he feels like it. If he still cannot get an erection and still wants to have sex then he can use any of the three techniques described in this chapter in the section, If the Man Ejaculates Before the Woman Climaxes. Doing so will let both the man and the woman experience sexual pleasure and satisfaction. It will also let the woman experience an orgasm. There is a myth that impotence or temporary impotence can be overcome by the man taking charge of his penis. The men who are the least potent are the ones who try to control their erection and force it to happen during sex. The men who are the most potent are the ones who do not try to control their erection at all during sex. The harder a person tries to get or maintain an erection the less likely he will get or keep one.

Both the man's and the woman's sexual arousal tends to build in waves during sex. There is a peak in sexual arousal followed by an ebb or diminishing of the intensity of feelings and then a new wave of sexual arousal that is more intense than the previous one. If a person does not worry about the decrease in sexual arousal when it happens and continues to enjoy the sexual encounter, then he or she will experience a new wave of sexual arousal that is more intense than the earlier one. However, if a person worries about the decrease in sexual arousal, that will stop his or her sexual response from occurring in its natural wavelike pattern. If this occurs to either the man or the woman, this will cause a decrease in his or her pleasure during sex. If this occurs to the man it, may prevent him from keeping an erection and orgasming. Also, if this happens to the woman it may prevent her from orgasming.

Do Not Accept Bad Sexual Behavior

In order for the sexual encounter to be pleasurable to the greatest extent to both partners, neither partner should submit to a sexual encounter where he or she is mistreated or unhappy. A person should never do anything during sex that he or she or his or her partner does not like to be done. A person should never let anything that he or she does not like to be done, be done to him or her during sex.

After Sex Play

After the man and the woman orgasm during sex, some people incorrectly believe that the sexual encounter is over with. The man or the woman, after orgasming, sometimes falls asleep, or jumps into the shower. Sometimes he or she just gets out of bed and goes on with his or her normal every day routine. The man and the woman should realize that after both of them orgasm during sex, the sexual encounter is not over with. They should realize that there is another stage to the sexual encounter. That stage is the after sex play stage.

The after sex play stage is necessary because some people's sexual tension is not released intensely and rapidly after sex. Rather it occurs gradually. The more gradual a person's body returns to its pre-stimulated state, the more a person is in need of the after sex play stage. The after sex play stage is a time where both people talk, touch each other, kiss each other, hug, cuddle, laugh together, and play together. This stage is important to help a person's body get rid of its vasocongestion and return to its pre-stimulated state. Usually a woman has a gradual release of her sexual tension after sex while the man usually has an intense and rapid release of his sexual tension after sex. That is why a man usually feels sleepy and goes to sleep after sex, while the woman stays wide awake, irritable and tense. She finds herself in need of being touched, kissed, hugged, and cuddled. She finds herself in need of affection. However, there are cases where the man has a more gradual release of sexual tension and the woman has a more rapid release of sexual tension.

After the man and the woman orgasm during sex, if a person has a gradual release of sexual tension, he or she will feel irritable and tense if there is not an after sex play stage. However, if a person has an intense and rapid release of sexual tension then he or she will feel satisfied without an after sex play stage. However, an after sex play stage will make a person that has an intense and rapid release more satisfied and fulfilled with the sexual experience. An after sex play stage makes both the person with a gradual release of sexual tension and a person with a rapid release of sexual tension feel satisfied with the sexual experience and makes them feel that the sexual experience was pleasurable to the greatest degree.

During the after sex play stage the couple could talk pillow talk, making the experience more exciting and pleasurable. Also, the couple could play together and laugh together, making the experience fun. The couple could hug and cuddle together, which makes both of them feel deep intimacy. The couple could touch and kiss each other, showing each other affection. Furthermore, during the after sex play stage, the man could remain next to the woman with his penis inside her for five minutes. Even though the man's erection subsides, he could keep his penis inside her vagina since this makes the couple feel amazing intimacy and lets them feel fulfilled from the sexual encounter. It lets both people feel fulfilled from the closeness of their body to each other.

The after sex play stage lets both people feel tenderness and closeness to each other. Also, it lets both people feel intense caring and affection to each other. Both people feel that they love each other and that they are important to each other as a result of the after sex play stage.

When Sex is Not Working in the Bedroom

Sex should be a wonderful thing that is an incredibly sensual and exciting experience for both partners. When sex is not working in the bedroom, it is either because of relationship issues or because of lack of sexual techniques that are pleasurable to both parties during sex. Understanding the source of the problem is the first step. The second step is to rectify it. If the source was a relationship issue then the relationship issue needs to be corrected. If the source was lack of sexual techniques that are pleasurable to both parties during sex then both parties should use sexual techniques that are pleasurable to both of them. Rectifying the problem will make the sex in the bedroom pleasurable, fulfilling, and satisfying to both parties. It will also lead to greater passion and intimacy entering the relationship.

Chapter 20

Variety During Sex

In a new relationship between a man and woman, the initial chemistry ignites passion and excitement during sex that is intense and requires no work. But after the initial excitement of being in a new relationship wears off, usually the sex becomes less pleasurable, dull, and boring. The reason the sex becomes less pleasurable, boring, and dull is because the sexual encounter usually becomes routine. The couple usually follows the same sexual script with each encounter. The sex usually occurs at the same time and at the same place. It also begins and ends the same way. A couple making the sexual encounters routine is like a person eating his or her favorite meal every day. After a while, a person no longer would salivate and desire his favorite meal because he or she gets bored and tired of eating it. Any pleasurable activity can become boring after a while if it is done the same way each time, even sex. This is because a response tends to decrease when presented with the same stimulus time after time. Scientists call it habituation. Sexual arousal is a response and it tends to decrease when presented with the same stimulus time after time. In the case of sex, the same stimulus is usually having the sex the same way time after time. Therefore, the key to great sex all the time is variety. By the couple having the sexual encounter differently each time, the sex remains exciting and pleasurable to the greatest extent. The sex remains pleasurable to the greatest extent and exciting no matter how long the relationship goes on, as long as the sexual encounter is done differently each time.

Variety is the spice of life and it can spice up a couple's sex life. Variety in all forms of sexual intimacy will lead to more pleasure during sex. Variety can be in many forms, including touching, talking, kissing, thrusting, and moving during sex. Variety can also be in using different sexual toys and different sexual techniques during sex. Variety can also be in using a different setting during sex. Changing one simple thing during sex is enough to cause great excitement and pleasure during sex. It can make a person feel like he or she is having sex with a new partner. For example, changing the angle of thrusting, the sexual position in a series of positions, the sequence of sexual positions, one sexual technique, or one way of moving during sex is enough to cause great excitement and pleasure during sex. It is important that a person does not hold rigid stereotypes of what is appropriate during sex. A person should be open to anything as long as it feels good to him or her and his or her partner.

Usually, once a person finds a method that gets him or her excited during sex, he or she does not usually experiment even though there may be alternatives available which work just as well or better. Having an exciting sex life is about exploring. A couple should find new ways to please each other during sex. There are numerous sexual techniques for a couple to use to please each other. Each couple is different. Some techniques work for a certain couple, but do not work for other couples. The couple should go with what is comfortable to both people during sex. A person should be versatile during sex because his or her partner's needs during sex are different from minute to minute and from one encounter to another. Also, no two people are alike. If a person's previous partner found a certain move pleasurable it does not mean that this partner will find the same move pleasurable. Sex should not be an acrobatic ordeal, nor an act requiring great strength and agility. If a technique is used from time to time, that is perfectly okay as long as it is not used consistently in each encounter. If a technique is used consistently in each encounter it tends to lose its effectiveness in producing pleasure during sex after a while. However, if a technique is used from time to time during sex, it does not lose its effectiveness in producing pleasure during sex. For example, a person could use the same technique during five sexual encounters in a row, then the next three encounters he or she does not use the technique, then after that he or she uses the technique three sexual encounters in a row, which causes the technique to remain effective because it is used from time to time and not consistently. If a technique is used from time to time during sex the person when he or she does it should have the attitude that it is new and act as if it is new and exciting. He or she should not act as if it is boring or routine.

Variety during a sexual encounter is most likely to occur when both people are free to enjoy each other's body with creativity and variety. It is the freedom in the relationship that allows both the man and the woman to experiment and try things sexually that they have not tried before. By trying new things they have not tried before a couple will add new sensations to their sexual experience, making them both feel amazingly sexually aroused. If there is variety in a sexual encounter, even if a sexual technique is used by a couple from time to time, it provides a feeling of newness during the sexual encounter. Also, a person can have variety during a sexual encounter by being flexible and spontaneous. The more sex techniques a person knows, the more fantastic his or her sex life will be, and the better of a lover he or she will be. This is so because he or she will have a greater amount of techniques available to create variety during a sexual encounter.

A person usually does not try new things during sex because he or she is embarrassed or afraid of rejection. Deep down the person may doubt his or her ability to be an exciting lover, so he or she shies away from trying new things during sex. Also, a person does not try new things during sex because he or she is afraid that they will fail to produce pleasure. In addition, the fact that a person is afraid to be guided by his or her own internal desires and urges during sex usually makes a person not try new things during sex.

Most couples have a very boring sex life. After being in the relationship together a while, they feel distanced or disconnected from each other. The relationship may lack sex and physical affection like touching and hugging. Sometimes one partner or both start looking for more exciting sex by trying to have an affair. This can be disastrous to a relationship and could lead to an end of it. All these negative effects of a boring sex life usually happen because eventually the couple develops a habit of making love with a certain pattern. Acquiring a pattern of making love is the start of boredom, and breaking that pattern can be the road to excitement, ecstasy, and new discovery. Once a person has been in a monogamous relationship for a while, he or she may begin to feel the need to spice things up in the bedroom. This is a perfectly normal feeling. It is not a sign of insecurity or that something is wrong with his or her partner. Great sex is no longer something that just happens on its own, but can still be experienced by a couple making a conscious effort to have it. A sexual relationship, like any relationship, needs maintenance and nurturing. A couple could maintain the sexual relationship so that it is pleasurable to the greatest extent to both people by having variety in the sexual encounters.

Variety not only allows a person to satisfy his or her partner sexually, but it also lets the partner beg for more sexual stimulation. It is important to have variety in a person's sex life because a boring sex life is the leading cause of divorces and relationship breakups. Variety will transform a boring sex life and loveless relationship into an exciting sex life and loving relationship. Variety lets a couple's sex life be adventurous. It makes a couple's love and lust for each other stay strong. Variety intensifies a person's sexual desire. Variety lets a couple build sexual intimacy and passion in their sexual relationship that is deep and fulfilling and that will last a lifetime.

Variety in the Location of the Sexual Encounter

If the couple changes the location where they have sex from time to time, that will make their sex life more pleasurable and exciting. It will energize their relationship and put a new spark into it. Just the fact that the couple is changing the locations where they have sex from time to time will make the sexual encounters seem new and not routine. The couple could take turns choosing the location to have sex from time to time. This adds the element of surprise to the sexual encounter since a person does not know where the sexual encounter is going to be until his or her partner tells him or her where it is going to be.

Unfortunately, most people incorrectly view the bedroom as the only place that is appropriate to have sex. They do not realize that their entire house can be a sexual playpen. They do not realize that other places other than their house can be a sexual playpen as well. They fail to realize that by them making the bedroom the only place that is appropriate to have sex in and having sex in the same room over and over for years, they make their sex life boring and monotonous. They fail to realize that it decreases their pleasure during the sexual encounters.

Virtually any room can be an erotic venue for the couple as long as they are assured their privacy. The couple could have the best sex when they have sex in a room other than the bedroom. The couple's sensations of being nude in another room other than the bedroom or bathroom and making love feels deliciously forbidden, making the sexual encounter more exciting and pleasurable. For example, if the couple has sex in the kitchen or in the living room it will feel deliciously forbidden, making the sex more exciting and pleasurable. The couple having sex in the bathroom can also feel deliciously forbidden. In the bathroom, the couple could have sex in different places, including inside the shower or bathtub. The couple can have sex in the shower with the water running on them. They could also have sex in the bathtub filled with soap suds as a result of a bubble bath. If the couple has sex in the shower or bathtub and water is involved, that is very romantic and intensifies the sexual pleasure of both people.

Regardless of which room the couple could have sex in, the couple does not have to have sex on a bed. They could have it on anything including on the floor, carpet, couch, table, or chair. In fact, sex that's not on the bed is the most fun and exciting sex that will occur. It is exciting and pleasurable because it is different than the usual sex on the bed. There are numerous things on which the couple could have sex on, however one place that is worth mentioning is the rocking chair. Using a rocking chair without arms, a woman can sit on top of the man either facing him or facing away from him and the couple could gently rock together as they have sex. This would produce wonderful sensations to the couple.

The couple could also have sex in places other than the house to add variety to the sexual encounters. There are numerous places other than the house where a couple could have sex. These include the beach, car, hotel, cruise, backyard, park, pool, Jacuzzi, and cabin in the woods. The couple could have sex in a tent while camping. However, wherever the couple has sex, they have to make sure that no one is around because they do not want to get arrested for indecent exposure.

The beach is a very exciting place for the couple to have sex at because both the man and the woman enjoy the sensations of the soft sand as they make love. They also enjoy the sound of the waves while having sex. If the couple cannot guarantee their privacy at the beach, they could have sex in a tent on the beach. They could have the bottom of the tent removed. That way they feel the sensations of the sand as they make love. The pool and Jacuzzi are also a favorite place for many couples to have sex because the water gives them a sense of weightlessness and increases the intensity of the sex. The water also acts as a natural lubricant, making insertion of the penis easier. An additional benefit of the water is that it is relaxing and soothing.

Many people have fantasies of making love in a parked car. They view it as very exciting. Today's cars have seats that will recline all the way back, making it quite comfortable to have sex in a car. By a couple having sex in a parked car, they can make those fantasies come true. The couple could also have sex in the backyard or park. The sensations of the grass in the backyard or the park as the couple makes love will make the sex extremely delightful. If the couple cannot guarantee their privacy in the backyard or park they could have sex in a tent in the backyard or park. They could have the bottom of the tent removed. That way they feel the sensations of the grass as they make love.

The couple could travel to different areas and have sex in a hotel. The fact that the couple is having sex in different areas makes the sex more erotic and interesting. For example, the couple could travel to Hawaii and have sex in a hotel room on the beach. Or the couple could travel to New York and have sex in a hotel room where it is snowing. The fact that the couple is changing the setting, once it is on the beach and the other time it is where there is snow the sex becomes extremely thrilling. The couple could take a cruise and have sex on a cruise. The fact that the couple is having sex while cruising in the sea makes the sexual encounter extremely pleasurable. The couple could spend time in a cabin in the woods, and have sex there. The fact that the couple is in the woods away from civilization with no distractions other than each other the sexual encounter becomes intensely delightful. The couple could have sex in a tent while camping. The fact that the couple is having sex while camping makes the sexual encounter more pleasurable.

When the couple travels and has sex, the couple frequently finds that their sexual interest in one another miraculously intensifies. This usually happens because they are away from their everyday routine and away from their usual setting. It also happens since they are on vacation and are not tired, stressed, or overworked. A couple cannot always afford to travel long distances to have a sex vacation. Therefore, the couple should consider taking one day and one night vacations that are not too far or too expensive several times during the year to revitalize their relationship and sex life. This will make the couple's sex life exciting, pleasurable and continuously fresh.

In conclusion, the couple could add variety to their sexual encounters by changing the location from time to time. The location could be a different location in the same house, or a different location outside the house. The couple could also change on what they have sex from time to time to add more variety to the sexual encounters. The couple, instead of having sex on a bed, could have sex on the carpet, floor, table, chair, or couch. The couple could take turns choosing the location and on what to have sex. This will add the element of surprise to the sexual encounter making it more thrilling. Finally, the couple could travel and have sex while on vacation making the sex intensely more pleasurable and exciting.

Variety in the Atmosphere of the Location

Even if a person is having sex in the same room over and over for a while, he or she can make the experience seem to be new each time it occurs by changing the atmosphere of the location from time to time. The lighting, smell, and sounds in a room could be changed from time to time to create variety in the sexual encounters. A relaxed, sensual atmosphere that varies from time to time makes the sexual encounters extremely pleasurable and exciting.

The easiest way to change the atmosphere of the location is to change the lighting of the room. Changing the lighting in a room not only changes the atmosphere of the room, but it also affects the mood of the couple. A person can use blue light bulbs in a room to create a mysterious and sensual atmosphere ideal for sex. He or she can use pink light bulbs to provide light that is soft, romantic, and flattering. The pink light makes most people look much younger than they actually are. A person can use red light bulbs to make the room seem like a brothel and to make him or her and his or her partner extremely horny. Another way to use lighting to change the atmosphere of the room is to change the brightness of the lights. A person sometimes can use bright lights in the room, and at other times he or she could use dim lighting. Dim lighting is a good source of a romantic and erotic mood. A person can create dim lighting by using a dimmer switch on the lights or he or she can use a bulb with low voltage. Another way a person can create dim lighting is to use candles in the room. Candlelight makes a person look more beautiful, so it is a good idea for a couple to position candles around the room from time to time. Varying the lighting in the room from time to time makes a couple's visual enjoyment of each other's bodies during sex enhanced. This leads to very delightful and thrilling sexual encounters.

The second way a person can change the atmosphere of the location is by changing the sounds in the room. The easiest way to change the sounds in a room is to play music in the room and change the music being played in the room from time to time. Music that is relaxing when played on a low volume provides a romantic and erotic mood. Soft music can be quite romantic. Music with a steady pulsing rhythm can inspire powerful, passionate lovemaking. A person should not play any music that is annoying or distracting. If he or she does so, it will reduce his or her pleasure during sex. Also, a couple can use environmental sounds in the room from time to time instead of music. An example of environmental sounds is a recording of the sounds of the river flowing. Another example of environmental sounds is a recording of waves of the ocean splashing against the beach. Each type of environmental sound when played in the room creates a different atmosphere in the room. Environmental sounds contribute to a romantic and sensual atmosphere. Furthermore, a person can use no sounds in the room from time to time. Silence during sex that is interrupted only by deep breathing and sighs of pleasure is the best sound imaginable during sex.

The third way a person can change the atmosphere of the room is by changing the scent in the room. The idea is to create a fragrance atmosphere that will turn both people on during sex, making the sex more arousing and exciting. Ylang-ylang, jasmine, sandalwood, rose, patchouli, cedar wood, lavender, or clary sage are some specific scents that have been shown to excite a person's senses and act as a sexual stimulant in the brain. There are other scents that a person could use also. A person can release scents in the room by lighting candles that contain these fragrances around the room. A second way a person could release scents in the room is by placing sachets that contain these fragrances around the room. A third way a person could release scents in the room is by using an aromatherapy diffuser. One type of aromatherapy diffuser a person could use is to place essential oils in a diffuser over a light bulb. The heat from the light bulb will release the fragrance into the air. A person also, could use the smell of incense burning to change the atmosphere of the room. In addition, a person could use perfumes or colognes to change the atmosphere of the room. However, a person from time to time could use nothing to change the scent of a room. The smell of two natural, freshly bathed bodies during sex is the best smell imaginable during sex.

There are other ways besides these three main ways for the couple to change the atmosphere in the room. The couple could have a pornographic movie play in the room from time to time, which would create an erotic atmosphere. However, a person should not use pornography in a sexual encounter if his or her partner finds it offensive. A person could also change the things present in the room from time to time to make the atmosphere in the room different. For example, the person could put a small water fountain from time to time in the room. The sound and sight of the water flowing is very romantic and erotic. Another example is the person could put flowers in the room from time to time. A large bouquet near where the couple is having sex will please both of them with its beauty and fragrance. An additional example is the person could change the sheets, blankets, or comforters in the room from time to time and use ones with different colors or different materials. The final example is a person could put a full length mirror in the room from time to time. The couple could make love in front of the full length mirror. The couple seeing each other in the mirror making love could find the encounter to be very sexually exciting and pleasurable.

Variety in Time of Day, Frequency, and Duration of Sex

A couple could spice up their sex by changing the frequency that they have sex from time to time. For example, if a couple usually has sex three times a week, they could change the frequency to two times a week or four times a week. The change in frequency, whether it is an increase or a decrease results in a more exciting and pleasurable sex life.

Also, a couple could spice up their sex by changing the time of day that they have sex from time to time. For example, if the couple usually has sex in the morning they could have it during the day or in the evening. There is no right or wrong time to have sex. A couple can have sex anytime during the twenty-four-hour period. Therefore, a couple from time to time can change the time that they usually have sex to make their sexual encounters more exciting and more pleasurable. In addition, if a couple is usually spontaneous about having a sexual encounter, then they could try planning a sexual encounter from time to time. However, if a couple usually plans for a sexual encounter, they could have it spontaneously from time to time. The change in how the sexual encounter occurs, whether it is spontaneous or planned, adds variety to the sexual encounter, making it more thrilling and delightful.

The couple can change the duration of time that they have sex from time to time to add variety to their sex life. For example, if the couple usually has sex for forty-five minutes they can usually change the duration of time either to thirty minutes or to an hour. Whether the couple increases or decreases the duration of time that they have sex from time to time, it will serve to make their sex life more exciting, pleasurable, and satisfying. Even though the sexual encounter should be at least thirty minutes to be fulfilling to both people, especially the woman, the couple could make it shorter from time to time. The encounter is usually at least thirty minutes because the woman needs at least 20 minutes foreplay, then at least five minutes is required for the actual sex act, and then at least five minutes is required for the after sex play.

When the couple has quick sex, affectionately it is known as a quickie. The quickie can feel amazing and thrilling because it breaks the predictability of the couple's sex life. A quickie can occur when one or both people are still wearing some of their clothes. It can be spontaneous. It adds some fast fun to the couple's sex life. However, the couple should have sexual encounters less than thirty minutes only occasionally, because they are usually not fulfilling and pleasurable to the greatest extent to both people. The only reason they are very exciting and very pleasurable is because they are done occasionally and offer a variation to the sexual encounter. However, if the quickie is done often, it no longer is thrilling and pleasurable.

Variety in What a Person Wears to a Sexual Encounter

A person can change what he or she wears to a sexual encounter from time to time to add variety to the sexual encounters. The man can sometimes wear a suit with a tie to a sexual encounter. The fact that he looks very nice with the suit on will cause great excitement to the man and the woman before and during the sexual encounter. The man can also wear tight jeans and a tight shirt to a sexual encounter. This will make him look very sexually attractive to his or her partner. This will cause great excitement to both of them before and during the sexual encounter. The man can also wear pants and be half naked on top. This makes him look very seductive to the woman. This will make the sexual encounter thrilling and delightful to the both of them. The man can also wear tight shorts with a tight shirt. This makes him look very sexually appealing to the woman. This will make the sexual encounter thrilling and pleasurable to the both of them. The man can also wear tight shorts only with nothing on top. This will drive his woman wild with desire, making the sexual encounter pleasurable to the both of them. The man can also wear to a sexual encounter just underwear. This will make him look irresistible to his woman, making the sexual encounter pleasurable to the both of them. The man can change the colors and styles of the clothes to add variety to the sexual encounter.

A woman can sometimes wear a suggestive night gown to the sexual encounter. This will make her look very sexually appealing to the man. This will result in a very exciting sexual encounter for both the man and the woman. A woman can wear a formal dress or a formal skirt and top to the sexual encounter. This will make the woman look very nice. The fact that the woman looks nice will make the man and the woman thrilled before and during the sexual encounter. A woman can wear a tight shirt and tight pants to the sexual encounter. The man will find that very sexy and the woman will feel sexy. This will make both the man and the woman excited before and during the sexual encounter. The woman can wear a bra and panties to a sexual encounter. This will make her look very sexually appealing to the man. This will make the man and the woman have a very thrilling sexual encounter. A woman can also wear nothing but a thong, which will make the man lust for her. This will make the sexual encounter extremely thrilling to both the man and the woman. A woman can wear black lacy lingerie to the sexual encounter, causing great sexual excitement to both the man and the woman. A woman can change the colors and styles of the clothes to add variety to the sexual encounter. Also, a woman can wear high heeled shoes to a sexual encounter. She can change the styles and colors of the high heeled shoes. The high heeled shoes will make the woman feel sexy, and will make the man see the woman as sexy. This will make the sexual encounter more pleasurable to both the man and the woman. As a matter of fact, there is a fetish that is called altocalciphilia. This fetish is a high heeled shoe fetish. This is the fetish where the male gets carried away by the sight of a woman's high heeled shoes before a sexual encounter.

There is another fetish called podophilia. It is very common among both men and women. It is a shoe fetish where a person derives sexual pleasure from seeing a certain type of shoes worn on his or her partner's feet. Therefore, a man and a woman can change the type of footwear that they wear to a sexual encounter to add variety to a sexual encounter. The footwear that a person wears to a sexual encounter does affect the sexual encounter. It is important that the man and the woman remember that the best outfit to be worn to a sexual encounter from time to time is for a person to be totally in the nude with no footwear. This is very exciting and thrilling to both the man and the woman.

Both the man and the woman can change the color of their hair or the style of their hair to add variety to a sexual encounter. The man or the woman can wear a wig to a sexual encounter to add variety to the sexual encounter. The man or the woman can use different designs and different colors of wigs to add variety to the sexual encounter.

It is important that the man and the woman do not overlook the fact that what they wear to a sexual encounter does affect the outcome of a sexual encounter. They should remember to change what they wear to a sexual encounter from time to time to add variety to the sexual encounters. As a matter of fact there are several fetishes in regards to what a person wears to a sexual encounter. One such fetish is wearing rubber clothes to a sexual encounter. The texture and odor of the rubber clothes are a great turn on for the rubber enthusiast. Also, rubber makes the wearer very hot and sweaty thereby adding to the sexual appeal of the wearer. Another fetish is wearing leather clothes to a sexual encounter. The texture and odor of the leather clothes are a great turn on for the leather enthusiast.

Covered with Stuff During Sex

Variety during sexual encounters can occur by one person or two people during intercourse being covered with stuff. A person can also change what he or she and his or her partner cover their bodies with during sex from time to time to add variety to the sexual encounters. There are many things that a person or two people could be covered with during sex. However, there are several worth mentioning. Flower petals could cover one person or both people during sex. The fact that a couple is having sex with flower petals makes the sexual encounter very romantic and pleasurable. A second thing that a person or both people could be covered with during sex is leaves. When a couple has sex with leaves being involved, the sexual encounter becomes very exciting. The feeling of the leaves during sex against a person's skin is very sensuous. A third thing that a person or both people could be covered with during sex is massage oil. If a person's body is covered all over with sweet smelling massage oil, then the sexual encounter will be very ecstatic. The massage oil will enhance the pleasure of both people's skin touching each other. It will give a creamy smooth feel to the skin when touched. A person's body will glide smoothly against his or her partner's body during sex if his or her partner has massage oil on it.

The fourth thing that a person or both people could be covered with during sex is shaving cream. Both people could jump in the shower and blast shaving cream on each other's body. The shaving cream will make both people's bodies slippery during sex. This will make the sex very thrilling. Once the couple finishes having sex with the shaving cream on them in the shower they could turn on the water and wash away the shaving cream from each other's body. The fifth thing that a person or both people could be covered with during sex is soap suds. The couple could put a shower curtain on the bed or floor, or they could get an inflatable mattress. One person or both people could lather their bodies with soap suds. One person would lie on his or her back and another person would lie on top of him or her. The person on top would swish up and down his or her partner's body during sex, making the sex extremely delightful and thrilling.

A person's body or both people's bodies could be covered with something that is edible. This makes the sexual encounter even more exciting and pleasurable because not only is a person's body covered with stuff which is different, but also the partner can eat and lick stuff off the person's skin during sex. One person or both people can cover the entire body, or just some parts of the body, or just the genital area with stuff that is edible. Usually, if a person's body or both people's bodies are covered all over with stuff that is edible, that makes the sexual encounter more exciting and pleasurable. It is more exciting and pleasurable because a person finds it exciting for his or her sexual partner to eat stuff from all over his or her body during sex. Anything placed on a woman's breasts and eaten is very erotic to both the man and the woman. Also, anything placed on a woman's genital area or the man's genital area and eaten is very sexually exciting for both the man and the woman.

There are many things that are edible that a person or both people could use to cover their bodies during sex. A person or both people could crush berries on their bodies and have their sexual partner clean it off with his or her mouth during sex. This is very erotic. A person or both people could squeeze grapes on their bodies, and have the juices run over their bodies. Then their sexual partner could lick or suck it off. This is very sexually arousing to the couple during sex, making the sexual encounter a lot more pleasurable and exciting. Furthermore, a person or both people could cover their bodies during sex with honey, chocolate syrup, maple syrup, jelly or whipped cream. These stuff are great for pouring onto the body and are great for licking off the body parts. They are also great for eating during sex. Not only do they make the sexual encounter pleasurable because they feel great against both people's skin during sex, they make the sexual encounter more exciting and pleasurable because they stimulate the sense of smell and taste during sex as well.

In addition, a person or both people could paint their bodies with yogurt, ice cream, or custard. Such foods are a special treat to lick off a partner's body during sex. Not only do they feel good against the skin during sex, but they also taste good during sex. Other edible stuff that could be used during sex to cover a person or both people's bodies are edible paints or cake icing. They can be used to decorate a person or both people's bodies during sex. They are pleasant to look at during sex. They feel good during sex. They also taste and smell good during sex. They make the sexual encounter extremely thrilling and delightful. A person or both people could put wine, liquor, or champagne on their bodies during sex. This will make their bodies slippery during sex, making the sexual encounter more exciting. Also, a person could lick the stuff off his or her partner's body during sex, which is very exciting. The taste of wine, liquor, or champagne during sex is very stimulating and intoxicating.

A person can put food on his or her partner's body before sex, during a sexual break, or after sex. The person can eat the food off his or her lover's body. He or she can put a variety of food on his or her partner's body. Grapes, figs, and sushi are some of the foods that could be used. However, it should never be forgotten that the most delicious thing that a person can bring to his or her sexual encounter is himself or herself. The taste of a person's bare skin during sex is the most delicious thing in the whole world to his or her sexual partner. Also, the taste of a person's lips during sex is very sexually arousing to his or her partner.

Variety in Touching During Sex

Some people incorrectly believe that the penis and the vagina are the sole source of sexual pleasure during sex. A person's whole body is the source of sexual pleasure during sex. As a matter of fact, the skin is the largest sex organ. The most pleasurable part of sexual intimacy and intercourse is the person's experience of touching and being touched by his or her partner all over his or her body. When a person is touched during sex it makes him or her feel loved, happy, accepted, calm, and reassured. It also promotes the release of oxytocin, which is a hormone that promotes bonding between two people. Touching during sex is a way for a person to show his or her love and affection to his or her partner. It is also a way to promote bonding between both people. If both people during sex only stimulate each other's genital area, without stimulating other parts of each other's bodies, then the sexual encounter won't be very pleasurable. However, if both people during sex not only stimulate each other's genital area, but also stimulate other parts of each other's bodies by touching them, then the sexual encounter will be pleasurable to the greatest extent to both people.

A person can use any part of his or her body to touch any part of his or her partner's body during sex. This intensifies the couple's sexual pleasure during sex. However, there are certain parts of a person's body that are more sensitive to sexual stimulation than other parts. They are known as erogenous zones. An erogenous zone is the part of the body which when touched will send pleasurable sensations throughout the body, and sometimes it might send pleasurable shivers throughout the body. When an erogenous zone is stimulated it will give a person a sense of intense relaxation. This will occur more likely if the erogenous zone is stimulated repeatedly. Erogenous zones exist because some spots on the skin have more sensory nerve endings than other areas of the skin, which allows greater stimulation when touched. Both men and women have erogenous zones on their bodies. The locations of the erogenous zones vary not just from gender to gender but from person to person. It is possible that an erogenous zone in one woman might not be an erogenous zone in another woman. It is also possible that an erogenous zone in one man might not be an erogenous zone in another man. However, there are several areas of the male and female body which are more likely than others to be an erogenous zone.

The erogenous zones that are common to most men are the mouth, tongue, penis, testicles, prostate, nipples, ears, anus, buttocks, scrotum, perineum, neck, shoulders, scalp, inner thighs, and toes. The erogenous zones that are common to most women are the mouth, tongue, vagina, clitoris, labia minora, labia majora, anus, buttocks, nipples, breasts, neck, shoulders, ears, perineum, scalp, mons pubis, inner thighs, and toes. In both the man and the woman, usually the ticklish spots are erogenous zones also. Examples of ticklish spots that might be erogenous zones are the palms of the hands, bottoms of the feet, armpits, and the ribcage. In both the man and the woman other erogenous zones that have not been discussed in this paragraph exist, but they vary from individual to individual. During sex, a person needs to find the other erogenous zones on his or her partner's body. A person can tell which areas are the other erogenous zones by seeing which areas produce more powerful pleasurable sensations than the rest of the body, when they are touched.

By a person changing the erogenous zones that he or she stimulates on his or her partner's body during sex from time to time, this will cause variety in the sexual encounters. This will cause the sexual encounters to be more pleasurable and exciting. Even during the same sexual encounter, a person needs to vary the erogenous zones that he or she stimulates to make the encounter more exciting and pleasurable. A person should not stick to one erogenous zone during the encounter, since the pleasure from stimulating the same area for too long will decrease and sometimes wear out.

During sex, a person should touch his or her partner's body gently, slowly, sensuously, and with feeling. By a person touching his or her partner's body gently and slowly, both people will experience the greatest pleasure from the touching. The slower a person touches his or her partner during sex, the more sensation is provoked. However, a person can touch his or her partner slowly during sex and then increase the speed. He or she could continue increasing the speed until the maximum speed that is pleasurable to his or her partner is reached. Then the person can maintain that speed. This technique is also a pleasurable way of touching, but not as pleasurable as going slowly and gently. However, using this technique from time to time will make the sexual encounter more pleasurable because it creates variety in the sexual encounter.

If a person touches his or her partner rapidly during sex, this will not be very pleasurable to both people. The partner will not experience the pleasure to the greatest extent because the touching is done rapidly. If the touching is done extremely rapidly then the touching might become irritating and sometimes cause numbness in the person touched. However, a person can touch his or her partner rapidly occasionally during a sexual encounter because it adds variety to the sexual encounter. Even though when a person touches his or her partner rapidly the sensations produced are not pleasurable to the greatest extent, the fact that the touching is done differently than usual causes great excitement, which is very pleasurable. However, a person should touch his or her partner rapidly and not extremely rapidly, since touching extremely rapid touching might cause a person's partner irritation and even numbness.

To add variety to the sexual encounters a person can also touch his or her partner's body with different stuff. The stuff can be many things including a piece of fake fur, fur, velvet, wool, rubber, silk, or leather. The stuff can also include a feather. When a person uses different stuff to touch his or her partner's body during sex, he or she is communicating his or her love in a different way. Also, he or she produces different sensations in his or her partner depending on the material being used. Since different sensations are produced, this causes variety to exist in the sexual encounters. A person using something soft like fur, fake fur, velvet, wool, or silk is very sensual to his or her partner. A person using leather or rubber is a real turn on to his or her partner. A person can touch his or her partner with a feather very lightly, so the feather just barely brushes against his or her skin. This will send shivers of pleasure throughout the partner's body.

Although the different ways that a person can touch his or her partner during sex are extremely numerous, there are several ways that are worth mentioning. The first way is the man can touch the woman's breasts slowly and gently during sex. When the woman's breasts are swollen with erect nipples as a result of sexual excitement, it is very arousing to the man to touch and play with them. The woman also finds it very arousing that the man touches and plays with her breasts and nipples during sex. As a matter of fact, a number of women stroke their own breasts during masturbation, proving that the woman does enjoy her breasts and nipples being stimulated during sex. There is a direct connection between the breasts and the woman's genital area. When the breasts are stimulated, the flow of blood increases in the genital area and the pleasurable sexual sensations in the genital area intensify. One method for a man to touch the woman's breasts during sex is for him to play with her breasts and devote generous attention to everywhere except the nipples. The teasing will drive her wild. Eventually, when the man touches the nipples, he should do so very gently and slowly giving the woman great sexual pleasure and fulfillment.

The second way that a person can touch his or her partner during sex that is worth mentioning is for the person to insert his or her tongue in and out of his or her partner's ear during sex. This will create great pleasure to the sexual partner. The third way is for the woman to touch the man's testicles during sex. Usually men feel their testicles do not get enough attention during sex. Therefore, while the man is thrusting, the woman can gently squeeze his testicles to the rhythm of his motion. This will give the man great pleasure. A man's testicles are highly sensitive and should be gently stroked. The fourth way is for the woman to touch the man's penis during the sexual act and during the sexual break with her hand. She could just touch it without moving her hand just for a second, several times during the sexual encounter. The man loves to have his penis touched during sex and during the sexual break that way.

The fifth way is for the man to use his penis to massage the woman's breasts and nipples during a sexual break. The woman finds it very erotic to have the man's erect penis massage her breasts and nipples. The man finds it very exciting to have his erect penis stimulate the woman's breasts and nipples. The sixth way is for the woman to use her breasts to touch and massage parts of the man's body, especially his nipples during sex or a sex break. The man and the woman find it very sexually exciting to have the woman's breasts massaging the man's body. The seventh way is for the person to grope, rub, and squeeze his or her partner's buttocks during sex. This will get the blood flowing all the right places, making the pleasure for the partner during sex more intense, and making the orgasm more intense. A person can also use his or her finger to gently rub the partner's outer rim of the anus during sex. The outer rim of the anus contains a large number of nerve endings, so stimulating this area will send pleasurable shivers up the sexual partner's spine.

The eighth way is for the person during sex to touch his or her partner's mouth gently and slowly with his or her fingers. This is very wild and sexy and intensifies the pleasure of the partner during sex. The ninth way is for the man, during sex, to stroke the woman's labia minora. This will send shivers of pleasure racing through the woman's body. The tenth way is for the woman to cup and stroke the man's testicles during sex. This will provide the man with pleasurable sensations, making the sexual encounter and the orgasm a lot more pleasurable for him. The eleventh way is for the man to stroke the woman's mons pubis during sex. The mons pubis contains many nerve endings and when the man strokes this area during sex, it intensifies the woman's pleasure and orgasm during sex. The twelfth way is for the person to touch his or her partner's perineum during sex. He or she could gently stroke it during sex to make the sex a lot more pleasurable and to make the orgasm more intense. When a person strokes his or her partner's perineum it causes more blood to enter the genital area.

Variety in Kissing, Licking, and Sucking During Sex

A person kissing, licking, or sucking his or her partner during sex is very important. It is very important because when a person does that passionately during sex he or she will feel pleasure all over his or her body all the way down to the toes. Also, his or her partner will feel pleasure all over his or her body all the way down to the toes when that is done to him or her. Not only does that contribute to pleasure during sex, it also lets a person express love and affection to his or her partner during sex. It lets both people become closer physically and emotionally.

A person can kiss, lick, or suck any part of his or her partner's body during sex or during a sex break. Any part of the partner's body when kissed, licked, or sucked will provide pleasure to both people. However, a person could also kiss, lick, or suck the erogenous zones of his or her partner. When a person kisses, licks, or sucks the erogenous zones of his or her partner the pleasure produced will be more intense than when other areas of the partner's body are kissed, licked, or sucked. A person can change the areas that he or she kisses, licks, or sucks during sex from one encounter to another, adding variety to the sexual encounters. This will make the sexual encounters more exciting and more pleasurable. Also, a person can change the areas that he or she kisses, licks, or sucks during the same sexual encounter, adding variety to the sexual encounter. This will make the encounter more delightful and thrilling. A person should not kiss, lick, or suck an area for too long during a sexual encounter since this decreases the pleasure produced and may even result in numbness in that area. When a person changes the areas that he or she kisses, licks, or sucks during sex, he or she should be unpredictable. By him or her being unpredictable, the sexual encounter is a lot more pleasurable and exciting. A person can alternate between kissing, licking, sucking, or touching the partner's body during sex to create variety in the sexual encounter. This will make the sexual encounter more thrilling and more pleasurable to both people.

When a person kisses, licks, or sucks his or her partner during sex, he or she should be slow and gentle. By a person being slow and gentle, both people will experience pleasure to the greatest degree. The slower a person kisses, licks, or sucks, the more sensation is provoked. When a person kisses, licks, or sucks his or her partner slowly, sensuously, and with feeling, that produces pleasure to the greatest degree in both people. A person can also start kissing, licking, or sucking slowly, then increase the speed until the maximum speed that is pleasurable to both people is attained. Then the person can maintain that speed while kissing, licking, or sucking during sex and during a sex break. This technique is pleasurable, but not as pleasurable as going slow and gentle all the time. However, since it is different it offers variety and makes the encounter exciting and pleasurable if done from time to time. Also, if a person kisses, sucks, or licks fast during sex, both people will not find the sensations produced very pleasurable. However, if a person kisses, licks, or sucks extremely fast during sex the sexual partner might find that irritating and it may cause numbness. Even though kissing, licking, or sucking fast during sex does not produce very pleasurable sensations, a person can do them occasionally since the fact that that is different offers variety and makes the encounter very exciting, which is very pleasurable. However, a person should not kiss his or her partner extremely fast, since that may irritate his or her partner, and may even cause numbness. If a person changes the speed of kissing from time to time, it makes the encounter different and more exciting.

The lips and tongue have numerous nerve endings all waiting to be stimulated during sex. There are many ways that a person can kiss, lick, or suck on his or her partner's body during sex to stimulate the nerve endings in his or her lips and tongue. However, there are several ways that are worth mentioning. One way that a person can lick his or her partner during sex is for him or her to put his or her wet slippery tongue inside his or her partner's ear. This produces very pleasurable erotic feelings in the partner during sex, making the sexual encounter more delightful. A way that a person can kiss or lick on his or her partner's body during sex is for the person to kiss or lick the closed eyelids of his or her partner. This is very exciting to both people, making the sexual encounter more exciting. A way that a person can kiss, lick, or suck on his or her partner's body during sex is for the person to kiss, lick, or suck on his or her partner's nipples. Both men and women find it extremely pleasurable to have their nipples licked, kissed, or sucked during sex. It intensifies the pleasure during sex. A person can kiss, lick or suck his or her partner's body from the head all the way down to his or her feet. This can be done during a sexual encounter. This is very erotic and sensually pleasing to both people.

In addition, a man can kiss, lick, or suck on the woman's breasts during sex. This is extremely sexually exciting for a woman, making the sexual encounter more pleasurable. Furthermore, a person can kiss, lick, or suck on his or her sexual partner's genital area during a sex break or during sex. When a person does so, he or she should do it to provide extra stimulation, but not to get the person to orgasm from the kissing, licking, or sucking. This produces extremely delightful sensations during sex, making the sexual encounter more delightful. As a matter of fact, a woman goes wild with pleasure if the man kisses her vagina the same way he kisses her lips. That is a big, soft, wet and warm kiss. She also goes wild with pleasure if a man sucks on her clitoris the same way he sucks on her tongue. On the other hand, the man goes wild with pleasure if the woman kisses his penis like she kisses his lips. The man also goes wild with pleasure if the woman puts his testicles in her mouth one at a time, and then both at the same time. The man goes wild with pleasure if the woman sucks or licks his testicles.

A person can suck on the fingers of his or her sexual partner during sex to make the sexual encounter more pleasurable to both people. Many people find it sexy to suck on their sexual partner's fingers during sex. When a person sucks the fingers of his or her sexual partner during sex it causes blood to increase in the partner's genital area, making the pleasurable sexual sensations more intense. A person can also suck on the toes of his or her sexual partner during sex to make the sexual encounter more pleasurable to both people. Many people find it erotic to suck on their sexual partner's toes during sex. When a person sucks the toes of his or her sexual partner during sex, it causes blood to increase in the partner's genital area, making the pleasure during sex and orgasm more intense.

A slightly open-mouth kiss on the partner's mouth during sex is more sexually arousing to both people than a closed-mouth kiss. Kissing using full mouth kissing (French Kissing) during sex is the most passionate form of kissing. A person can alternate kissing his or her partner with different types of kisses on the mouth to add variety to the sexual encounter.

Variety in Sexual Positions

The most obvious change a person can do to his or her sexual routine is altering the sexual position or positions that he or she usually has sex in. If a person does that from time to time, his or her sexual encounters will have variety. This will make his or her sexual encounters exciting and pleasurable to the greatest degree. A sexual position has a very great effect on the quality of the sexual encounter. As a matter of fact, if a person has been with the same lover for years, a new position or a new sequence of positions can make the couple feel like they are having sex with a new person. This is so because by the couple having a new position or a new sequence of positions they are coming at each other from all new angles.

Sadly, some people have never tried any sexual position besides the missionary position during sex because it was comfortable and they were afraid to try anything new for fear that it might be uncomfortable. A person can change sexual positions from one sexual encounter to another from time to time. A person can do so to add variety to the sexual encounters. This will intensify the pleasure during sex and orgasm to both people. A person can change sexual positions during the same encounter to add variety to the encounter. This will make the sexual encounter more pleasurable to both people. When a person changes positions during the sexual encounter, he or she should do it slowly and gently. This makes the sexual encounter pleasurable to the greatest degree. The slower a person changes positions during a sexual encounter, the more sensation is provoked. If the couple changes sexual positions quickly, this will decrease the pleasure during the sexual encounter.

There is no set number of positions for a couple to use during one sexual encounter. The couple can use one position during a sexual encounter or they can use more. The couple usually uses two or three positions during one sexual encounter, moving from one position to another. The couple finds the sex pleasurable and exciting if they change from one position to another during the same sexual encounter. The number and type of positions used during a sexual encounter should grow out of the feelings of both people at the moment. Different positions produce different sensations during sex to both the man and the woman, so the couple should alternate positions to alternate the sensations felt during sex to keep the sex exciting. There is a wide variety of positions that a couple could use during sex.

One position that a person can use to add variety to the sexual encounters and intensify the pleasure during sex and orgasm is for him or her to turn his or her head so that it falls over the edge of the bed. Any time a person turns his or her head upside-down he or she will feel a rush as blood pours in his or her head and oxygen is depleted. This head rush during sex will intensify the sexual pleasure and orgasmic pleasure during sex. There are three ways that the head upside-down during sex can be achieved. In the first way, the woman can lie on her stomach on the bed with her feet straight and she can bend her head over the edge of the bed forward. The man can lie on top of her with his chest on her back and his feet straight. Then he can penetrate her vagina from behind. A second way is the woman can lie on her back on the bed with her feet straight, but turn her head so that it falls over the edge of the bed. The man can lie on top of her with his chest touching her chest and his feet straight. This is the missionary position. The man can penetrate the woman's vagina from the front. A third way is the man can lie on his back on the bed with his feet straight. The woman can straddle his hips with her bent knees and sit on top of him. She can face his face or his feet. She can have his penis penetrate her vagina while she sits on top of him. The man can turn his head so that it falls over the edge of the bed. This is the woman on top position.

Variety in Thrusting During Sex

The couple could change the thrusting that occurs during a sexual encounter to create variety in the sexual encounters. The way of thrusting during a sexual encounter could change from one sexual encounter to another. It can also change during the same sexual encounter. This will create variety during the sexual encounters. This will make the sexual encounters more pleasurable and exciting.

There are many ways that a couple could change the thrusting that occurs during a sexual encounter. One way is the person who is doing the thrusting could change. For example, if the man usually does the thrusting during a sexual encounter, the woman can do the thrusting from time to time. If the woman usually does the thrusting during sex, the man can do the thrusting from time to time. If one person usually does all the thrusting during a sexual encounter, the couple could have both people doing the thrusting equally during a sexual encounter from time to time. If both people usually do the thrusting equally during a sexual encounter, one person could do all the thrusting from time to time.

A second way is the depth of the thrusting could change regardless of whether the man or the woman is doing the thrusting. If the thrusting is usually deep, then the couple could do shallow thrusting from time to time. If the thrusting is usually shallow, then the couple could do deep thrusting from time to time. If only shallow thrusting or deep thrusting is done in a sexual encounter, then the couple could have thrusting that is a combination of both shallow and deep thrusts during the same encounter from time to time. If the couple usually does the shallow and deep thrusts during the same encounter, they could do only shallow thrusting or deep thrusting during the sexual encounter from time to time.

The third way is the movement of the thrusting could change from time to time. Whether the man or the woman is doing the deep or shallow thrusting, the movement is usually in and out. However, a person can produce different sensations during thrusting by thrusting in and out while moving in a circular motion. Also, while thrusting in and out, a person can move from side to side. That will also produce different sensations. In addition, while thrusting in and out, a person can move from top to bottom or in a diagonal direction. However, the easiest way to do deep or shallow thrusts is to simply move in and out. There is another type of thrusting called grinding that a person could also do to add variety to the sexual encounters. Grinding does not involve thrusting in and out. It involves keeping the penis inside the vagina at the same depth, but having the man or the woman thrusting in a circular motion. The circular motion can be done in any direction. The person doing the circular thrusting is the person that is in control in that particular position. The clitoris will be stimulated through such action by the man's pelvis stimulating it. This usually causes the woman to orgasm. The man's penis is usually stimulated by such action causing him to orgasm. Also, there is another variation of grinding. As a variation, while keeping the penis at the same depth in the vagina the man or the woman can move up and down. He or she could move up towards the face of his or her partner and then down towards his or her feet. He or she is not moving in and out like regular thrusting. This is usually a rocking motion. This will also cause the man's pelvis to stimulate the woman's clitoris, causing the woman to orgasm. The man usually orgasms from having his penis stimulated during such motion.

The fourth way is the angle of the thrusting could change from time to time. Changing the angle of the thrusting during sex creates different pleasurable sensations. The secret to great sex can be as small as a slight change of angle during thrusting. A person should not stimulate one spot for too long during thrusting since that area may become less sensitive to the stimulation. A person should change the areas that are being stimulated by thrusting. The fifth way is the speed of the thrusting could change from time to time. Usually, the thrusting is pleasurable to the greatest degree if the thrusting is slow and gentle regardless of whether the man or the woman is thrusting. However, the thrusting speed during sex could be altered by having the thrusting start slow and increase in speed gradually until the maximum speed that is pleasurable to both people is attained. Once attained, that speed could be maintained throughout the encounter. This way is pleasurable also, but not as pleasurable as thrusting slowly. Thrusting fast, but not extremely fast, is a third way the speed during sex could be altered. When a person thrusts fast, the sensations produced are not very pleasurable. However, a person can thrust fast occasionally since that is different than usual, which creates variety and makes the sexual encounter very thrilling and very pleasurable, even though the sensations produced from going fast are not very pleasurable. A person should not thrust extremely fast since that may cause the area to go numb, and it may irritable to both people. By changing the speed of the thrusting during a sexual encounter from time to time, the person creates variety in the sexual encounters. As a matter of fact, varying the speed and intensity of the thrusting will vary the stimulation of the penis. This will allow a man to maintain an erection for a longer period of time.

A person can change the way sex feels to both people in any position by changing the thrusting. Regular sex can become sensational sex just by a person changing the thrusting during a sexual encounter from time to time. This is true whether the man or the woman is doing the thrusting.

Variety in Movements During Sex

During sex, both the man and the woman should relax and let their body move the way it wants to. This will make the sex intensely as pleasurable as possible to both people. This is so because both people have variety in their movements during sex if they let their body move the way it wants to. A person should never lack variety in movements during sex because that decreases the pleasure during sex. It also shows that a person is not letting his or her body move the way it wants to. By a person having variety in movements during sex, he or she will intensify his or her orgasm.

Varying Speed During Sex

Varying the speed during sex is a way to make the sexual encounters have variety. The speed can be varied from one sexual encounter to another. It can also be varied during the same sexual encounter. This makes the sex more pleasurable and exciting. It also makes the orgasm more pleasurable and exciting. The speed of everything during sex can be varied, including the thrusting, kissing, hugging, cuddling, touching, and moving.

There are three main speeds that a person could utilize during sex. There is going very slowly and gently during sex. This produces pleasure during sex to the greatest extent. The second type of speed that there is, is going slowly and then increasing the speed to the maximum speed that is pleasurable to both people, then maintaining that speed throughout the encounter. This is pleasurable but not as pleasurable as going slow throughout the encounter. The third type of speed is going fast. This is not very pleasurable to the couple because the sensations produced are not pleasurable to the greatest degree. However, doing it from time to time is very exciting and pleasurable because it is something different, despite the fact that the sensations produced are not pleasurable to the greatest degree. It is important that when the couple goes fast during sex, they go fast but not extremely fast, because going extremely fast can sometimes be irritable and cause numbness in the areas of the body being stimulated.

The couple can vary the speed during sex from one sexual encounter to another from time to time. The couple can also vary the speed during the same sexual encounter from time to time. Varying the speed during sex adds a lot of excitement, pleasure, and zest into a couple's sex life. It also revives a couple's sex life after the sex life no longer exists. It is a very important technique that should not be overlooked.

Variety in a Sexual Encounter Using the Pubococcygeus Muscle (PC Muscle)

Both the man and the woman have a PC muscle. Both the man and the woman can use the PC muscle to create variety in the sexual encounters. The man and the woman can use the PC muscle to create variety from one sexual encounter to another. The man and the woman can also use the PC muscle to create variety during the same sexual encounter. Creating variety in a sexual encounter using the PC muscle makes the sexual encounter more thrilling and more delightful.

When the woman contracts the PC muscle, it improves the blood flow to the vagina and perineum, which increases her sexual responsiveness, sexual energy, and lubrication. It also makes her clitoris and genital area more sensitive. When the woman contracts the PC muscle during sex, the increase in blood flow to the genital area and pelvic area also makes the woman's sexual arousal greater and allows her to experience a greater depth of skin sensation. It also allows the woman to enjoy prolonged stamina during sex. All this makes the sex more pleasurable and makes the orgasm more pleasurable to the woman. When the woman contracts the PC muscle during sex, it is more likely that she will experience an orgasm, and it is more likely that she will experience multiple orgasms. When the woman contracts the PC muscle during an orgasm, the orgasm becomes a lot more intense and pleasurable.

The woman can contract the PC muscle during sex as if she is trying to stop the flow of urine. She can contract her PC muscle during sex and during an orgasm any time she likes and as much as she likes. She can contract it once or several times. There is no set number to follow, but the more the woman contracts it during sex, the more pleasurable the experience will be for her.

The PC muscle controls the size and tension of the vaginal opening. The woman can tighten her vagina during sex by tightening the PC muscle. This will increase both her pleasure and the man's pleasure. The man will love it as the woman grips, strokes, and caresses his penis during sex with her tightened vagina. The vagina's ability to grip the penis during sex increases when the woman tightens the PC muscle. Both the man and the woman will experience increased sexual sensations as a result of the woman tightening her vagina during sex. Also, as a result of the woman tightening her vagina during sex, both the man and the woman will experience more intense orgasms. In order to make the sex more pleasurable the woman can tighten her vagina during sex as many times as she likes.

A woman can contract her PC muscle during sex not only to tighten the vaginal opening, but also to stimulate the man's penis. A woman can contract the PC muscle during sex to grip and massage the man's penis. This produces exquisite sensations to the man's penis. There are several ways that the woman can contract her PC muscle during sex to stimulate the man's penis, regardless of who is doing the thrusting. The first way is the woman can contract her PC muscle rhythmically as the man's penis enters her vagina during thrusting. This causes the man to feel that his penis is being sucked into the woman's vagina while thrusting. This causes thrilling sensations to both the man and the woman. The second way is the woman can squeeze the PC muscle rhythmically when the penis withdraws during thrusting. This creates suction against the woman's vaginal walls, which can be quite pleasurable to both people. The third way is the woman can squeeze the PC muscle rhythmically when the penis enters and withdraws during thrusting. This method is a combination of the first two methods. This is very exciting and pleasurable to both the man and the woman. The fourth way is the penis can remain deep inside the woman's vagina and remain still. Then the woman can contract her PC muscle rhythmically. The woman can bring the man to orgasm just with the contractions of her PC muscle. The woman will make the man feel as if the ejaculate is being pulled from his body. This is delightful and thrilling to both people. The fifth way is when the man is close to climaxing and is climaxing, the woman can contract her vaginal muscles rhythmically to intensify his pleasure. The sixth way is when the woman contracts her PC muscle only while the shaft of the penis is in the vagina during thrusting. This causes the contractions to squeeze around the shaft of the penis only. This will energize the man's whole body and allow him to experience very high levels of pleasure during sex. It will also cause the man's ejaculation to delay because her PC muscle is squeezing the shaft of the penis while it is erect. This causes the amount of time that the couple makes love together to be prolonged, making the sexual experience more pleasurable to both people. A woman can use any of these methods to stimulate the man's penis during sex from time to time. She can do so to add variety to the sexual encounters.

A man can contract the PC muscle during sex to increase the blood flow to his genital area. This makes his genital area more sensitive and increases his sexual responsiveness. This also makes the man's sexual arousal and depth of skin sensation greater. It also lets the man enjoy prolonged stamina during sex. All this makes the sex more pleasurable and makes the orgasm more pleasurable to the man. When the man contracts the PC muscle during an orgasm, the orgasm becomes more intense and more pleasurable.

The man can contract the PC muscle during sex as if he is trying to stop the flow of urine. He can contract his PC muscle during sex and during an orgasm any time he likes and as much as he likes. He can contract it once or several times. There is no set number to follow, but the more he contracts it during sex, the more pleasurable the experience will be for him.

A man can contract his PC muscle during sex to make the erection firmer, and thicker. This will make the sensations more pleasurable to the woman. Also, the fact that the erections are firmer and thicker increases the sensations for the man making the sexual encounter more pleasurable to the man. During sex, a man can make his erection firmer and thicker using the PC muscle as many times as he feels like it.

A man can contract his PC muscle during sex to make the penis move inside the woman's vagina. When a man contracts the PC muscle during sex it makes the penis move up and down. If the penis moves up and down while inside the vagina during sex it feels good to both the man and the woman. Most women respond to the man's penis moving by tightening inside their vagina which makes it more pleasurable to both of them. A man can make his penis move inside the vagina during sex using the PC muscle as many times as he feels like it.

A man and a woman can use the PC muscle to create variety from one sexual encounter to another or during the same sexual encounter. A man can use the PC muscle to make the erections firmer and thicker or to make the penis move up and down inside the vagina in order to add variety to the sexual encounter. A man can also use the PC muscle to make the blood flow increase in his genital area, to add variety to the sexual encounter. Although the man contracting the PC muscle during sex causes these three reactions described, when the man contracts the PC muscle during sex he can have in mind only one reaction. He can use that reaction to create variety in a sexual encounter. For example, when a man has sex he can have in mind only to move his penis up and down inside the woman's vagina, and he can contract his PC muscle only concentrating on that reaction to create variety. In another sexual encounter when the man has sex he can have in mind only to make his erection thicker and firmer, and he can contract his PC muscle only concentrating on that reaction to create variety. A woman can use the PC muscle to make the vagina tighter, or to increase blood flow to her genital area. She can also use the PC muscle to stimulate the penis in different ways during sex. Although when a woman contracts the PC muscle during sex it causes all three reactions described, when she contracts the PC muscle during sex she can have in mind only one reaction in order to create variety in a sexual encounter.

Variety in a Sexual Encounter Using Dominance and Submission

Issues of dominance and submission are part of almost every relationship to some degree. When a person argues with his or her partner and one party gives in to another, that is dominance and submission playing in a relationship. Likewise, issues of dominance and submission are part of almost every sexual encounter to some degree. When a person holds his or her lover's hand back or controls the thrusting during sex that is dominance and submission playing during sex. Excitement during sex is experienced by the couple from control and the loss of it. Control and the loss of it add variety to the sexual encounters, making them more pleasurable and exciting. Every person derives erotic pleasure from assuming temporary consensual control over another person during sex from time to time. Also, every person derives erotic pleasure from temporarily consensually relinquishing control to another person during sex. A person can use control and the loss of it during sex to add variety to the sexual encounters.

There are several ways during sex that a person can exercise control over his or her partner, putting his or her partner in a submissive position. The first way and most obvious way is by the person telling his or her partner what to do during sex. The fact that one person is taking control of the encounter and another person is fulfilling his or her wishes is pleasurable to both people.

The second way is by a person putting a blindfold on his or her partner's eyes, covering his or her eyesight during sex. For comfort a person could use soft material for a blindfold. The material could include a sleep mask or a silk scarf. The partner that can see is in a dominating position and the partner that cannot see is in a submissive position. The partner that is blindfolded can get in a number of positions, including lying on his or her stomach, back, side, sitting, or standing. He or she can remain still or move a little. The partner that is not blindfolded can kiss, cuddle, hug, caress, and have sex with his or her partner. He or she can have sex with his or her partner by making sure that the penis is in the vagina and thrusting is occurring. Either the blindfolded partner or the one that is not blindfolded can do the thrusting during sex. The blindfolded partner can also kiss, cuddle, hug, and caress his or her partner. Usually, the partner that is not blindfolded takes charge of the encounter and the blindfolded partner follows his or her lead. The fact that one partner is extremely dominating in the situation because he or she can see and the other partner does not have the ability to see during sex because of the blindfold makes the sexual encounter more exciting and pleasurable to both people. Since the sense of sight is gone, the rest of the blindfolded person's senses are heightened. This makes every touch that the blindfolded person feels extremely exciting and erotic. The sex becomes a completely different experience to him or her. Plus, the fact that the person never knows what his or her partner is going to do next because he or she is blindfolded adds excitement to the sexual encounter. Using a blindfold during sex adds variety to the sexual encounter.

The third way is the person can tie his or her partner up during sex. The person can use soft material including a silk scarf, a silk tie, or a silk cord from a gown. A person can also use handcuffs designed especially for the purpose of sex play. A person can tie his or her partner up by tying both of his or her hands behind his or her back or in front of his or her stomach. The partner can be in any position including sitting, lying on his or her back, standing, or lying on his or stomach. A person can also tie his or her partner's hands to the bedposts or other furniture while standing, sitting, or sleeping. Plus, a person can tie his or her partner's feet during sex. In addition, a person can tie his or her partner's whole body to a bedpost or other furniture. A person can do so by wrapping soft fabric around his or her partner's chest and arms and around the piece of furniture. The person would also wrap soft fabric around his or her partner's stomach and arms and around the piece of furniture. A person can have sex with his or her partner tied in any of these ways. This makes the sex exciting and adds variety to the sexual encounter. Bondage releases the tied person's inhibitions on the grounds that there is nothing he or she could do to prevent the sexual activity that is occurring. This is very important for people that are uptight during sex and find it very hard to let go during sex to enjoy their sexuality. This is important because a person can enjoy sex because his or her inhibitions are released. Also, the person that is not tied enjoys the encounter more because he or she has more power over the restrained person during sex. Once the sexual partner is tied, the person can tease him or her with a feather, light licks, or kisses all over his or her body before having sex, during sex breaks, or during sex.

The fourth way is for the person to spank his or her partner playfully during sex. A person could spank his or her partner playfully during sex from time to time to make the sex more pleasurable and exciting. A light slap of the hand can bring the blood pleasantly to the surface of the partner's skin, making the pleasant sexual sensations felt more intense.

A person can use any of these techniques involving control and loss of control during sex from time to time to spice up the sexual encounters. A person can use them to add variety from one sexual encounter to another and to add variety during the same sexual encounter. Both partners can alternate during sex in taking the controlling role when using any of these techniques. A person can use a combination of these techniques at the same time from time to time to add variety to a sexual encounter. For example, a person can tie, blindfold, and spank his or her partner during a sexual encounter from time to time. While at other times he or she can only blindfold him or her. These techniques should be used with the consent of both partners. A person should never inflict any pain on his or her partner.

These techniques allow both people to experience being totally in control during sex and being totally submissive during sex. The person in the controlling position finds it very sexually arousing that his or her partner trusts him or her enough to put himself or herself in a helpless position during sex. A person in the controlling position finds it very exciting to be sexually aggressive and getting whatever he or she wants sexually. The person in the submissive position feels very desired and wanted, making the encounter more thrilling for him or her. Also, the person in the submissive role finds it very exciting to relinquish responsibility for his or her sexual acts.

The exchange of power during sex is so erotic and pleasurable that some people practice sadomasochism or S/M. Sadomasochism refers to receiving pleasure, often sexual pleasure, from the exchange of power or pain between consenting adults. In sadomasochism, one person agrees to take control and the other agrees to be submissive. In sadomasochism, sometimes one person agrees to inflict pain and the other agrees to receive it. The S in S/M stands for sadist and M stands for masochist. The sadist usually is in control and inflicts the pain, while the masochist likes to be submissive and receive pain. Usually both partners take turns being the sadist and the masochist. When people practice S/M sometimes they engage in intercourse. Sometimes they have sex after the S/M behaviors are finished. There is a group of people that practice sadomasochism. There is a wide range of equipment and clothing that they use to practice it. Sadomasochism is a lot more advanced than the techniques described in this section. However, the fact that sadomasochism exists proves the point that the exchange of control during sex makes the sexual encounter more pleasurable and exciting to the couple.

Creating Variety During Sex through Teasing

A person could create variety during sex through teasing. There are two teasing techniques that could be employed during sex. The first teasing technique could be used by the man or the woman. It is usually done by the person doing the thrusting. If the woman is doing the thrusting, she uses this technique. If the man is doing the thrusting, he uses this technique.

This technique starts by having the penis and the vaginal lips touch and stimulate each other with the penis being outside the vagina. This is done until both people are sexually aroused greatly. Then the penis should enter the vagina slightly with the first thrust. Then each thrust that follows should allow more of the penis to be taken inside the vagina. This causes the partner that is not thrusting to beg and yearn for deeper penetration. When full penetration occurs, the partner on the receiving end of the thrusting will be groaning with relief and pleasure. At that point a person should continue thrusting until his or her partner orgasms. Both people will find the encounter a lot more exciting and pleasurable than usual because of the teasing. The thrusting done in this technique should be very slow and gentle to cause teasing. If a woman is using this technique the woman on top position is very suitable. The woman can tease the man effectively in the woman on top position. If the man is using this technique the missionary position is very suitable.

A person can use this teasing technique from time to time in his or her sexual encounter. This makes a sexual encounter different than other sexual encounters. This technique is simple but very effective. It builds the intensity of the sexual pleasure felt during sex and during an orgasm. In women, it increases the likelihood that the woman will orgasm and also increases the likelihood that the woman will experience multiple orgasms. In men, this technique increases the likelihood that the man will get an erection and will maintain it. It also increases the duration of the erection.

A second teasing technique is for a person to stimulate his or her partner during sex by thrusting until his or her partner is close to orgasming. Then he or she should stop thrusting and have the penis withdrawn from the vagina for a minute or more until his or her partner's sexual arousal has decreased. He or she should wait until his or her partner's sexual arousal decreased about halfway, but not completely. Then he or she should resume thrusting and continue the same process several times. Each time the process is done, the pleasurable sexual sensations will be more intense. After the process is done several times, the partner on the receiving end will be yearning and begging for stimulation until orgasm. When the person thrusting decides to end the encounter by thrusting until orgasm, the person on the receiving end of the thrusting will climax feeling great joy, satisfaction, and fulfillment. He or she will be satisfied that the teasing is over with. This technique makes the sexual encounter more pleasurable and more exciting to both people as a result of the teasing effect. The thrusting should be very slow and gentle so that teasing occurs. This technique is done by the person doing the thrusting. The person doing the thrusting can be either the man or the woman. If the woman is doing the thrusting the woman on top position is suitable. If the man is doing the thrusting the missionary position is suitable. This technique could be used from time to time to create variety in a sexual encounter.

Sex Toys

A person can create variety in his or her sexual encounters by using sex toys from time to time. Sex toys can enhance a person's sex life, making it more exciting and fun. Sex toys are never a substitute for a sex partner. They are only an addition to a person's sex life.

There are many sex toys. They come in a vast variety of colors, shapes, sizes and materials. However, there are some sex toys that are worth mentioning. The first one is the vibrator. A vibrator is a vibrating device intended to pleasurably stimulate various parts of a person's body. It could be used inside the vagina and on the clitoris as well. The vibrators come in a wide range of shapes and sizes. There is the penetrative vibrator that measures five to seven inches in length and one to two inches wide that mimics the size of the average penis. The woman usually uses that to stimulate her vagina and the clitoris. There is the anal vibrator that is designed to be inserted into the rectum to pleasure the man's prostate, or to give the woman a feeling of fullness. There is the G-spot vibrator that is curved at one end to facilitate stimulation of the female G-spot. There is a bullet vibrator that is a small, bullet-shaped vibrator that can be used for direct stimulation or inserted into other sex toys to increase stimulation. There is the vibrator wand that is large and is marketed as a back massager. It is typically used for clitoral stimulation.

A vibrator could be used by the woman if she is multi-orgasmic to get her to orgasm. Then the man can have vaginal sex with the woman, causing the woman to experience multiple orgasms and causing the couple to experience simultaneous orgasms. The vibrator could be used by the woman if she is not multi-orgasmic to get her sexually aroused, but not to get her to climax. Once the woman gets sexually aroused then the man can have vaginal intercourse with the woman. This allows the couple to experience simultaneous orgasms. The man can also use the vibrator on the woman to implement any of the techniques described. The couple finds it erotic when the man uses the vibrator on the woman. The couple could also use a vibrator on different parts of their bodies, including non-sexual parts during sex to produce pleasurable sensations, and to make the sexual pleasure more intense. The couple could also use a vibrator on different parts of their bodies, including non-sexual parts, during a sex break to produce pleasurable sensations, and to make the sexual pleasure more intense during sex.

The second sex toy is the dildo. The dildo is a non-vibrating device which is used for sexual stimulation of the vagina or the anus. It is usually made of silicone rubber, but can be made of other materials like metal or glass. It is usually made to resemble a penis. It could be used before sex or during a sex break to stimulate the woman to orgasm, or to get her sexually aroused but not to the point of orgasm. Then the man can have vaginal sex with her. It can also be used to stimulate the woman's anus before sex or during sex for added pleasure.

The third sex toy is the artificial vagina. It is modeled to accept a penis for simulated intercourse. It is shaped like a vagina with a hole for penetration. Some artificial vaginas have sex machine capabilities that usually stimulate the penis to orgasm. This sex toy could be used during encounters when the couple is not having vaginal sex, but the man is stimulating the woman to orgasm using oral sex or manual stimulation. The man could use this device or have the woman use this device to stimulate him to orgasm. Using this device from time to time can add variety to the encounters.

The fourth sex toy is the cock ring. The cock ring functions by restricting the flow of blood out from the penis and results in the man having a firmer and longer lasting erection. It also has the effect of creating a feeling of pressure that many men find very pleasurable. It is usually worn by the man during sex to enhance his sexual pleasure and to enhance the woman's sexual pleasure. Most cock rings are made of rubber and leather and are worn at the base of the penis and behind the scrotum. A cock ring should never be worn more than 30 minutes. A man can also wear it to fight erectile difficulties. Some cock rings have a protruding clitoral stimulator designed to stimulate the clitoris during sex. Some cock rings also vibrate.

The fifth sex toy is the penis sleeve. The penis sleeve is a cylindrical device that is placed on the shaft of the penis. It is used to increase the stimulation of the woman being penetrated with the penis. Sometimes it has soft bumps intended to provide further stimulation. It is usually worn by the man during sex. The sixth sex toy is the penis extension. It is like a very short dildo, and is placed on the penis to increase the length of the penis. This is done to increase the pleasure of the woman being penetrated during sex. It is usually worn with a condom to prevent it from falling off during sex. The seventh sex toy is the nipple clamp. It is used to stimulate the nipples by applying varying degrees of pressure. This can be worn by women before or during sex to enhance their sexual pleasure.

The eighth device is the nipple suction device. It is usually used by the woman before sex to make her nipples more sensitive to stimulation. It fits around the woman's nipple. It is usually made of glass or plastic and uses a pump to create suction. The suction causes the nipples to become more sensitive due to engorgement, or increased blood flow to the surface of the skin of the nipple. This causes the woman to experience greater pleasure during sex. The ninth device is the butt plug. It usually resembles the dildo but is shorter, and is intended for anal insertion. It has a flared base that prevents it from being sucked into the rectum. The butt plug can be used by either the man or the woman during sex. It gives the person a feeling of fullness in the anus, which contributes to greater sexual pleasure during sex, and contributes to an incredibly powerful orgasm.

The tenth device is the Ben Wa balls. The Ben Wa balls are hollow metal balls that are inserted in the vagina. They can be inserted in the vagina for an extended period of time. The penis will move the balls inside the vagina during sex. The internal rolling of the balls during sex is claimed to enhance the woman's sexual pleasure and pleasure during orgasm. It also enhances the man's pleasure during sex and during an orgasm. The eleventh sex toy is anal beads. Anal beads is a string of beads designed for anal penetration. The beads create pleasure when they are pulled out of the anus, and pass along the two ringed sphincter muscles. The beads could be pulled out at any point during sex to enhance the sexual pleasure felt during sex. They also, could be pulled out at the point of orgasm to enhance the pleasure of orgasm. They could be used by both the man and the woman during sex.

The twelfth sex toy is a popsicle. A popsicle is an edible sex toy. The man or the woman can use a popsicle during sex to stimulate different parts of his or her partner's body. He or she could use the popsicle to stroke his or her partner's body in order to stimulate it. The coldness from the popsicle will enhance the stimulation of the area touched. This will make the sex more pleasurable for the person who is being touched by the popsicle. Then the person using the popsicle can lick the melted liquid off his or her partner's body during sex, making the sex more exciting for both people.

A man can also put the popsicle in the woman's vagina or on her clitoris during a sex break for a couple of seconds. This will make her sexual arousal increase greatly, making the sexual encounter more pleasurable for the woman. The man can also lick the liquid from the popsicle from the woman's vagina and clitoris during a sex break, which both the man and the woman find erotic. From time to time when the couple is having an encounter that does not involve vaginal sex, but involves the manual or oral stimulation of the man and the woman, the man can manually stimulate the woman with a popsicle. He can insert the popsicle inside the vagina and move it in and out and can use the popsicle to rub the clitoris. He can do so until the woman orgasms. The woman will find it very thrilling and pleasurable to be manually stimulated with a cold popsicle. The man could lick the liquid from the popsicle from the woman's vagina and clitoris after she orgasms which both people find very exciting and erotic.

Other Ways to Add Variety in a Sexual Encounter

There are several other ways to add variety to a sexual encounter that have not been discussed. One way is for the woman to spread her vaginal secretions on her breasts prior to having sex with the man from time to time. This makes the man's erection larger and harder during sex, thus adding variety to the sexual encounter. Normal vaginal scents from a woman's vaginal secretions are very sexually stimulating to the man and make the sexual experience more pleasurable to both the man and the woman. The natural odor of the vaginal secretions can best be described as a pleasant musky scent, however each woman has her own signature scent. A second way is for the person to change what he or she says to his or her partner during sex. By a person changing what he or she says to his or her partner during sex from time to time, a person creates variety in the sexual encounter. This makes the sexual encounter more pleasurable and exciting.

The third way is for the person to use sensitizing cream from time to time. Sensitizing cream is a lubricant which promotes genital blood flow. There are sensitizing creams available for both men and women. The ones designed for women promote blood flow in the clitoris and the genital area. The woman's sensitizing cream is usually applied to the vaginal lips and clitoris. This increases the woman's sexual sensitivity, making the man's every touch very arousing. The increased genital blood flow as a result of the sensitizing cream makes it easier for the woman to a achieve an orgasm. It also makes the sex and orgasm more pleasurable for the woman. The sensitizing cream helps the woman achieve the ultimate pleasurable sensations during sex. The sensitizing cream for men promotes blood flow in the genital area. The man's sensitizing cream is usually applied to parts of the penis. The increased blood flow in the genital area as a result of the sensitizing cream increases the size and the hardness of the man's erection. It also increases the man's stamina during sex. This causes the sex and the orgasm to be more pleasurable for both the man and the woman. When a person uses sensitizing cream during sex from time to time he or she creates variety in the sexual encounter, making the sexual encounter more thrilling.

The fourth way is for the person to drink alcohol before the sexual encounter from time to time. Alcohol relaxes a person and lowers his or her inhibitions. This lets his or her natural sexy side emerge, making the sex a lot more fun for both people. A person should only drink one or two glasses of alcohol before sex, because if he or she drinks more than two glasses it will ruin the encounter. If a person drinks more than two glasses of alcohol before sex, his or her sex drive will decrease, and he or she will feel sleepy and uncoordinated. In men, it also has the effect of making it difficult for the man to get and maintain an erection. Using alcohol to create variety in the sexual encounter is very exciting. The fifth way is for the couple to sleep in separate bedrooms for a couple of weeks, even though they have sex regularly. They can do so from time to time. Many couples find that sleeping in separate bedrooms for a period of time that is temporary and not permanent can increase their charge and attraction to each other making the sexual encounters more pleasurable for both people. This is a very effective way to add variety to the sexual encounters.

Other Ways to Have Sex

There are other ways that a couple could have sex to add variety to their sex life. The first way is for the couple to have sequential orgasms. Sequential orgasms are when one person at a time is sexually stimulated and experiences an orgasm. The person can stimulate his or her partner through oral sex or manual stimulation. The woman could also stimulate her partner to orgasm by stimulating the prostate. The man could also stimulate the woman by stimulating the G-spot. Sequential orgasms are preferable at times rather than regular sex, since that allows a person to enjoy the intensity of his or her own sexual experience rather than being distracted by thinking of his or her partner's enjoyment. This makes the person's pleasure during sex more intense and exciting. If a couple experiences sequential orgasms from time to time it adds variety to the sexual experience.

The second way is for the man to bring the woman to orgasm using manual or oral sex. Then the man could have vaginal intercourse with the woman by inserting his penis into her vagina and thrusting. This technique should be done only if the woman is multi-orgasmic, meaning that she can experience more than one orgasm in a sexual encounter without a refractory period. This technique will allow the woman to experience multiple orgasms. This technique will also allow the couple to experience simultaneous orgasms, making the sexual encounter more pleasurable and exciting to both. The woman's sexual pleasure and orgasms as a result of the multiple orgasms are more intense. A woman finds that one of the most enjoyable sensations is to let the man continue thrusting after she has climaxed. There is nothing sexier to a woman than to feel the man's penis moving inside her vagina as she experiences contractions from multiple orgasms. A woman also feels liberated that she no longer has the anxiety of making sure that she climaxes. This makes her feel greatly responsive to sexual pleasure. It also makes her sexual pleasure intense. If the woman climaxes before the man that will give the man great confidence and will get rid of any fears that he might have during the sexual encounter. This will make the sexual encounter a lot more pleasurable for him. Those five or so minutes between the woman's first orgasm and the man's orgasm are the best and most pleasurable to both people. This technique, if done from time to time, adds variety to the sexual experience.

The third way is for the man to stimulate the woman using oral sex or manual stimulation until she is very aroused sexually but not close to orgasming. Then he should stop stimulating her manually or orally but should insert his penis into her vagina and start having vaginal sex with her. This will allow the man and the woman to experience simultaneous orgasms. Most women need more stimulation than the man in order for both the man and the woman to climax simultaneously. Therefore, the man should excite the woman first using manual or oral sex until she reaches a point of arousal that appears to match his own. This will make the sexual experience exciting and very delightful because the woman is being stimulated manually or orally then she is stimulated with vaginal sex. This technique adds variety to the sexual encounter if done from time to time.

The fourth way is for the couple to simultaneously manually stimulate each other until orgasm. This, if done from time to time, adds variety to the sex life of the couple. The fifth way is the couple to simultaneously perform oral sex on each other. They could do so in the 69 position. In this position, the man lies flat on his back on the ground with his legs straight. The woman lies on top of him on her stomach. She should be facing his feet. Her mouth should stimulate his penis while the man's mouth should stimulate her vagina and clitoris. This also adds variety to the sex life of the couple if done from time to time. For a variation, the couple could do the 69 position with the man on top. Also, for a variation, the couple could do the 69 position with both people side by side with their mouth at their partner's sex organ. The sixth way is for the couple to have anal sex. If the couple has anal sex from time to time, that adds variety to the couple's sex life. Any of these techniques described in this section could be done by the couple from time to time to spice up their sex lives.

Outercourse

A person, in order to have variety in his or her sex life, can participate in outercourse, since it is totally different than intercourse. Outercourse is when the man's penis is stimulated until orgasm without penetrating the vagina. Outercourse will make a person's sex life more pleasurable and more interesting since it is different from intercourse. A couple can use outercourse if the woman is menstruating and either the man or the woman does not like penetration when the woman is menstruating.

A woman could begin the first outercourse technique by lying on her back with her legs straight and applying a water-based lubricant to her labia, clitoris, and inner thighs. The man could also apply lubricant to the head and shaft of his penis. Then the man lowers himself on top of the woman so that he is flat on top of her with his face facing her face and his chest on top of her chest. The woman separates her legs just enough to allow his penis to slide between her thighs, and against her vulva and clitoris. A woman can spread her labia, as the man lowers himself on top of her so that he has better access to her clitoris. The woman can then close her legs trapping the penis between her thighs and vulva. The man should be lying on top of the woman with his legs straight. The man should thrust in and out while sliding his penis against the woman's vulva and clitoris. At no time does the penis enter the woman's vagina. In this technique both the man and the woman can orgasm because the woman's clitoris is being stimulated while the man's penis is being stimulated. A word of caution: during this outercourse technique, the penis does not enter the vagina, but that does not mean that the man does not need contraception. If the man ejaculates anywhere near the vagina it is possible for the sperm to swim up into the vagina and for conception to occur. Likewise it is possible during this outercourse technique for the man or the woman to get a sexually transmitted disease even though the penis does not enter the vagina. So it is important that a man wear a condom during this outercourse technique to prevent transmission of a sexually transmitted disease and to prevent the woman from becoming pregnant.

A second outercourse technique lets only the man orgasm because only the penis is being stimulated and the clitoris is not stimulated. The second outercourse technique involves having the woman lie down on her back with her legs straight. Her hands should be squeezing her breasts close together. The man can straddle her breasts with both of his knees bent so that he is in a kneeling position. The man should be facing the woman's face. Then he can insert his penis between her breasts and move his penis forward and back between her breasts. Both breasts should cause friction against the man's penis causing him to ejaculate and experience an orgasm. This technique brings the woman great pleasure because she finds it erotic to have her breasts stimulated with the man's penis. This technique also brings the man great pleasure because he finds it erotic to have his penis stimulated by the woman's breasts.

A third outercourse technique involves the woman lying on one of her sides and the man kneeling behind her. Then the man can insert his penis under one of her armpits, the armpit that she is not lying on. She should adjust the angle of her hand so that her hand is squeezing his penis underneath the armpit. The man should move his penis forward and back until he experiences an orgasm and ejaculates. This third outercourse technique also lets only the man orgasm. This technique, even though it lets only the man orgasm, could be used by the couple because it adds variety to the things that they can do together. Even though the woman is not orgasming as a result of this technique, the woman enjoys the experience because it is something different and finds it erotic to have her armpit stimulated by the man's penis.

Conclusion

Many ways of creating variety from one sexual encounter to another have been discussed. A couple might use some techniques to create variety and might not use others. A couple might use only one technique in each sexual encounter. The technique used could be different each time. Or the couple might use a combination of techniques in each sexual encounter. The combination of techniques used could be different each time. A couple should never wear out a technique by using it over and over until it is not pleasurable any more. The couple should use a technique, but change it after using it a couple of times. The couple could go back and use the technique after using another technique a couple of times. By the couple doing so, both techniques remain pleasurable to the greatest degree and are not worn out. However, a couple should always create variety in their sexual encounters to keep their sex life alive and exciting.

Chapter 21

The Climax Dilemma

The climax dilemma is that an average man during sex does not orgasm at the same time that an average woman during sex orgasms, leaving the woman sexually unsatisfied. The average man can orgasm in 4 to 5 minutes while the average woman needs at least 12 to 15 minutes to orgasm. An average woman needs around an average of 8 to 10 minutes longer than an average man to orgasm during sex. The average man orgasms in 4 to 5 minutes, and after that has a refractory period of an average of 20 to 30 minutes where he cannot have an erection nor orgasm. This makes it impossible for the average man to bring the average woman to climax during sexual intercourse. It is impossible for the average man to bring the average woman to climax during sexual intercourse because the average woman needs around an extra 8 to 10 minutes to orgasm during sex, but the average man cannot provide her with those extra 8 to 10 minutes of thrusting to orgasm during sex because of the refractory period. Therefore, the sexual encounter is usually from the time the average man inserts his penis inside the vagina until he orgasms, leaving the average woman sexually unsatisfied.

Causes of Climax Dilemma

Although the average woman can orgasm in at least 12 to 15 minutes during sexual intercourse, around 30 percent of the women can orgasm regularly during sexual intercourse, in 4 to 5 minutes. Of the seventy percent of the women that can orgasm in at least 12 to 15 minutes during sexual intercourse, one half of them have never experienced an orgasm during sexual intercourse, and the rest experience an orgasm during sexual intercourse from time to time. During sexual intercourse the penis does not come in contact with the clitoris, thus the clitoris is not stimulated directly. Some women always have an orgasm during sexual intercourse because the thrusting of the penis in the vagina during sexual intercourse moves the labia minora. The labia minora moves the clitoral hood that it is attached to it against the clitoris, indirectly stimulating the clitoris. It is the movement of the clitoral hood against the clitoris that usually creates the orgasm. For some women, this slight stimulation is enough to orgasm. But for most it is not.

Some women have an orgasm during sexual intercourse from time to time for two reasons. The first reason is sometimes before sexual intercourse the man may have stimulated the clitoris physically, greatly exciting it, and then the movement of the clitoral hood against the clitoris during sex is enough to get the woman to orgasm, when usually it is not. The second reason why some women orgasm from time to time during sexual intercourse is because sometimes before sex the man may have stimulated the G-spot physically, greatly exciting it, and then the thrusting of the penis against the G-spot during sex is enough to get the woman to orgasm, when usually it is not.

Some women have never had an orgasm during sexual intercourse for several reasons. The first reason is the woman never had her clitoris physically stimulated enough before intercourse in order for the movement of the clitoral hood against the clitoris during sexual intercourse to be enough to get the woman to orgasm. The second reason why a woman never had an orgasm during sexual intercourse is because the woman never had her G-spot physically stimulated enough before intercourse in order for the movement of the penis against the G-spot during sexual intercourse to be enough to get the woman to orgasm. Also, not all women have a G-spot. Women that do not have a G-spot cannot orgasm if where the G-spot is supposed to be is stimulated. In addition, the movement of the penis during sex does not always stimulate the G-spot, it depends on the sexual position.

It is unrealistic to expect all women to orgasm from vaginal sexual intercourse. This is true regardless whether the man or the woman is doing the thrusting. Expecting the woman to orgasm from the repetitive penetration of the male penis into the female vagina during thrusting is like expecting the man to orgasm from the rubbing and movement of the scrotal sac that causes the skin on the upper tip of the penis to move. Stimulating the tip of the penis by moving the scrotal sac will take a long time for the man to orgasm if he orgasms at all. Likewise, repetitive penetration of the penis into the vagina during thrusting during sexual intercourse will cause a woman to take a long time to orgasm, if she orgasms at all. Female orgasm during sexual intercourse usually results not from vaginal sensitivity but from indirect stimulation of the clitoris by the movement of the clitoral hood against the clitoris. A woman's climax depends primarily on the amount of stimulation her clitoris receives. The clitoris is the woman's main organ of sensation during sex. The climax dilemma occurs during sexual intercourse because when a man's penis repeatedly penetrates into a woman's vagina during thrusting the man has his most sensitive sexual organ, the head of his penis, being stimulated, but the woman's most sensitive sexual organ the clitoris is not directly being stimulated. The clitoris is not being directly stimulated during sexual intercourse because the penis does not come in contact with the clitoris during sexual intercourse. The clitoris is only indirectly being stimulated during sexual intercourse, by the clitoral hood moving against it during sexual intercourse because of the repetitive penetration of the penis into the vagina during thrusting.

All women can orgasm. There is not a woman that cannot orgasm. Most women can achieve an orgasm in 4 to 5 minutes when masturbating. The average woman during masturbation can climax in 4 to 5 minutes, the same amount of time it takes the average man to climax during sexual intercourse or masturbation. Given the fact that the average woman can climax during masturbation within 4 to 5 minutes, that means that she can also climax during sexual intercourse within 4 to 5 minutes. The average woman can achieve orgasm consistently during sexual intercourse within 4 to 5 minutes by receiving direct clitoral stimulation during sexual intercourse. The woman can receive direct clitoral stimulation during sexual intercourse by her or the man manually stimulating the clitoris during sexual intercourse.

The mistake that many couples make is assume that the woman and man should not manually touch the clitoris during sex. They incorrectly believe that if the woman cannot orgasm during vaginal intercourse without any added manual stimulation to the clitoris, that means that there is something wrong with the woman. They are also ignorant of the fact that the stimulation of the clitoris is the primary source of orgasms. Rather, they incorrectly believe that the stimulation of the vagina is the primary source of orgasms. There is no reason why a woman should not have an orgasm the same time as the man during sexual intercourse, provided there is direct stimulation of the clitoris. It is only ignorance of the true sexual facts that causes the climax dilemma.

The average man and woman should know that if the woman does not climax during sexual intercourse without added manual stimulation to the clitoris, there is nothing wrong with the woman. It is perfectly normal. The average man and woman should also know that it is perfectly normal for the woman to receive added manual stimulation to her clitoris during sex in order to orgasm. Furthermore, the average man and the average woman should know that the clitoris and not the vagina is the primary source of female orgasms. As a matter of fact, they should know that when women masturbate, 90 percent of them climax by stimulating the clitoris exclusively. Only 10 percent of the women stimulate their vagina while masturbating, and even then they usually stimulate their clitoris at the same time.

The Effects of the Climax Dilemma

The climax dilemma has several effects. The first effect is that a man may feel that there is something wrong with his sexual performance since the woman did not orgasm during sexual intercourse. This causes the man to feel guilty and uncomfortable and deprives him of much enjoyment during sexual intercourse. This also causes the man to suffer a lot of pain. A man may sometimes incorrectly believe that he failed to orgasm the woman during sexual intercourse because of the size of his penis. The second effect is that a woman may feel that there is something wrong with her because she did not orgasm during sexual intercourse. This will cause the woman to sacrifice her sexual satisfaction by faking an orgasm during sexual intercourse. The sexual unsatisfaction of the woman will cause a woman to want sex less. This will cause the man to think that the woman is less attracted to him, causing him to feel resentful and to withdraw. This leads to a vicious cycle where the woman also feels resentful that the man is distant from her and she will withdraw more. This vicious cycle will cause the relationship to break apart sooner or later.

The third effect is that a woman may feel unsatisfied sexually because she did not climax during sex to the degree that after sex she cannot rest and fall asleep. Rather after sex she may sneak into the bathroom to masturbate to relieve herself of physical discomfort for not climaxing and to satisfy herself sexually. The fourth effect is that many women would rather watch television than have sex, because they are frustrated that they cannot climax during sexual intercourse. The woman might resent the fact that the man can orgasm during sex and that she cannot, leading to disharmony in the relationship. This disharmony might lead to the end of the relationship sometimes. The fifth effect is that a woman may feel inadequate for not experiencing an orgasm. Not having an orgasm for most women is worse than having no sex at all.

The man and the woman should not feel guilty, nor inadequate because of the climax dilemma. They should know that it is perfectly normal and find a way to overcome it. They should overcome the climax dilemma because good sex is the key to good health and the glue in any monogamous relationship. If the woman overcomes the climax dilemma and experiences an orgasm during sex she would enjoy the sex and would want it frequently. This will cause the man to feel desired and loved by the woman, thus drawing both closer to each other. This closeness would cause the couple to have a happy successful relationship.

Overcoming the Climax Dilemma— By Manually Stimulating the Clitoris

There are numerous things that a couple could do to overcome the climax dilemma. The first thing for the couple to do to overcome the climax dilemma is to have the woman masturbate so that she overcomes the ignorance of her body's sexual response and learns how to climax. A woman can quickly learn how to have an orgasm through masturbation. Masturbation lets the woman learn exactly what sorts of moves will bring her to a peak and makes her comfortable with those sensations. It lets a woman know her own body and what is most satisfying for her sexually. It lets a woman know how to get the clitoral stimulation she needs to experience an orgasm and lets her become comfortable with her own body. A woman's ability to have an orgasm during masturbation is widely regarded as one of the best ways of determining her sexual potential.

All sexologists agree that masturbation is simply a highly effective means for the woman to learn to experience an orgasm reliably. Virtually all women who masturbate can do so to orgasm, thus enabling virtually all women to overcome the climax dilemma. Women who have never managed to have an orgasm with a partner can almost always have one on their own quite easily and quickly. Also, masturbation lets many women orgasm within 4 to 5 minutes, about the same time it takes a man to orgasm, which helps the woman overcome the climax dilemma. If a woman is slower than average in climaxing, she can improve with practice. Most sex therapists recommend that a woman masturbate until she can reliably have an orgasm by herself. The woman learning to masturbate with ease and flexibility is the right way to success in overcoming the climax dilemma. Until a woman is a real expert at climaxing on her own she cannot be sure of climaxing with another person. Most sex therapists emphasize the fact that a woman should masturbate to learn her sexual response, while they do not emphasize that fact in regards to the man because inability to orgasm during sex is a common complaint of women, but it is rare for a man not to experience an orgasm during sex.

After the woman can orgasm reliably by herself during masturbation, then she can have an orgasm while masturbating in front of the man. This is the second thing that a couple could do to overcome the climax dilemma. There is nothing better than for the man to watch the woman masturbate to help him understand where and how she needs to be stimulated during sex in order to climax. Many women are embarrassed to ask their male partner to watch them masturbate. However, most men would like to watch the woman masturbate, since that turns them on. Not only does it usually turn the man on, but it also lets the man know what feels good to the woman as sexual stimulation. It lets a man learn a great deal about how she likes to have her clitoris stimulated during sex. This improves the man's technique a thousand percent when he makes love to the woman afterward.

After the woman can orgasm reliably by herself during masturbation in front of the man, then she can have the man manually stimulate her clitoris, for him to make certain he knows what places she likes stimulated and how she likes them stimulated. The man could make certain as to the speed and the rhythm the woman likes her clitoris stimulated. He could also make certain as to the pressure that she likes to have her clitoris stimulated. This will also improve the man's ability to satisfy the woman during sexual intercourse. Every woman's preference in regards to clitoral stimulation differs, so a woman can communicate to the man how she likes to have her clitoris stimulated manually by guiding his hand with her hand or by verbal communication. The woman having the man manually stimulate her clitoris is the third thing that a couple could do to overcome the climax dilemma.

After the woman can orgasm reliably by the man manually stimulating her, then it is time for the woman to orgasm during sexual intercourse either by the man manually stimulating her clitoris, or by her manually stimulating her clitoris. This is the fourth thing that couple could do to overcome the climax dilemma. It is better for the man or the woman to stimulate the clitoris when the woman's vagina is being penetrated by the man's penis because having the penis to contract around when climaxing is far more satisfying than climaxing with an empty vagina. Climaxing without anything in the vagina might take three or four times before a woman is satisfied sexually, whereas climaxing with the penis inside the vagina a woman is satisfied with just one time. Also, a woman finds the fact that the penis is inside her during sex and when climaxing to be arousing, increasing her pleasure during sex.

It is important whether the man or the woman is manually stimulating the woman's clitoris that the person stimulating the clitoris uses a lubricant. Using a lubricant on the finger will make the stimulation a lot more pleasurable. When manually stimulating the woman's clitoris during intercourse, the man should see whether the woman likes direct contact with the clitoris or whether she likes indirect stimulation of the clitoris by having the area around the clitoris touched. Whether the woman likes direct stimulation of the clitoris or indirect stimulation of the clitoris differs from woman to woman. It depends on the sensitivity of each woman's clitoris. As a matter of fact, direct contact with the clitoris by touching it with a finger, vibrator, or a tongue can cause more discomfort than pleasure for some women. Many women report that the most pleasurable place to receive stimulation is around the clitoris not directly on it. Some women also like indirect stimulation of the clitoris, through the clitoral hood. This is done by having the man or woman's finger use the clitoral hood to rub against the clitoris.

Some women that like direct stimulation of the clitoris prefer only stimulation of the clitoral head during sexual intercourse, while other women that like direct stimulation of the clitoris only prefer stimulation of the clitoral shaft during sexual intercourse. A number of women that like direct stimulation of the clitoris prefer stimulation of both the clitoral head and the clitoral shaft during sexual intercourse. The clitoral shaft is less sensitive than the head of the clitoris.

All women, whether they like direct or indirect manual stimulation of the clitoris, prefer the stimulation when it is slow and gentle because it provides the most pleasure. The other type of clitoral manual stimulation that they like is for the stimulation to start extremely slow and keep on increasing in speed as long as it feels amazing to the woman. Once the maximum level or speed that feels amazing to the woman is reached, the man should maintain that speed until the woman orgasms. This technique is pleasurable, but not as pleasurable as going very slow. Several common discomforts for most women are the man's tendency to manually stimulate the clitoris too roughly, too quickly, too intensely, or for a long period of time. Usually the man has no idea that what he is doing is uncomfortable or painful for the woman and the woman might be embarrassed to say anything. However, the woman should gently lift the man's hand to reduce the pressure, or move his hand to another location that feels hungry for touching. The woman could also tell him verbally that she feels uncomfortable being touched like that.

Whether the man or the woman is manually stimulating the clitoris during sex, the stimulation of the clitoris should have a consistent rhythm, not changing too often. Many women, in order for them to climax, have to get the man to establish a consistent rhythm when manually stimulating their clitoris. During sex, if the man breaks the rhythm of the manual stimulation of the clitoris, the woman's arousal will drop and she won't be able to climax unless the man again maintains a consistent rhythm. When creating a rhythm for the manual stimulation of the clitoris during sex, a man can read the woman's facial expressions varying his movements until he reaches a rhythm that is ideal. Whether the man or the woman is stimulating the clitoris during sex, clitoral stimulation should continue while the woman is orgasming, right through to the last spasm. This should be done since that makes the orgasm more intense and more pleasurable.

By using manual stimulation of the clitoris during intercourse, whether the man or the woman herself stimulates the clitoris, an average woman can climax in a matter of 4 to 5 minutes. It also usually takes the man 4 to 5 minutes to orgasm during intercourse. Thus, by using manual stimulation of the clitoris during intercourse, an average woman can overcome the climax dilemma by orgasming the same time that the man orgasms during sexual intercourse. Therefore, during intercourse the main concern should be the manual stimulation of the woman's clitoris. Another reason why the main concern during intercourse should be the manual stimulation of the woman's clitoris is because 90 percent of women, when they masturbate, only stimulate the clitoris. Also, 10 percent of the women that stimulate their vagina during masturbation also stimulate the clitoris during masturbation. The clitoris is the woman's real sexual pleasure center, and stimulating it should be the main concern during sexual intercourse.

Women that can orgasm from the penile thrusting during intercourse only find the stimulation of the clitoris by the clitoral hood as a result of the thrusting during intercourse to be weak compared to direct or indirect manual stimulation in the clitoral area. Women that can orgasm from the penile thrusting during sex only find that the manual stimulation of the clitoris during sex adds a lot more excitement and pleasure during sex. For all women, manual stimulation of the clitoris during sexual intercourse not only provides the woman with an orgasm, but it also gives the woman great sexual pleasure. It intensifies the sexual pleasure that the woman usually feels during sex. Women who have manual clitoral stimulation during intercourse are more likely to climax consistently during sexual intercourse. It is more than okay for the woman to stimulate her own clitoris during sex. Most men find it highly erotic to see the woman stimulating her clitoris to orgasm during sex. If the man stimulates the woman's clitoris during sex, she will love him forever as the world's greatest lover.

Different Techniques to Stimulate the Clitoris by Hand During Intercourse

There are numerous techniques to stimulate the clitoris by hand during intercourse. A person can get ideas by reading the Masturbation chapter in this book, and by reading the Manual Stimulation chapter in this book. A person can also be creative and come up with his or her own techniques of stimulating the clitoris during sex. Whether the person stimulating the clitoris during sex is the man or the woman, several techniques are worth mentioning. As to which technique or techniques to use depends on the woman, since each woman likes a different form of clitoral stimulation.

If the woman likes direct clitoral stimulation, one technique that could be used is for the man or the woman to stroke the sides of the clitoris slowly and softly with his or her fingertips during sexual intercourse until the woman is aroused. Once the woman is aroused greatly and her orgasm is near at hand, the man or the woman can rub the whole clitoris. It won't take long before the woman is moaning with ecstasy. If the woman likes direct clitoral stimulation, a second technique that could be used during intercourse is for the man or the woman to touch the clitoris shaft and circle his or her fingertips gently around it in a clockwise and counterclockwise motion while touching it. This will cause the clitoral shaft to be stimulated. Doing this during intercourse will induce intense pleasure. If the woman likes direct clitoral stimulation, a third technique that could be used during intercourse is for the man or the woman using his or her fingers to rub up and down the clitoris, and then vary the movement from side to side, or to a circular movement.

If the woman likes indirect clitoral stimulation, one technique that could be used during intercourse is for the man or the woman to use a finger or two to rub the clitoral hood to indirectly stimulate the clitoris. The man or the woman could move the finger or fingers in a circular motion, since that is the motion that most women use when masturbating. If the woman likes indirect clitoral stimulation, a second technique that could be used during sexual intercourse is for the man or the woman to use a finger or two to rub the area around the clitoris in a circular motion. A circular motion could be used because most women when pleasuring themselves use a circular motion

Overcoming the Climax Dilemma— By Stimulating the Clitoris Not Manually

There are other ways to stimulate the clitoris during sexual intercourse without using manual stimulation in order to overcome the climax dilemma. One way is to rub the clitoris against the man's pelvis area during sexual intercourse. This is easiest with the woman on top position. In this position, the man is lying on the floor with his legs straight and the woman is straddling his hips with her legs in a kneeling position with her on top. The woman in this position can rub her clitoris against the man's pelvis as she thrusts up and down his penis. In this position, the woman can also rub her clitoris against the man's pelvis without thrusting up and down while the penis is inside the vagina. It is easiest to rub the clitoris against the man's pelvis area with the woman on top in a kneeling position because she can control where she can get the best clitoral stimulation. Also, with the woman on top she can direct the amount of pressure she wants. Rubbing the clitoris against the man's pelvis area can also be accomplished with the man on top, in the missionary position, provided an adjustment is made to the missionary position. The adjustment is that the man's pelvis is tilted close to the woman's pelvis so that he can rub her clitoris on his pelvis. This can be done if the woman lies straight on the floor and the man lies on top of her, placing his pelvis against her clitoris. He would part her labia with his fingers to expose her clitoris before he enters her. Then he can glide his penis inside her, tilting his pelvis close to hers so he can rub her clitoris on his pelvis area as he thrusts. The man can also use only a grinding or rocking motion in this position to stimulate the clitoris while keeping the penis inside the vagina without thrusting.

A second way to stimulate the clitoris during sexual intercourse without using manual stimulation in order to overcome the climax dilemma is to rub the clitoris against the base of the man's penis during sexual intercourse. The easiest way for the woman to do that is for her to get in the woman on top position. The man would lie flat on the ground with his legs straight and the woman would sit on top of him, straddling his hips with her legs with his penis inside of her. Then she could part her vaginal lips and lean forward to the man's chest, bringing her clitoris directly into contact with the base of his penis. Then she could rub softly from side to side or in a circular motion the exposed shaft of the man's penis against her clitoris. Rubbing the clitoris against the base of the man's penis during sexual intercourse can also be accomplished with the man on top. This could be accomplished using the Coital Alignment Technique. The woman would lie flat on the ground with her legs straight and then the man lies on top of her with his legs straight. Then the man inserts his penis inside her vagina and moves his pelvis forward so that his pelvis overrides the woman's pelvis. In this position, the base of the man's penis is pushed up against the woman's clitoris. The man can rub the base of his penis against the clitoris in this position by moving forward towards the woman's face and back towards her feet and from side to side. He would do a rocking motion and not a thrusting, in-and-out motion.

Rubbing the clitoris during sex with the man's pelvis or base of the penis is very pleasurable to the woman because it produces a motion that is similar to when the woman masturbates. When a woman masturbates she uses a rubbing motion, often circular, on her clitoris. Rubbing the clitoris in a circular motion with the man's pelvis or base of the penis during sex produces close intense contact that is very intimate to the couple, and lets the woman overcome the climax dilemma by letting her climax the same time that the man climaxes. Every woman can orgasm during sexual intercourse if rubbing of the clitoris against the man's pelvis area or base of the penis occurs, thus allowing every woman the ability to overcome the climax dilemma.

Overcoming the Climax Dilemma— By Stimulating the G-Spot

It is possible for some women to overcome the climax dilemma during sexual intercourse by having the G-spot stimulated by the penis during thrusting. However, since the G-spot does not appear to be present in all women, overcoming the climax dilemma through G-spot stimulation is not possible for all women. However, for those women who can climax through G-spot stimulation, overcoming the climax dilemma through G-spot stimulation is possible. This is possible whether the man or the woman is thrusting.

The G-spot is a small spot that is located about one and a half to two inches from the opening of the vagina. It is located on the front wall of the vagina, between the pubic bone and the cervix. It is a tiny bean-shaped area. Its size varies from woman to woman. The amount of time that the G-spot has to be stimulated in order for the woman to orgasm varies from woman to woman. During sexual intercourse, some women can climax the same time as the man as a result of G-spot stimulation from the penis during thrusting because they are sufficiently aroused before sex. In some women that are not sufficiently sexually aroused before sex, it may take up to 15 minutes of G-spot stimulation in order for them to climax, while in others that are not sufficiently sexually aroused before sex it may take up to half an hour of G-spot stimulation for them to climax. Therefore, in order for a woman to climax from G-spot stimulation during sexual intercourse, she and the man should make sure that she is sufficiently sexually aroused before sex. They should make sure that she is greatly sexually aroused before sex, to the point that she is very close to an orgasm. They should do so, so that during thrusting during intercourse the G-spot will receive enough stimulation from the penis in order for the woman to climax within 4 to 5 minutes of sexual intercourse the same time that the man climaxes. Also, getting the woman sufficiently sexually aroused before sex will make the penetration of the vagina with the penis very pleasurable because the vagina will respond intensely to even the smallest thrusts. The man or the woman herself could get the woman sufficiently sexually aroused before sex by manually stimulating the G-spot.

Sometimes a woman cannot orgasm from G-spot stimulation during sexual intercourse because the man's penis may not hit her vagina in the right spots during thrusting. The woman should know where her G-spot is located. She should let the man know how to move in order to stimulate her G-spot during penile thrusting, if she wants to climax from G-spot stimulation and the man is doing the thrusting. If the woman is doing the thrusting, she should make sure that the penis is hitting her vagina in the right spots in order for her G-spot to be stimulated. The couple could also try different sexual positions and thrusting angles, to find the most pleasurable positions and the most pleasurable thrusting angles for the woman to climax from G-spot stimulation. A slight change in the angle of the penile thrusting could make a great difference in the degree of stimulation of the G-spot.

Deep penile thrusts during sexual intercourse tend to stimulate the G-spot the most. The G-spot responds best to a steady rhythm of thrusting. During thrusting, the pace, pressure, and motion should be maintained as much as possible, because that provides for the best possible G-spot stimulation. The G-spot is stimulated best when there is consistency. Thrusting to stimulate the G-spot should be very slow and gentle because that provides the most pleasurable sensations. A second way to thrust in order to stimulate the G-spot is to start thrusting slow then slowly increase the intensity and speed of the thrusting until the maximum speed and intensity that is pleasurable for both the man and the woman is reached. That maximum speed and intensity of thrusting, once reached, should be maintained until the woman orgasms. This is pleasurable but not as pleasurable as going slow and gentle. The G-spot responds best to firm pressure that is often not achieved during normal sex. Therefore, if the man or the woman press on the G-spot from the outside while thrusting is occurring, the woman's erogenous zones in the vagina, including her G-spot, will come into fuller contact with the man's penis and will trigger a very powerful orgasm. The exact location of the G-spot varies from woman to woman. Therefore, during sex the man or the woman will have to find out where to put their hand on the woman's stomach by playing it by feel. The man or the woman should start by gently pressing the heel of his or her hand into the woman's belly button. If the woman squeals with delight then the right location has been found. If the woman does not squeal with delight, the man or the woman should gradually move his or her hand down below the belly button until the woman squeals with delight. Once the woman squeals with delight the right spot where the G-spot is located has been found. Pressing the stomach with a man's hand or woman's hand during sexual intercourse gives the woman the most incredible orgasms.

Positions that Could Be Used to Overcome the Climax Dilemma

There are numerous sexual positions that could be used to overcome the climax dilemma. In order to allow the couple to overcome the climax dilemma, the sexual position should allow the man or the woman easy access to stimulate the clitoris by hand during sexual intercourse. If the woman has a G-spot that allows her to climax from it being stimulated, then the couple could overcome the climax dilemma by using sexual positions that allow the penis to easily stimulate the G-spot during sex. The chapter about Sexual Positions discussed many different sexual positions. The couple could try those sexual positions and see which ones allow them to overcome the climax dilemma. Also, the couple could be creative and try other sexual positions that they think of, and try to overcome the climax dilemma using those sexual positions. Although there are many sexual positions that could be used to overcome the climax dilemma, there are several sexual positions that are worth mentioning.

The first and most important sexual position worth mentioning is the woman on top sexual position. In this sexual position the man lies flat on his back with his legs straight. The woman sits on top of him facing his face, with her knees bent straddling his hips. This sexual position allows the couple to overcome the climax dilemma because it gives the woman complete control of how her G-spot and clitoris are stimulated during sex. In this position the woman can ensure that she gets the movements during sex that will bring her the most pleasure and may even bring her to a climax. In this sexual position, the woman can ensure that the G-spot is stimulated easily during sexual intercourse to the point of orgasm if she can orgasm from G-spot stimulation. In this sexual position the woman and the man have easy access to stimulate the clitoris by hand during sexual intercourse to overcome the climax dilemma. This position is a very comfortable and convenient position for the woman to have her clitoris stimulated manually either by the man or by herself. In this sexual position, the penis penetrates the vagina deeply during sex, giving a woman great pleasure and giving her a feeling of fullness during orgasm. The feeling of fullness makes the orgasm satisfying and fulfilling to the woman. In this position the woman can easily rub her clitoris against the man's pelvis area while thrusting up and down on his penis, thus stimulating her clitoris during sex to the point of orgasm without any manual stimulation. This allows the woman to overcome the climax dilemma. In this position, the woman can also grind her clitoris against the man's pelvis area while keeping the penis inside the vagina, without thrusting in and out in order to stimulate the clitoris during sex. This also lets the woman overcome the climax dilemma.

The second sexual position worth mentioning is a variation of the woman on top position. In this position, the woman while in the woman on top position facing the man could lean backwards until both her hands are touching the ground. She would lean backwards at an angle that allows the man's penis to lie against the front wall of the vagina. Even the most minor thrusts made by the woman will cause the penis to automatically rub against the G-spot in this position. This position also gives the man easy access to manually stimulate the clitoris during sex, thus allowing the couple to overcome the climax dilemma. This position also gives the woman control of how deep and how fast she will thrust, which will make the sex extremely pleasurable and relaxing for her, thus helping her overcome the climax dilemma.

The third sexual position that is worth mentioning is the side-by-side position with the man facing the back of the woman's head. In this position, the woman lies on her side and the man lies on his side behind her facing her back, and penetrates her vagina from behind. In this position the woman's G-spot is easily reached by the man's penis during intercourse, thus allowing a woman to easily overcome the climax dilemma during sex if she can orgasm from G-spot stimulation. In this position, the woman or the man can easily stimulate the clitoris by hand during sex, thus allowing the woman to overcome the climax dilemma.

The fourth sexual position that is worth mentioning is the doggy style position. In this position, the woman is on her knees and the palm of her hands, like a dog. The palms of the woman's hands are flat on the floor, helping support her weight. A woman can overcome the climax dilemma in this sexual position if she climaxes from G-spot stimulation because the man's penis presses against the front wall of her vagina during sex, thus providing stimulation of the G-spot. This position allows deep penile penetration during sex, thus giving a lot of pleasure to the man and the woman during sex, which allows the woman to overcome the climax dilemma. In this position, the man or the woman can stimulate the clitoris manually during sex, thus allowing the couple to overcome the climax dilemma.

The fifth sexual position that is worth mentioning is a variation of the rear entry position. In this position, the woman lies flat on her stomach with her legs slightly apart and the man lies flat on top of her and penetrates her vagina from behind. In this position, the walls of the vagina will be compressed and this will make it virtually unavoidable for a man's penis to evade the G-spot during sex. In this position, the G-spot can easily be stimulated from penile thrusting during sex, thus letting a woman that can climax from G-spot stimulation overcome the climax dilemma. Also, in this position the woman can stimulate her clitoris manually during sex, thus overcoming the climax dilemma.

The sixth sexual position that is worth mentioning is a variation of the missionary position. In this position the woman lies flat on her back with a pillow under her buttocks, and lifts her legs in the air resting them on the man's shoulders. The man lies on top of her flat with her legs resting on his shoulders. In this position the man can stimulate the G-spot during penile thrusting thus letting the woman that can climax from G-spot stimulation, overcome the climax dilemma. In this position the woman can manually stimulate the clitoris during sex, thus letting her overcome the climax dilemma.

Overcoming the Climax Dilemma with Multiple Orgasms

Multiple orgasms are defined as one orgasm spilling into another without a refractory period in between. A multi-orgasmic woman has the ability to attain more than one orgasm in succession without a refractory period in between orgasms. Most women can experience multiple orgasms. However, some women cannot. If a woman can experience multiple orgasms that does not mean that she is a better lover than the woman that cannot. There is nothing wrong with a woman that cannot experience multiple orgasms. That is only normal. Even some women that can experience multiple orgasms are fully satisfied with one orgasm and need nothing more. However, some women that can experience multiple orgasms prefer two or three orgasms to just one. That is perfectly normal and does not make them better lovers than women that are satisfied with only one orgasm. A woman only needs one orgasm during a sexual encounter to be happy, healthy, fulfilled, and content.

Women that can experience multiple orgasms can use that ability to overcome the climax dilemma and make sex more pleasurable for them. Multiple orgasms are a lot of fun for a woman to have, but a woman should not ruin the orgasm that she is already capable of having by pressuring herself to have more. When multiple orgasms become a goal rather than a natural reflex response during sex, the multiple orgasms are less likely to happen. A woman can experience multiple orgasms by continuing to breathe when she feels an orgasm starts to build. She should continue to breathe through an orgasm also, in order for her to experience multiple orgasms. She should not give in to her instinct to hold her breath as she approaches an orgasm and during an orgasm. She should not do so because if she holds her breath before an orgasm and during an orgasm, it makes it difficult for her to keep going from one orgasm to another. Also, as a woman approaches an orgasm and during an orgasm excited, erratic, shallow breathing is usually instinctual. However, the woman should not give in to her instincts and breathe that way. Rather, she should breathe deep breaths to make it easy for her to keep going from one orgasm to another. Breathing deep breaths will make the woman relaxed, and will make the orgasm more intense and pleasurable.

The woman can make it easier for her to experience multiple orgasms by using a lot of lubricant during sex. The woman would also, make it easier for her to experience multiple orgasms by her having her clitoris stimulated manually by her hand or the man's hand during intercourse. The manual stimulation of the clitoris during sex will ensure that the woman's clitoris will get sufficient stimulation for her to move from one orgasm to another. Another way that would help the woman experience multiple orgasms is for her to continue the sexual stimulation, including clitoral stimulation, after the first orgasm. She should do so because it is very hard for her to regain sexual sensation and attain an orgasm without a refractory period if sexual stimulation, including clitoral stimulation, stops. By her continuing the sexual stimulation, including clitoral stimulation, after the first orgasm, she will experience multiple orgasms. She will experience a second, maybe even a third, or even a fourth orgasm. As each orgasm occurs, it becomes more intense and more pleasurable than the previous orgasm.

If a woman is multi-orgasmic, the couple could use that to their advantage to overcome the climax dilemma. A man can have the woman climax once or several times through oral sex or by manually stimulating her. After she climaxes once or several times, then he can penetrate her vagina with his penis and have sexual intercourse with her. Doing this will make it most likely that the woman will climax at the same time that the man climaxes during sex because the vagina and clitoris will respond intensely to the smallest thrusts. Not only does the woman overcome the climax dilemma, but she experiences more pleasure during the sexual encounter, and experiences the orgasm during sex as more intense and more pleasurable than usual.

Some women cannot experience multiple orgasms because they find that their genital area and clitoris are extremely sensitive immediately after an orgasm and they can no longer tolerate any more contact due to this increased sensitivity. A man can find out during sex whether the woman is multi-orgasmic by assessing her physical reaction after an orgasm to his touching of her clitoris. If she is reluctant to be touched, the man can assume that she is not multi-orgasmic. However, if she groans with pleasure and is seriously responsive to his touch then she is multi-orgasmic.

Overcoming the Climax Dilemma— By Making the Sex Longer

Usually, the average man climaxes before the average woman in a sexual encounter, and that is why the climax dilemma exists. Some people believe that the climax dilemma could be overcome by the man continuing the sexual encounter after he ejaculates. But this belief is incorrect since usually the man, after he ejaculates, has a refractory period of 20 to 30 minutes where he cannot get another erection, nor orgasm. However, there are an extremely small number of men that can get an erection and resume sex right after ejaculating. They do so because they have no refractory period or a refractory period lasting less than a minute. But since the average man has a refractory period of 20 to 30 minutes where he cannot get another erection, nor orgasm, there are ways to make sex longer for him so that he climaxes the same time as the woman climaxes, overcoming the climax dilemma.

The first way that the couple could make the sex longer is if the man is thrusting, he could stop thrusting while keeping the penis inside the vagina when he feels he is close to climaxing. He would wait until the urge to climax subsides. Then he would resume thrusting. He would continue this process until the woman is close to orgasming. When the woman is close to orgasming, then he would continue thrusting so that both he and the woman climax simultaneously. This process works because the man's sexual arousal decreases far more quickly than the woman's sexual arousal. Therefore, when the man stops thrusting, his sexual arousal decreases far more quickly than the woman's sexual arousal, allowing the woman to be able to maintain her gradual buildup towards a climax. The second way the couple could also make the sex longer is by having the man stop thrusting when he is close to climaxing and having him withdraw the penis from the vagina. The man would wait until the urge to orgasm subsides. While waiting if the man chooses he could press the tip or base of the penis with his thumb and fingers and that can decrease his urge to ejaculate and orgasm more quickly. The man could also have the woman press the tip or base of the penis with her thumb and fingers. Then when the man feels that his urge to climax has subsided he would resume thrusting. He would continue this process until the woman is close to climaxing. When the woman is close to climaxing, then he would continue thrusting so that both he and the woman climax simultaneously.

A third way that the couple could make the sex longer is if the woman is thrusting, when she feels the man is close to orgasming she could stop the thrusting and keep the penis motionless in her vagina. She would do so until the man's urge to orgasm goes away. Then she could resume thrusting. She would continue this process until she is very close to orgasming. When she is very close to orgasming then she would continue thrusting so that both she and the man climax simultaneously. A fourth way that the couple could make the sex longer is if the woman is thrusting, when she feels the man is close to orgasming, she could stop the thrusting and withdraw the penis from inside her vagina. She would do so until the man's urge to orgasm goes away. While waiting for the man's urge to climax to go away, the woman could press the tip or base of the penis with her thumb and fingers to decrease his urge to ejaculate and orgasm more quickly. The man could also press the tip or base of the penis with his thumb and fingers. Then when the man feels that his urge to climax has subsided, the woman could resume thrusting. She would continue this process until she is very close to orgasming. When she is very close to orgasming then she would continue thrusting so that both she and the man climax simultaneously.

A fifth way the couple could make the sex longer to overcome the climax dilemma, is when a man is close to ejaculation the woman can tug on the testicles gently downward with one of her hands. She would do that because when a man is about to ejaculate, the testicles tend to retract to the body and move up. If the woman keeps the testicles down, the man cannot ejaculate, because if the testicles do not undergo at least a partial elevation during sex, then ejaculation won't happen. The woman would keep the testicles tugged gently downward until the man's urge to ejaculate goes away. The man can also pull down his testicles either by holding them between his legs or by gently tugging them down with one hand until the urge to ejaculate subsides. Once the urge to ejaculate has subsided, the sex could resume. The couple could keep this process until the woman is close to orgasming. When the woman is close to orgasming the man could continue thrusting until they both climax simultaneously.

The final way that the couple could make the sex longer to overcome the climax dilemma is when a man is close to orgasm, the couple alters the sexual encounter so that the man is not stimulating his penis, but is only sexually stimulating the woman until his urge to climax subsides. He could stimulate the woman sexually without stimulating his penis through oral sex or manual stimulation. Once the man's urge to climax subsides, the couple could resume the sexual encounter with the man stimulating his penis. The couple could keep this process going until the woman is close to orgasming. Once the woman is close to orgasming, the man could continue the sexual encounter with his penis being stimulated so that they both climax simultaneously.

If the couple make the sex longer using any of these methods the sexual encounter will be very pleasurable. Also, the sexual encounter would result in extremely more intense pleasurable sexual feelings than usual, because when the sexual arousal is high, then decreases, and then increases again, the intensity of the feelings is increased. Also, the sexual encounter would result in extremely more intense and longer lasting orgasms than usual for both the man and the woman.

Other Factors that Affect the Climax Dilemma

There are many factors other than clitoral stimulation affecting whether the woman climaxes the same time as the man. The first and most important factor affecting the climax dilemma other than clitoral stimulation is the emotional state of mind of the woman. The woman needs both the proper physical stimulation and the proper emotional state of mind during sex in order to climax. Even if the woman receives the proper physical stimulation during sex but does not have the proper emotional state of mind during sex, she will not climax, thus causing the climax dilemma. A man needs the proper emotional state of mind to orgasm, and not having the proper emotional state of mind prevents a man from orgasming. However, a woman is affected a lot more by her state of mind in order for her to orgasm than the man. A man can tolerate a larger level of an improper emotional state of mind than the woman and still experience an orgasm. Stress, anxiety, being depressed, a history of emotional or physical abuse, anger, a sense of failure, and feelings of inadequacy all could prevent a woman from experiencing an orgasm during sex, thus promoting the climax dilemma. Even if the woman's clitoris is manually being stimulated during sex, the woman may not orgasm because she does not have the right emotional state of mind. The woman might desire her partner, might want to have sex with him, but her body cannot orgasm because of her state of mind.

The woman might resort to several ineffective strategies to try and deal with the problem. She might seek out a younger, sexier partner or she might give up on sex altogether. But the real answer lies not with seeking more arousal by seeking out a younger, sexier partner, nor by giving up on sex altogether. The real answer lies in having the proper state of mind by making sure that stress, anxiety, anger, feelings of inadequacy or failure, and feelings of past emotional and physical abuse do not exist anymore. The woman could overcome those feelings by talking about them with someone including a professional therapist. She could also overcome them by rationalizing to herself why they should not exist anymore. She could also overcome those feelings by focusing during sex on the physical pleasure that she is feeling, and not on those improper feelings. There will be always be the occasional day when the woman does not climax because she is not in the right state of mind. She might be feeling anxious, tired, painful, or she might have had too much to drink. The man and the woman should not worry about these days, they are only normal.

The second factor other than clitoral stimulation affecting whether the woman can overcome the climax dilemma is the woman worrying about having an orgasm or a simultaneous orgasm with the man. If the woman worries about having an orgasm or a simultaneous orgasm with the man she will put pressure on herself and this will only hinder her from experiencing an orgasm or a simultaneous orgasm with the man. This will ruin her enjoyment of the sexual experience. The woman should just enjoy herself during sex, not worrying about whether she orgasms and not worrying whether she has a simultaneous orgasm with the man. If the woman does that, she is more than likely to have a simultaneous orgasm with the man. A woman cannot force an orgasm nor will it. An orgasm is a natural reflex that occurs as a result of sexual stimulation. If the woman tries to force or will an orgasm she is more likely to prevent it from happening. A woman should just relax, enjoy the sexual sensations during sex, and let the natural reflex response of orgasming occur. The man should not pressure the woman to have an orgasm or have a simultaneous orgasm with him, since that will also hinder the woman from having an orgasm.

The third factor other than clitoral stimulation affecting whether the woman can overcome the climax dilemma is the woman letting go during sex. The woman should do what is comfortable to her and her lover during sex. She should not do anything that is uncomfortable to her or her lover during sex. It is crucial for the woman to let herself fully experience the normal physical responses during sex. The physical responses during sex include body movements, facial grimaces, groans, and intense breathing. The woman should not stop those physical responses from happening because they seem unladylike, since they are necessary for the woman to orgasm. If the woman tries to inhibit these natural physical responses during sex she may hinder her ability to orgasm and her ability to overcome the climax dilemma. The woman should let herself go during sex by not controlling her body, and by letting her body's normal physical responses manifest themselves. An orgasm is a reflex response that is triggered when there is enough sexual stimulation and the freedom to pursue the orgasm without inhibition or fear of being out of control. A number of women who have had difficulty climaxing find that they stop their natural intense breathing when they get highly aroused. A woman should concentrate on keeping her intense breathing during sex by breathing deeply during sex and not holding her breath. She should do so, so that she relaxes during sex and increases the likelihood that she will climax.

The fourth factor other than clitoral stimulation for the woman to overcome the climax dilemma is to understand that her sexual arousal is experienced in waves. The waves are experienced as a peak in arousal and then an ebb, or diminishing of the intensity of the sexual feelings, followed by a new wave of sexual arousal. The woman should not become anxious when she feels her level of sexual arousal decrease because that will stop her from climaxing and overcoming the climax dilemma. The woman rather should enjoy the waves of sexual arousal when they go up as well as when they go down, until she climaxes. By the woman enjoying the waves of sexual arousal when they go up as well as when they go down the intensity of each sexual arousal wave will be more intense and pleasurable than the previous one.

The fifth factor other than clitoral stimulation for the woman to overcome the climax dilemma is for the woman to know what an orgasm is and feels like. She should know that an orgasm is an intense pleasurable sexual sensation that results from sexual stimulation. She should know that not all women show outward physical signs like writhing and moaning as a result of a climax. She should know so, so if she does not moan or writhe she does not worry that she did not experience an orgasm, or a full orgasm. She should also know that the intensity and length of the orgasm can vary from one sexual encounter to another. Sometimes the orgasm may be strong and long and other times it may be barely perceptible. It might be barely perceptible because it might be short and mild. If she knows that then when she experiences a short and mild orgasm she will know that she experienced a full orgasm and overcame the climax dilemma.

The sixth factor other than clitoral stimulation for the woman to overcome the climax dilemma is for her to know that the man's erection during sex can come and go several times. If she knows that, then she won't worry when the man's erection decreases during sex. If she worries during sex about the man's erection decreasing, then that anxiety might prevent her from orgasming and overcoming the climax dilemma. By her not worrying during sex when the man's erection decreases, then she will not be anxious and will experience an orgasm, overcoming the climax dilemma. The seventh factor other than clitoral stimulation for the woman to overcome the climax dilemma is for her to communicate her sexual needs to her male partner. Each woman wants something different during sex in order for her to receive sexual pleasure and orgasm. Also, what each woman needs during sex changes from one sexual encounter to another. Therefore, in order for the woman to orgasm and overcome the climax dilemma she needs to communicate to her sexual partner what her sexual needs during that particular sexual encounter are.

The eighth factor other than clitoral stimulation for the woman to overcome the climax dilemma is for her to receive sufficient foreplay. Unlike men, who can be ready and willing at a moment's notice for sex, most women need some time of foreplay to be ready for sexual intercourse. It takes a woman on average about 15 to 20 minutes of foreplay to become sufficiently aroused and sufficiently lubricated for sexual intercourse, while it takes a man one minute to two minutes of foreplay to be ready to have sex. If the couple rushes the foreplay stage, then the woman will not be ready for sexual intercourse and will feel invaded by the man's penis during sex. This may cause her not to be able to experience an orgasm and not to overcome the climax dilemma.

The ninth factor other than clitoral stimulation for the woman to overcome the climax dilemma is for the man not to focus only on the woman's vagina during sex, but to focus on her whole body during foreplay and during sex. Men have the tendency during foreplay to focus only on one part of the woman's body, and they have the tendency to focus only on the woman's vagina during sex. If this occurs, the woman is most likely not going to orgasm because she needs her whole body to be stimulated during foreplay and during sex. During foreplay, her whole body could be stimulated through kissing and touching. During sex, her whole body could be stimulated through kissing and touching as well. If the woman's whole body is stimulated during foreplay and sex, then she will orgasm and will overcome the climax dilemma.

The tenth factor other than clitoral stimulation for the woman to overcome the climax dilemma is the speed of the bodily movements during sex and during foreplay. The bodily movements during foreplay and during sex need to be slow, including the thrusting during sex. Bodily movements during foreplay and sex include kissing, touching, and changing from one position to another. Men have the tendency to have their bodily movements go fast during foreplay and during sex. However, the bodily movements during foreplay and sex should be slow so that the woman's pleasurable sexual sensations and her sexual tension build up gradually and slowly. Also the bodily movements during foreplay and sex should be slow so that the woman remains relaxed. Rushing during foreplay and sex totally disrupts the woman's buildup of sexual tension and pleasurable sexual sensations causing the woman to feel less pleasure, and making it more likely that the woman will not orgasm. Also, rushing during sex will make the woman feel that she is taking too long to climax which causes her to worry, thus hindering her from climaxing. As the woman approaches orgasm the bodily movements during sex including the thrusting should remain the same pace with the same intensity. They should not increase in speed, at all.

The eleventh factor other than clitoral stimulation for the woman to overcome the climax dilemma is the rhythm during sex. Many women, in order for them to climax, have to have a consistent rhythm established during sex. This is the case because if the rhythm breaks during sex, their arousal will drop and they won't be able to climax unless again a consistent rhythm is maintained. Failure to maintain a consistent and acceptable rhythm during sex is one of the main causes of the woman's failure to climax during sex. A steady rhythm during sex results in great pleasure during the sexual encounter. A steady rhythm during sex could be maintained by not varying the pace, pressure, or activity during sex.

The twelfth factor other than clitoral stimulation for the woman to overcome the climax dilemma is for the man to show her affection during sex and foreplay. Men usually view the sex act as showing affection and love to the woman. However, the woman usually does not view the sex act as showing affection and love to her. Usually during sex, the woman wants the man to show her affection and love by compliments, kind words, and by soft loving touching all over her body. The man should not make the woman feel just like a piece of meat during sex by not showing her affection. Rather, the man should make her feel as if she is important to him and loved by him by showing her affection during sex. It is important that the man shows the woman affection during sex and not just focus on the sex act in order for the woman to experience an orgasm and overcome the climax dilemma.

The thirteenth factor other than clitoral stimulation for the woman to overcome the climax dilemma is for the woman to be able to handle the disappointment if the man orgasms before she does during sexual intercourse. If the woman is upset that the man orgasmed before her during sex, and that resentment is carried over to the next sexual encounter then the woman will not orgasm in the next sexual encounter, and will not overcome the climax dilemma. However, the woman should accept the fact that the man orgasmed before her during sex and still be happy with the sexual encounter. She should do so, so that way her contentment with the sexual encounter carries over to the next sexual encounter making it most likely that she will orgasm during the next sexual encounter and overcome the climax dilemma. The woman can still be happy with the sexual encounter even though the man orgasmed before her, by having the man leave his limp penis inside her vagina as she stimulates her clitoris manually until she orgasms. She will still feel satisfied to climax with a limp penis inside her, and will find herself having a strong orgasm around his penis. The woman will find having an orgasm with the man's limp penis still inside her more fulfilling and pleasurable than orgasming with no penis inside her. A soft penis can still provide a multitude of wonderful sensations for a woman during sex.

The final factor other than clitoral stimulation for the woman to overcome the climax dilemma is whether the woman should have sex when she does not want to have sex. If the woman has sex when she does not want to then she will not climax and overcome the climax dilemma. However, if the woman has sex only when she wants to have sex, then she will most likely climax and overcome the climax dilemma. Therefore, the woman should only have sex when she wants to have sex in order for her to climax and overcome the climax dilemma.

In conclusion, even though the woman is receiving sufficient clitoral stimulation during sex, all the other factors mentioned in this section should exist in the sexual encounter for the woman to overcome the climax dilemma. If one of these factors is missing from the sexual encounter, then this will hinder the woman from overcoming the climax dilemma. It will cause the woman to experience less pleasure during sex and may cause her not to overcome the climax dilemma by not orgasming at the same time as the man.

Chapter 22

Non-Physical Aspects of Sex

Sexual intercourse is much more than just physical movements. It includes non-physical aspects that make it pleasurable. For sex to be truly great it must include the proper physical techniques and the proper state of mind. Inattentiveness to the emotional wellbeing of both partners will cause the sex not to be satisfying. The proper state of mind or emotional wellbeing of a person does not just happen, but a person must make it happen by being deliberate about it. The proper state of mind that a person should have during sex does not just happen at the time of sex. Rather, it starts long before a person reaches the bedroom. The amount of time a person invests in cultivating the proper state of mind will result in tremendous pleasure that a person receives during sex and will make the connection between both sexual partners stronger. It is not easy for a person to identify the things affecting his or her state of mind or emotional wellbeing. Sometimes they are subconscious and a person does not know that they exist. The only way for a person to know that they exist is by careful analysis. Other times, a person knows the things affecting his or her state of mind or emotional wellbeing but does not know how to rectify the situation. This chapter will let a person know the non-physical things that affect his or her state of mind for sex, and how to rectify the situation if something is affecting him or her negatively.

Relationship Issues

The first non-physical aspect of sex is the relationship. Sex is meant to give two people that are in a relationship a way to express their love and commitment through deep pleasure. It is a manner of human expression. Since the couple is expressing their love and commitment through deep pleasure during sex, if there are difficulties in a relationship then they are bound to show up in bed, decreasing the couple's sexual pleasure. The difficulties show up in many forms. The most obvious way is through rejection. Another way is through contempt or total disregard for the other partner's sexual needs during sex. Discord in a relationship will manifest itself in the sabotaging behaviors that a couple uses to destroy the possibilities of a satisfying sexual experience together. In other words, discord in a relationship will cause both partners not to have the proper state of mind for pleasurable sex. Therefore, the first step for pleasurable sex for the couple is for them to resolve any relationship problems that they might have.

Low Self-esteem

The second non-physical aspect of sex is low self-esteem. The way a person feels about himself or herself is his or her self-esteem. If a person has a low opinion of himself or herself then he or she has a low self-esteem. A person's self-esteem directly affects his or her sexuality. If a person has a low self-esteem then it will affect his or her sexuality negatively. It will make a person feel unworthy to be able to receive and give pleasure during sex, thus limiting his or her pleasure and the pleasure of his or her sexual partner. Usually these feelings of unworthiness are unrealistic and not based on reality. A person can overcome these feelings of unworthiness by analyzing the attitudes that cause them and replacing those negative attitudes with positive ones. For example, a person might feel that he is unworthy of pleasure because he is does not have a certain level of education, or a certain dollar value in his bank account. However, a person can change his attitude by seeing himself as worthy of pleasure despite his level of education or dollar value in his bank account because he is a caring person and can offer his or her sexual partner a lot in a relationship.

If a person has a low self-esteem he or she will usually also have a negative body image. In other words, a person will view his or her body negatively. A negative body image will cause a person to feel that he or she is not sexually attractive, and can make the person shy away from sex. A negative body image will also hinder a person's ability to relax and enjoy the sex. Rather, it will cause a person to feel insecure, anxious, and distracted during sex. This will cause the sex to become less pleasurable and satisfying. One way for a person to overcome a negative body image is for him or her not to compare himself or herself to other people especially movie stars or athletes. He or she should remember that his or her body is unique. He or she should also appreciate, accept, and like himself or herself for what he or she is. A person can appreciate himself or herself and change a negative body image to a positive body image by changing the attitudes that cause the negative body image. For example, if a man views his nose as ugly because of its shape, he should change his attitude and see his nose as beautiful because of its shape. He should remember that beauty is in the eyes of the beholder and that what might seem undesirable to one person might be desirable to another.

An example of beauty being in the eyes of the beholder is if a woman views herself as unattractive because she is flat chested, she could change her attitude and view herself as attractive for being flat chested, since a number of men are attracted to women that are flat chested. Once a person changes his negative attitudes about his or her body to positive ones, he or she will have a positive body image and the sex and the relationship will improve for the better. A person should remember that being sexy and attractive starts in the mind. A person does not have to be physically gorgeous or handsome to be attractive and sexy. A person just needs to have an attitude that he or she is attractive and sexy, and people will view him or her as so, because his or her attitude is apparent in his or her behavior.

It is important that a person has a high self-esteem and loves himself or herself because he or she cannot really love another person until he or she loves himself or herself. Therefore, it is important to cultivate self-love by changing negative attitudes about oneself to positive ones in order to have a healthy sex life. Self-love is different from egotism or narcissism. It is simply the feeling of loving, accepting, and having a positive attitude towards oneself. Once a person loves himself or herself and has a positive body image, the sex will be more pleasurable and the relationship will be more cohesive, having a greater chance of succeeding.

A person tends to attract people he or she thinks he or she deserves. This means that if a person likes himself or herself, he or she is more likely to attract someone who respects him or her and treats him or her well. This will most likely lead to a pleasurable sex life. If a person does not like himself or herself he or she is more likely to attract someone who does not like him or her and does not treat him or her well. This will most likely lead to a sex life that is not satisfying and pleasurable. A person should know that the first step to being loved by others is to love himself or herself and others will follow the lead. Therefore, whether a person's self-esteem or self-love was damaged because he or she was sexually abused, physically abused, emotionally abused, criticized, or mocked by others a person needs to rectify the situation by cultivating self-love.

Inhibitions

The third non-physical aspect of sex is inhibitions. Inhibitions hinder a person's sexual satisfaction. These inhibitions are a result of negative incorrect input a person received about sex and negative experiences a person had with sex. The negative experiences that a person might have had with sex that cause his or her inhibitions include sexual abuse and rape. They also include having sex with a partner who is complaining about the person's performance in bed, or a partner who is criticizing any of the person's body parts during sex. Incorrect input a person received about sex includes incorrect messages a person received from his or her parents when he or she was young that sex was dirty, something to be ashamed of, and something not to be enjoyed. Incorrect input a person received about sex includes misguided and incorrect teachings from religious figures in a person's childhood that sex was dirty, something to be avoided, and something not be enjoyed.

Inhibitions can cause feelings of guilt, anger, shame, anxiety, and depression that have a catastrophic effect on a person's ability to have a healthy sexual relationship. Inhibitions result in a decreased sexual desire and less pleasure during sex. Inhibitions make it difficult for a person to express sexual feelings. As a result of his or her inhibitions, a person may rush during sex, not experiencing his or her sensuous feelings. The person does not allow himself or herself to receive sexual pleasure to the fullest extent and feel good about it. The person and his or her partner feel frustrated and unfulfilled as a result of the sexual encounters. The person finds the sex boring and a waste of time. He or she does not find it exciting and pleasurable. To the person, sex is a burden to be endured or a duty to be accepted with grace. It is not viewed as a source of great fulfillment and not as a way to express love to the partner. Rather a person's inhibitions cause sex to be an unpleasant ordeal.

A person has the right to enjoy his or her sex life so he or she should never be embarrassed or ashamed by the fact that he or she is a sexual being. Sex is a good healthy part of person's life. A person has the right to get the most pleasure out of his or her sexuality. A person has to be comfortable with his or her sexuality so that he or she does not miss on one of life's greatest pleasures: sexual pleasure. A person should never feel guilty or embarrassed about wanting to improve his or her sex life and make it as pleasurable as possible.

The first step in overcoming inhibitions is for the person to accept sex as something that is normal, healthy, pleasurable, and beautiful. The person has to accept that there is nothing embarrassing or repulsive about sex. The second step in overcoming inhibitions is a person should believe that he or she has the right to enjoy the sex. The third step in overcoming inhibitions is for the person to identify the negative attitudes that are inhibiting him or her. Then he or she should change these negative attitudes to positive ones. Then he or she needs to accept those attitudes and adopt them as his or her own. Removing the negative inhibitions from a person's mind will open up a whole new world of freedom for the person and his or her partner. Once a person overcomes his or her inhibitions he or she will be free to experience sex to a far greater intensity than ever before.

Romance

The fourth non-physical aspect of sex is romance. Romance does not equal sex. Being romantic means expressing love or strong affection. Having sex is not considered being romantic. A person needs to show affection during the sexual act in order for romance to exist in the sex. Sex which involves mere thrusting of the penis in and out of the vagina without any affection is not romantic in any way. When a person in the relationship wants more romance that does not mean he or she wants more sex. It means that a person wants his or her sexual partner or future lover to show affection in bed and out of bed. Romance is an important ingredient for great sex. If there is romance in the relationship, then the sex will be satisfying, fulfilling, and greatly pleasurable. If there is not romance in the relationship then the sex will not be satisfying, and will be less pleasurable.

Romance in the relationship excites both people and builds passion in them towards each other. Passion is a strong desire for each other. It also includes a strong sexual desire for each other. If the passion has gone in the relationship, it is usually because the romance has gone. A person tends to be less willing to be sexual if the romance is not there, since the passion or strong desire for each other does not exist.

The way for a person to be romantic is to let his or her partner feel very special. He or she should show that he or she cares for his or her partner. A person could make his or her partner feel special by doing romantic acts. These acts include giving his or her partner flowers, chocolate, or love notes. These acts also include washing his or her partner's car, taking walks together, and most important of all saying the words, "I love you." If a person calls his or her partner during the day and expresses terms of affection to him or her that is also a very romantic act. If a person makes a gourmet meal with wine and candlelight for his or her partner or tells his or her partner that he or she cares for him or her, that is also a very romantic act. Touching, kissing, and expressing terms of affection during the day is very romantic and builds sexual passion in both partners. As a matter of fact, touching during the day is essential for a couple to maintain their bond together, because it conveys love and affection.

In order for a person to be romantic he or she must make sure that there is equality in the relationship and friendship. The friendship should be based on honesty, openness and trust. Manipulative game playing and being loose with the truth does not show that the person cares for his or her partner and does not allow romance to exist in the relationship. In order for a person to be romantic he or she must show that his or her partner's needs are as important as his or her own.

Usually, a couple is romantic at the beginning of a relationship, but after a while the romance goes. It is important to maintain the romance in the relationship all the time, even after many years. This is important because the minute the romance goes, it is just a matter of time before the relationship goes sour. Also, without romance in the relationship, the quality of the sex goes down and so does the quantity. In conclusion, a person should maintain romance in the relationship for a healthy sex life.

Intimacy

Intimacy is the fifth non-physical aspect of sex. If the couple has intimacy in the relationship, then the sex will be very pleasurable and satisfying. If the couple lacks intimacy in the relationship, then the sex will not be very pleasurable and will not be satisfying. If the couple lacks intimacy in the relationship, both people will not feel secure enough to relax and enjoy sex. Intimacy is when the couple feels close and familiar with each other, characterized as a form of friendship. It is when both people can be themselves and know it will be okay with their partner. It is when both people are comfortable with each other. Intimacy means that both people are understanding to each other and accept each other for what they are. It means that people are tolerant of each other's differences. True intimacy means that both people experience a sense of connectedness with their sexual partner that is deeply felt. It causes both people to experience a greater freedom and joy in the relationship. As time passes by and the intense sexual excitement about the newness of the relationship goes away, the intimate feelings between both people act as a reminder of the early days of the relationship and continue to bond them. Intimacy is vital for a healthy long-term relationship, helping to reinforce feelings of affection, attachment, love, and sexual interest.

Intimacy is not something that a couple instantly and automatically acquires when they become a couple. Rather it is something that a couple acquires gradually over time. A couple could acquire intimacy from daily hugs, kisses, touching, and terms of endearment. The couple could also acquire intimacy by daily talking about their feelings, their likes, and their dislikes. When a couple is open and honest with each other about how they feel and what they think, they become familiar with each other. Being sympathetic and sensitive to each other's feelings daily allows a couple to acquire intimacy. Intimacy can be also acquired if the couple spends time together sufficiently. Sharing experiences together like working together, playing together, swimming together, or walking together definitely will help a couple acquire intimacy. Intimacy is also acquired by the couple, as the couple becomes familiar with each other and trust between them develops. Intimacy is closely linked to the overall trust that is gradually built up in a relationship. It is important to note that intimacy in a relationship could disappear if the couple stops doing what it was doing to acquire the intimacy. It is not surprising that some relationships after many years end because the intimacy that the couple once had disappeared.

Love

Love is the sixth non-physical aspect of sex. Love is a feeling of warm personal attachment or deep affection, while sex is about physical pleasure and lust. Sex is separate from love. For a number of people, sex and love can be easily separated and do not have to exist at the same time. They can have sex without being in love. However, for others being in love is a requirement for having sex. In order for a person to be happy with his or her sex life and have a meaningful relationship, he or she has to sort out the issue whether love is a requirement for having sex, or if sex and love can occur separately. By sorting out this issue, a person can decide whether monogamy or casual sex with no commitments is for him or her. There is no right or wrong answer. It all depends on the individual. However, for great sex, love between both partners is a requirement. It is a requirement because without love, both partners cannot have great passion for each other and cannot be interested in each other. If both partners are in love, then the sex will be enjoyable for both of them to the greatest extent.

Sex with love is better than sex with no love because if both people are in love and are having sex, they feel that they are practically melding together during sex. They feel like they are really making love. However, if both people are having sex with no love then it just a mechanical act and they are not making love. They are just doing it. Most people prefer sex with love. They find it very pleasurable. They like their partner looking into their eyes during sex and saying "I love you." It makes them feel amazing. They view sex as a means of expressing their love for their partner. They find the sex more satisfying if they are in love, and doing it with someone they have built up an emotional bond with.

Anger and Resentment

Anger and resentment are the seventh non-physical aspect of sex. If a person has these two emotions in the relationship, they limit his or her affection and attraction towards his or her partner. Also what goes on in the bedroom is not separate from the rest of a person's life. So if a person has anger or resentment towards his or her partner it will carry over into his or her sexual relationship. These two emotions create disharmony in the relationship that spills over into the bedroom. These two emotions make sex less desirable to a person. Also, they make the sex less pleasurable and make it harder for the woman to orgasm during sex. They also make it harder for the man to get and keep an erection during sex.

The good news is that there is a method of overcoming anger and resentment to help things heal. The way to improve the relationship and free it from anger and resentment is sociability. The couple should spend time together socializing, talking to each other. They should discuss anything that concerns them. If there is something that is angering or causing resentment to a person, he or she should let his or her partner know. When the person has gotten what is bothering him or her off his or her chest, he or she could forgive the partner for any wrong that was done by him or her. If there was no wrong committed by the partner against the person, the misunderstanding could be clarified when the person talks about his or her irritation. In both cases the anger and resentment should disappear. Furthermore, if the person is suffering anger or resentment towards his or her partner because of a problem, then both people should come up with a solution that is pleasing to both of them.

Anger and resentment are toxic to a relationship and a person's sex life. So in order to avoid having such emotions in the relationship a couple should avoid lover's quarrels and fiery confrontations that happen in some relationships. Instead the couple should try being gentle, compassionate, and empathetic with each other.

Stress

The eighth non-physical aspect of sex is stress. Stress is mental or emotional strain or tension as a result of everyday life. All people lead stressful lives. They all juggle many roles like father, employer/employee, chauffeur for kids, tutor, friend, son, husband, and so forth. However, not everyone can handle the stress in everyday life. If a person cannot handle the stress in his or her everyday life, the stress will affect his or her sex life. The stress will decrease a person's desire for sex. The person may become tense and irritable as a result of the stress and not want sex as much as before. Stress notoriously lowers testosterone levels and depletes sex drive if it is not managed properly. Stress during everyday life, if the person cannot manage it, will carry over into the bedroom, making the sex less pleasurable to the person. It will also make it more difficult for the woman to orgasm during sex, and it will make it more difficult for the man to get and keep an erection during sex. It will also make it more difficult for the person to freely express himself or herself during sex and be himself or herself during sex.

When stress causes a person's sexual desire to decrease and the sexual encounters in the relationship become fewer, the partner may incorrectly confuse this with loss of love. The partner may incorrectly think that the person does not love him or her anymore because he or she does not have sex with him or her as often as before. The partner may also incorrectly think that the person has lost sexual interest in him or her. The partner needs to understand that the person has not lost sexual interest in him or her, nor has he or she stopped loving him or her. The partner should understand that the person is under stress and he or she cannot handle the stress properly so the stress is temporarily diminishing his or her sexual desire. The partner should understand that just because there is less sex it does not mean that he or she is loved less. The partner should understand that the decrease in the person's sexual desire does not have anything to do with him or her. If a person's sexual desire decreases as a result of stress that he or she cannot handle, he or she should tell his or her partner that he or she loves him or her and that he or she is still attracted to him or her. He or she should do so, so that the partner knows that the person still loves him or her and is still attracted to him or her.

If a person has stress he or she cannot handle, he or she should learn how to handle the stress. There are several things that a person could learn to handle the stress. The first thing that a person should learn is not to let anything cause him or her anxiety, since anxiety leads to stress. If there is something that is bothering a person and causing him or her anxiety the person should deal with it right away. The second thing that a person should learn is to get enough sleep, because stress that a person cannot manage can cause a person to get less sleep than usual. Getting less sleep than usual causes the person to become irritable, moody, lack energy, and lack desire to have sex. Being irritable, moody, and lacking energy make a person enjoy sex less than usual. Therefore a person should make sure to get enough sleep despite stress he or she cannot manage so that he or she enjoys sex as much as possible and not lack sexual desire. The third thing a person should learn is to make a list of his or her daily tasks and ask others for help in doing them. This way he or she could manage the stress. The fourth thing a person should learn that if he or she has a stressful life because of his or her living standard, he or she could scale down his or her living standard. A person would do so, so that he or she gets a less stressful job or works less hours. The fifth thing a person should learn is to take out a few minutes every day for meditation, relaxation, and breathing. These activities reduce stress. The sixth thing that a person should learn is to think positive thoughts only and no negative thoughts. If most of the time a person is feeling anxious or tired it might be because of negative thinking, including anxiety filled thoughts. The seventh thing that a person should learn is to do hobbies that he or she likes like dancing, sports, or socializing with friends. A person should do so since that tends to decrease stress and makes it more manageable. In conclusion, when a person learns to manage stress his or her sex life will be greatly pleasurable.

Insecurity and Jealousy

The ninth non-physical aspect of sex is insecurity and jealousy. Jealousy is an extreme form of insecurity. Insecurity and jealousy sometimes exist in a relationship and cause tension and stress to both people. This tension and stress is carried into the bedroom, making the sex less pleasurable. A person might be insecure about the relationship. He or she might worry that his or her partner might leave him or her for someone else. A person might be insecure about his or her education, income, or looks, and think that he or she is not good enough for his or her partner. A person might be very jealous over his or her partner not wanting him or her to talk or deal with members of the opposite sex. The way to overcome insecurity and jealousy is for the person to notice what he or she is insecure about, or if he or she is jealous. Whatever the person is insecure about, he or she should seek reassurance from the partner so as not to be insecure about it. If the person is jealous, he or she should have the partner reassure him or her not to be jealous. The person should have the partner reassure him or her, that he or she wants him or her and will never leave him or her. If the partner provides reassurances to the person the insecurities and jealousy will be overcome and the sex will be very pleasurable.

Depression

The tenth non-physical aspect of sex is depression. Depression is when the person is sad and gloomy. When a person is depressed he or she has difficulty sleeping, a pessimistic outlook, difficulty concentrating, low self-esteem and loss of pleasure in life. One of the main side effects of depression is the inability of the person to enjoy normal pleasurable activities such as eating, socializing, and making love. The depressed person has a low sexual desire. The sex becomes less pleasurable if a person is depressed. Experiencing an orgasm during sex becomes more difficult to the woman if she is depressed. Getting and keeping an erection for a man during sex becomes more difficult if the man is depressed. If a person starts to suffer from depression the dark cloud not only hangs over his or her head, but it often floats to his or her partner, having a negative effect on everyone in the household. Depression often causes an otherwise good sex life to dwindle or cease altogether. If a person suffers depression and becomes less interested in sex the partner often thinks that the person has lost interest in him or her. The partner should realize that the person is depressed that is why he or she is not interested in sex with him or her. The partner should know that it is not his or her fault that the person has low sexual desire.

The good news is that a person can overcome his or her depression several ways. The first way a person can overcome his or her depression is to find out what is bothering him or her and get it out of his or her life. If what is bothering him or her is something he or she can not get rid of then he or she should learn to accept it. For example, if a person is depressed because of the atmosphere at work, he or she could quit his or her job and get another job. However, if a person is depressed because he or she was diagnosed with cancer, he or she cannot change that fact, but he or she could accept that fact and not be depressed about it. By a person accepting what he or she cannot change and not be depressed about it a person overcomes depression. The second way a person can overcome his or her depression is talk to his or her friends. Socializing does help a person overcome his or her sadness. The third way for a person to overcome his or her depression is to keep busy. By keeping busy a person has no time to think depressing thoughts so he or she overcomes his or her depression. The fourth way for a person to overcome his or her depression is to maintain a positive mental attitude by thinking positively through the day. The fifth way for a person to overcome his or her depression is to cut out depressant drugs such as alcohol. The sixth way for a person to overcome depression is to exercise regularly. Once a person overcomes his or her depression his or her sex drive slowly returns and the couple resumes their sex life. The joy and pleasure during sex return to their normal levels.

Guilt

The eleventh non-physical aspect of sex is guilt. Guilt is the feeling of remorse for some wrong, whether real or imagined. Usually when a person feels guilty there is a feeling that he or she did something, or is doing something that he or she should not. Guilt is a good thing at times, making a person act properly. However, guilt at other times is a bad thing, ruining the passion and sexual pleasure during sex. A person may feel guilty during sex because of an erroneous idea that he or she has that sex is evil or nasty. Also, a person may feel guilty during sex because he or she cheated on his or her partner. Another reason a person may feel guilty during sex is because he or she does not know how to please his or her partner well during sex. Finally, a person may feel guilty during sex because he or she wants sex more frequently than his or her partner.

In order to overcome the feelings of guilt a person needs to find out the attitudes that are causing his or her guilt feelings. When he or she finds those attitudes he or she should change them to positive attitudes that do not cause him or her guilt feelings during sex. Then the person should accept those attitudes and adopt them as his or her own. For example, if a person feels guilty during sex because he or she thinks that sex is evil and nasty, he or she should change his or her attitude to view sex as good and pleasurable. If a person feels guilty because he or she cheated on his or her partner, he or she should forgive himself or herself so that he or she no longer feels guilty. If a person feels guilty because he or she does not know how to please his or her partner then he or she should find out how to please his or her partner. If a person feels guilty that he or she wants sex more frequently than his or her partner, then he or she should realize that there is nothing wrong for him or her to want sex more frequently than his or her partner. Overcoming feelings of guilt so that no guilt exists will make sex extremely pleasurable and satisfying for a person.

Grief

The twelfth non-physical aspect of sex is grief. Grief is the mental suffering over affliction or loss. Grief is usually experienced by a person over the loss of a partner, either through death or because the partner left him or her for another person. Usually a person that is suffering from grief withdraws from intimacy and avoids getting another sexual partner. After a while the person suffering from grief gets another partner if he or she is interested in having another relationship but the person finds it hard to have sex with the new partner although he or she is attracted greatly to the new partner. If the person is a man he would find it hard to get and keep an erection during sex with the new partner as a result of grief. If the person is a woman she would find it hard to orgasm during sex with the new partner as a result of grief. Whether the person is a man or a woman he or she would find sex less pleasurable because he or she is suffering grief. These occurrences with a grieving person demonstrate how attached he or she is to the person he or she lost. These occurrences are a sign that there is still a need for the person to let go of the sadness inside.

If a person is in a relationship and cannot perform well sexually as a result of the grief he or she could overcome the grief several ways. The first way he or she could overcome it is by accepting the loss and deciding to move on with his or her life happily enjoying it to its maximum. A person should avoid talking or thinking about the partner he or she lost. The second way he or she could overcome grief is by him or her having loving and non-penetrative physical contact with his or her partner. The non-penetrative physical contact could include touching, kissing, sleeping on top of each other, hugging, and cuddling. A person should continue to have non-penetrative physical contact with his or her partner until he or she is ready for sex. It might take a couple of days, weeks, or months before the person is ready for sex. However, when the person feels ready for sex he or she should resume having intercourse. When the person resumes having intercourse the intercourse should be as pleasurable as before and a person should have overcome his or her grief.

Mutual Respect

The thirteenth non-physical aspect of sex is mutual respect. Respect is when a person is held in high esteem or honor and is treated courteously as result of it. Mutual respect should exist in a relationship in order for the sex to be pleasurable to the greatest extent and for the sex to be satisfying. Lack of mutual respect in a relationship causes the sex to be less pleasurable and less satisfying. Lack of mutual respect is a source of sexual problems. It is difficult for a person to make love to someone he or she does not respect. It is difficult for a person to have someone he or she does not respect make love to him or her.

Respect may exist at the beginning of the relationship but then it diminishes because the partner does not measure up to the person's expectations. Lack of respect towards the partner will usually have to do with either his or her competence in his or her occupation, his or her integrity and honesty as an individual, or his or her competence in other aspects of his or her life. Other aspects of the partner's life include managing the household, dealing with the children, dealing with friends and relatives, and, most important of all, being a good lover.

In order to overcome lack of respect in a relationship a person should see what is causing it. If the person is not respected by his or her partner a person should find out why. Once he or she finds out the reason then if it is something he or she can change then he or she should change it so that his or her partner respects him or her. If it is something that he or she cannot change then he or she should have the partner change his or her attitude towards him or her and respect him. If the person does not respect his or her partner then he or she should find out why. If it is something that could be changed and changing it is for the benefit of the partner then the person could have his or her partner change it. If the partner does not want to change it, the person just has to change his or her attitude towards it, accept it and be respectful to his or her partner. If the partner cannot change it the person has to just accept it, change his or her attitude towards it and be respectful to his or her partner. Once lack of mutual respect in a relationship is overcome the sex will be pleasurable and satisfying to both people to a great degree.

Communication

The fourteenth non-physical aspect of sex is communication. Communication between the couple is necessary for a healthy relationship and a healthy sex life. The communication can be about anything. It can be about aspects of the relationship, what happened at work, the kids, sex, or anything else. It is important to have communication between the couple because people tend to have better sex with people they know and understand. The more a couple talks together, the more enjoyable the sex and the relationship are to both of them. Communication allows a couple to solve their problems. Communication allows the couple to adjust the differences that they have between each other. If the couple do not communicate sufficiently then they cannot solve their problems. As a matter of fact lack of communication is responsible for ending many marriages and relationships. The more a couple talks together the fewer the number of complications that will arise later on in the relationship and sex life.

The communication must be made in an atmosphere of freedom and openness. When a person shares himself or herself openly with his or her partner he or she has to know that he or she will be received with understanding and warmth, and that he or she is not going to be criticized or judged. Criticism is a common way of killing a good relationship. It may destroy the criticized person's confidence to such an extent that he or she retreats inward, is incapable of enjoying the relationship, and is incapable of being himself or herself. The communication must be honest so that it brings the couple closer together, and makes them more intimate. This will lead the couple to have more pleasurable and satisfying sex. If a person is dishonest in his or her relationship he or she will be anxious that his or her partner will find out that he or she was dishonest, which will take away from the sexual pleasure during sex.

Understanding Sexual Matters

A large number of people assume that sex comes naturally. They think that they do not need to learn how to have sex. Unfortunately sex, like math, reading and other skills, has to be learned. So when a person has sex and relies on his or her natural instincts, the sex is not satisfying and he or she feels that he or she is an inadequate lover. Others rely on the sexual knowledge they learned from everyday experiences. They rely on what they hear from family members, friends, television, and movies. Unfortunately only some of the information that they hear is accurate most of it is inaccurate. The information in the media and in movies about sex is very emotionally charged and very misrepresented. The information from family members and friends is inaccurate based on their misconceptions. Since most of the information acquired from everyday life is inaccurate, many adults, when they reach the point of readiness for sexual intercourse, they have a very inaccurate idea about sex. This inaccurate information leads to inhibitions during sex, making the sex less pleasurable and less satisfying.

Sex is supposed to be fun. Many people do not enjoy sex because a lot of them do not know all the accurate details about sex. They do not know how to enjoy their partner's body. They do not know where the clitoris is. They do not know how to get the most pleasure out of a sexual encounter. They have unrealistic expectations of what should happen during sex. Also, they do not know what are certain natural bodily responses during sex. Thus, they shy away from them during sex, as if they are abnormal, inhibiting their natural body responses. This makes the sex less pleasurable and satisfying. It is crucial that a person have an accurate idea about sex. When a person has an accurate idea about sex, he or she will understand the normal physical responses during sex and will let himself or herself fully experience them. He or she will not inhibit his or her natural sexual expression. When a person has an accurate idea about sex, he or she will have greater freedom, relaxation, enjoyment and satisfaction during sex. The way for a person to acquire accurate information about sex is to read books about sex like this one.

Right Age for Sex

The sixteenth non-physical aspect of sex is to have sex at the right age. Some people have sex too early, before they are the right age. Doing so causes the sex to be less pleasurable and not satisfying. Well, what is the right age? There is no number that is the right age to have sex. The right age to have sex is when a person can deal with the physical and emotional consequences of sex. A person can deal with the physical consequences of sex if he or she can use condoms and birth control responsibly. A person can also deal with the physical consequences of sex if he or she knows what to do if an unintended pregnancy or sexually transmitted disease did occur. A person can deal with the emotional consequences of sex if he or she can talk with his or her partner about any aspect of sex responsibly. A person can also deal with the emotional consequences of sex if he or she can cope with the situation if his or her partner breaks up with him or her. The right age to have sex is when a person feels ready and is confident that sex is the right thing for him or her. Some 18-year-olds can deal with having sex and on the other hand some 30-year-olds still cannot. Having sex at the right age will provide very pleasurable and satisfying sex.

Right Time in a Relationship to Have Sex

The seventeenth non-physical aspect of sex is to have sex at the right time in the relationship. If a person does not have sex at the right time in the relationship, then the sex will be less pleasurable and not satisfying. Well, when is the right time in the relationship to have sex? Some people believe that the right time in the relationship to have sex is when they get to know their partner well. They believe that if they have sex before they get to know their partner it would be too soon and it will cause the relationship to be based only on sex. This they believe will diminish the potential for a long-term relationship. They believe it will be confusing if they become physically intimate with someone before they have established emotional intimacy with him or her by getting to know him or her. They believe that they need to get to know their partner to determine if this next sex partner is someone they would like outside of bed before becoming physically intimate.

Others, on the other hand, believe that it is the right to have sex before they get to know their partner well. They believe that if they do not have sex by the third date, the person they are dating will lose interest all together and dump them. They believe that physical intimacy with a new person that they do not know well will teach them more about him or her than if they had hours of conversation. There is no right or wrong answer. A person needs to determine his or her own set of rules about when it is right to have sex with someone. A person has to decide whether he or she needs to know the person well before having sex with him or her, or not. Whatever a person decides, he or she should stick to it. In the long run if a person makes a decision about when to have sex with a new partner and he or she sticks to it, he or she will be happier than if he or she just improvised. Having sex in the relationship when the person feels is the right time will make the sex very pleasurable and very satisfying.

Monogamy

The eighteenth non-physical aspect of sex is monogamy. Monogamy is a sexually exclusive relationship between two people. Monogamy can work only if both people are completely committed to be sexually exclusive with each other. The advantage of a monogamous relationship is that the couple gets to know each other's body and sexual response. They know exactly how to make each other feel great during sex. A second advantage of a monogamous relationship is that the couple develops trust between each other. A third advantage of a monogamous relationship is that a couple feels uninhibited around each other, thus leading to more freedom and pleasure during sex. A fourth advantage of monogamy is that a person feels satisfied and fulfilled after sex. A large number of people who are not in a monogamous relationship usually feel lonely, depressed, and unsatisfied after sex. A fifth advantage about monogamy is that a person does not have to worry about sexually transmitted diseases during sex making the sex pleasurable. However, sex in a monogamous relationship can get boring if it is always done the same way. The way to keep the sex from becoming boring in a monogamous relationship is to have variety during sex.

Human beings tend to naturally pair. Pair bonding is a trademark of the human animal. It is interesting to note that all over the world it is the norm for the man and the woman to bond together in a monogamous relationship. This is true even in societies where polygamy is allowed. In societies where men are allowed to take multiple wives the majority still take only one wife. People in a monogamous relationship are usually happier than people that are not in a monogamous relationship. Some people practice serial monogamy, which is they are monogamous with a person for a while, then they change and get another person and are monogamous with the other person. It is interesting to note that the longer a person is in a monogamous relationship, the more pleasurable the relationship and the sex will be. Finally, monogamy is a non-physical aspect of sex that will cause the sex to be pleasurable and satisfying.

Conclusion

This chapter has provided knowledge about the important non-physical aspects of sex. It also, provided information on how to cultivate the proper state of mind for sex, so that sex is satisfying and pleasurable to the greatest extent. A person should cultivate the proper state of mind for sex, since that is as necessary for a pleasurable sex life as the sexual physical techniques are. It is important to remember that the wrong state of mind during sex will interfere with the pleasure and satisfaction of the sexual encounter.

Chapter 23

Does Size Matter?

The penis comes in many shapes and sizes. Likewise, the vagina comes in many sizes. The size of the penis has nothing to do with the size of a man. Large men can have small penises and small men can have large penises. Likewise, the size of the vagina has nothing to do with the size of the woman. Large women can have small and tight vaginas, while small women can have large and wide vaginas. The average size of the flaccid penis is 3.4 to 3.7 inches in length, and 3.7 to 3.9 inches in circumference. The average size of the erect penis is 5.1 to 5.9 inches in length, and 4.5 to 5 inches in circumference. The average size of the unaroused vagina is 3.5 inches to 4 inches in length, and less than an inch in diameter. The average size of the aroused vagina is 5 to 6 inches in length, and 1.5 to 2.5 inches in diameter. The vagina stretches a lot more. It stretches to such an extent, that it can accommodate a baby coming out of it.

Many men wonder whether the size of their erect penis affects their sexual pleasure and their partner's sexual pleasure. They also wonder whether the size of the woman's aroused vagina affects their sexual pleasure and the woman's sexual pleasure. Many women also wonder whether the size of their aroused vagina affects their sexual pleasure and their partner's sexual pleasure. They also wonder whether the size of the man's erect penis affects their sexual pleasure and the man's sexual pleasure. Many men and women wonder whether the size of the clitoris affects the woman's sexual pleasure. Unfortunately, some women incorrectly believe that a large erect penis will produce more pleasure for them during sex than a small erect penis. Likewise, some men incorrectly believe that a small, tight vagina will produce more pleasure for them during sex than a large, wide vagina. Also, some men and women incorrectly believe that a large clitoris will produce more pleasure to the woman during sex than a small clitoris. Also, some people incorrectly believe that a small limp penis means that a man will have a small erect penis.

Size Does Not Matter

The size of a limp penis does not matter, since it gives little indication of the size it will eventually grow to when erect. A small limp penis can grow to become a large erect penis. A large limp penis can grow to become a small erect penis. Usually the size of the man's erect penis and the size of the woman's aroused vagina do not matter in regards to the sexual pleasure that both the man and the woman experience during sex. This is the case because regardless what size the erect penis is, the aroused vagina adjusts well to it. The woman's aroused vagina can change to accommodate any size erect penis. The vagina can expand to allow the passage of a newborn baby, so there is no need to worry about an erect penis being too large, either in length or in circumference. Also, there is no need to worry that the erect penis is thin or that the aroused vagina is wide, since the woman's PC muscle can tighten to completely close the opening of the vagina. Thus, a thin erect penis can still have firm sensations, and pressure on the aroused vagina.

Another reason why the erect penis size and the aroused vagina size do not matter is because the majority of the nerve endings of the vagina are located near the vaginal opening. They are located within the first one and a half to two inches of the vaginal canal. Any size of an erect penis can stimulate the first one and a half to two inches of the vaginal canal, providing ample stimulation to the woman to have sexual pleasure. As a matter of fact, the primary contact the erect penis has with the walls of the vagina during intercourse occurs in the first one and a half to two inches of the vaginal canal. The first two inches of the vaginal canal stimulating the erect penis is all the man needs to orgasm. Furthermore, the size of the man's erect penis and the woman's aroused vagina does not matter because the man can move his erect penis during intercourse, or the woman can move her aroused vagina during intercourse. Such action by the man or the woman allows a large amount of the sensitive spots, on the first one and a half to two inches of the vaginal canal, to be stimulated, and allows the man's erect penis to be stimulated sufficiently.

The size of the man's erect penis and the size of the woman's aroused vagina do not matter because the best sex involves both the man and the woman involving their whole bodies for sexual pleasure and not just concentrating on the penis and vagina interaction for sexual pleasure. The man and the woman involve their whole bodies during sex for sexual pleasure by rubbing their body parts against their partner's body parts. For example, the man could rub his stomach against the woman's stomach or his legs against the woman's legs during sex. The man and the woman involve their partner's whole body during sex for sexual pleasure by caressing or kissing their partner's whole body. Regardless what the penis size is, all penises produce sufficient pleasure for the man and the woman. The size of the man's penis does not affect the man's virility, fertility, or skill as a lover. Regardless what the vagina size is, all vaginas produce sufficient pleasure for the man and the woman. The size of the woman's vagina does not affect the woman's fertility or skill as a lover.

The size of the woman's external clitoris varies from woman to woman. It ranges from a few millimeters to an inch or more. The average length of the external clitoris is a quarter of an inch. Despite the variety of sizes of the external clitoris, all the clitorises contain the same number of nerve endings. Each clitoris contains 8000 nerve endings. Thus, all clitorises, whether large or small, produce the same amount of pleasure when stimulated, and produce an intense orgasm when stimulated correctly. The size of the woman's clitoris does not matter in regards to the sexual pleasure that the woman experiences during sex. However, it is important to note that the sensitivity of the clitoris varies from woman to woman. But the sensitivity of the clitoris, has nothing to do with the size of the clitoris. Some women have a very sensitive clitoris and find direct stimulation of the clitoris uncomfortable or painful. While other women have a less sensitive clitoris and find great pleasure in prolonged direct stimulation of the clitoris.

Penis Shape

Besides penis size, another variation is the penis shape. Some men have limp penises that curve down, some men have limp penises that curve either to the left or right, and others have limp penises that do not curve at all, but are pointed straight. They are pointed straight because they are too short. Some men have erect penises that point up, some men have erect penises that point down, some men have erect penises that point straight, and others have erect penises that are slightly curved to the left or the right. Some people wonder whether the shape of the man's penis and the way it curves during an erection affect the pleasure for the man and the woman during sexual intercourse. The shape of the man's penis and the way it curves during an erection do not affect the pleasure for the woman and the man during sexual intercourse. The shape of the man's penis does not affect the man's virility, fertility, or skill as a lover.

Many people wonder if a man might have done something to make his penis curve. For example, some people might think that the reason a man's penis curves is because of the way he places his penis in his underwear. Other people might think that the reason a man's penis curves is related to the way he masturbates. The way a man's penis curves has nothing to do with what he has done to it. The way a man's penis curves is because of genetics.

Note that there is one condition in which a man should worry if his penis curves. That condition is if an adult man has always had a straight erect penis, but then notices a bend or curve forming in it. This may be Peyronie's disease. Peyronie's disease is a condition caused by a buildup of fibrous plaque in the walls of the blood chambers of the penis. This plaque buildup causes the penis to develop a bend in it. It can also be very painful to the man until it is treated. If a man notices such a condition, he should see a doctor right away.

Deeper Penetration

Although the size of the erect penis and the size of the aroused vagina do not matter for sexual pleasure, sometimes a woman with an aroused vagina canal longer than the erect penis of her lover would like deeper penetration during sex. For example, if the woman's aroused vagina measures 6 inches in length and the man's erect penis measures 5.1 inches in length, then a woman sometimes would like a deeper penetration of her vagina during sex. There are several ways for the woman to have a deeper penetration of her vagina during sex. The first way for the woman to have a deeper penetration of her vagina during sex is for her to lie on her back and then pull her knees all the way up against her chest. Then the man would lie on top of the woman with his face facing her face and have his penis in her vagina while his legs are kept straight or bent. The woman would keep her legs during sex against her chest, either under the man's chest or around his back. This position might be uncomfortable to some women, but other women find it very exciting. However, this position does increase the penile penetration of the vagina.

A second way to increase the depth of the penile penetration of the vagina is for the woman to lie down on the bottom in the missionary position with the man on top of her, but the woman should place a pillow under her buttocks. By elevating the buttocks of the woman, the penile penetration of the vagina is deepened. As a combination, in this position a woman can place a pillow under her buttocks and pull her knees all the way up against her chest as the man penetrates her vagina with his penis. The woman would place her legs either under the man's chest or around his back. This combination will make the depth of the penile penetration of the vagina increase greatly. A third way to increase the depth of the penile penetration of the vagina during sex is for the couple to get into the woman on top position. Since in this position the woman is sitting on top of the man with her legs straddling his hips as the man lies flat on his back, the depth of the penile penetration is the greatest in this position.

A fourth way to increase the depth of the penile penetration of the vagina during sex is for the woman to have sex in the doggy style position. In this position the woman is on her hands and knees like a dog and the man penetrates her vagina from the rear while kneeling. This allows the penis to deeply penetrate the vagina. A fifth way to increase the depth of the penile penetration of the vagina during sex is for the man to lose weight if he is fat. For every 35 pounds above the man's ideal weight, a man effectively loses an inch of penis length, due to fat encroaching on the penis shaft. In other words, the leaner the man is, the longer the penis is, thus allowing the penis to penetrate the vagina deeper.

Shallower Penetration

Although the size of the erect penis and the size of the aroused vagina do not matter for sexual pleasure, sometimes a woman with a small, tight aroused vagina, who has a partner with a large erect penis, would like to have shallow penile penetration of her vagina. For example, a woman with an aroused vagina 5 inches in length, who has a male partner with an erect penis 5.5 inches in length would like sometimes to have shallow penile penetration of her vagina. There are several things that a woman could do to have shallow penile penetration of her vagina, if her aroused vagina is small and the man's erect penis is large. The first thing that the woman could do is to make sure that she is relaxed. The woman should make sure that she is relaxed because tense muscles can interfere with the ability of the vagina to stretch. Also, if the woman is not relaxed during sex, she won't lubricate adequately.

The second thing that the woman could do is to make sure that the penile penetration by her male partner is gentle and mild. If the penile penetration by her male partner is not gentle and mild, then the woman will tense and her vagina will not stretch. However, if the penile penetration by the male is gentle and mild, then the woman will not tense and her vagina will stretch. The third thing that a woman could do is to get into the woman on top position. In the woman on top position the man lies flat on the floor with his legs straight, and the woman sits on top of the man, straddling his hips with her legs. This position allows the woman to control the depth of the penile penetration into her vagina and keep the penetration shallow.

The fourth thing that a woman could do is to get in the missionary position with her legs straight close to each other, since when the woman keeps her legs straight close to each other, that limits the depth of the penile penetration. In the missionary position, the woman would be lying flat on her back on the bottom and the man would be lying flat on top of her, facing her. The fifth thing that a woman could do is to get in the side-to-side position, either facing the man or with the man facing the back of her head. In the side-to-side position the woman should have her legs straight close to each other, but allowing enough space for the penis to penetrate the vagina. When the woman keeps her legs straight close to each other in the side-to-side position that limits the depth of the penile penetration. The sixth thing that a woman could do is to have the man during sex not move his penis in and out like a piston, but rather she could have him move his penis in a circular or side-to-side motion, while keeping the penile penetration of the vagina shallow. The seventh thing that a woman could do is to have the man during sex keep his thrusting of the penis shallow.

Chapter 24

Faking an Orgasm

Faking an orgasm is usually a woman problem and not a man problem. The reason it is not a man problem is because for the man an orgasm is accompanied with external incidents like an erection and an ejaculation, so it is difficult to hide that they did not occur if they do not occur. So there is no need for the man to fake an orgasm if he does not have one. However, if the man tries to fake an orgasm when he does not have one, the woman can easily know that he is faking it, because he does not have an erection and does not have an ejaculation. (Note rarely a man experiences an orgasm without an ejaculation, and that is possible only if he knows how to experience multiple orgasms.) Men do not fake orgasms. Rather, men pretend to suddenly pull a groin muscle or get a stomach ache to hide the fact that they cannot get an erection and an orgasm.

Why Faking an Orgasm is a Woman Problem

Faking an orgasm is a woman problem because a man cannot tell whether a woman has climaxed or not. Since a man cannot tell that a woman has climaxed or not, the woman is tempted to fake an orgasm. It is easy for a woman to fake an orgasm. She can fake an orgasm easily by writhing, thrashing around, moaning, and throwing her head back and forth in mock ecstasy as she breathes deeply and rapidly. The fact that it is very easy for the woman to fake an orgasm makes it very tempting for the woman to fake an orgasm.

Some men claim that they can tell if the woman is faking an orgasm, from her breathing during an orgasm. The truth is that no man can tell if a woman is actually orgasming or faking an orgasm from her breathing, because there is no one way for the woman to breathe during an orgasm. During an orgasm, the woman's breathing is not rhythmic and the pace varies from minute to minute. Also, women vary in their breathing during an orgasm from day to day. So if a woman breathes heavily and rapidly during sex, even though she is faking an orgasm, there is no way for the man to know that her breathing is not a result of an actual orgasm.

Some men claim that they can tell that the woman is faking an orgasm by seeing her nipples. They claim that if she has erect nipples, then she is really orgasming. They claim that if the woman does not have erect nipples, then there is no orgasm. However, this is far from the truth. There is no specific breast or nipple reaction to a woman experiencing an orgasm. In other words, whether the woman's nipples are erect or not does not give a man a clue if she is experiencing an orgasm or not. As a matter of fact, those women who show nipple erection at orgasm also show nipple erection when they are first sexually aroused. Also, temperature plays a role in how the woman's nipples behave. On a cold day the nipples of the woman will be erect, regardless of whether she is experiencing an orgasm or not. Some men claim that they can tell if the woman is faking an orgasm from her vaginal contractions. The truth is, they cannot. Finally, the way a woman displays her orgasm varies from woman to woman. Also, the way a woman displays her orgasm varies from day to day. Therefore, unless a man has a flashlight and some measuring devices with him, there is no way he can tell for certain whether the woman's orgasm is genuine or not.

Reasons Why Women Fake an Orgasm

Many women fake an orgasm. They do so for several reasons. The first reason that some women fake an orgasm is because they do not want to seem inadequate because they could not climax. They do not want to seem less adequate than the other women that their partner has been with. They are afraid of being labeled frigid and are embarrassed of the fact that they could not climax. A second reason why some women fake an orgasm is because some men insist that the woman climax during sex. The men do so, either because they are genuinely concerned about the woman's pleasure, or in order to satisfy their vanity and prove that they are good lovers. These women are afraid that the man might feel inadequate and have his feelings hurt if they do not climax during sex. These women are afraid that their male partner would become angry and upset with them for not climaxing. These women are afraid that the man's anger towards them would lead to the man leaving them.

A third reason why some women fake an orgasm is because they want to be polite and not ruin a good time in bed. Some women, after a nice evening out with their male partner, find it rude and ungrateful not to indicate that they enjoyed the sex that goes with it. A fourth reason some women fake an orgasm is because after a while of having sex they get tired and just want to go to sleep. They find it easier to fake an orgasm than to deal with the problem of not having an orgasm. A fifth reason some women fake an orgasm is because they believe that it is only necessary for the man to experience an orgasm. They think that it is not necessary for the woman to experience an orgasm. They do not think that it is the woman's right to expect to have an orgasm during sex.

Reasons Why Faking an Orgasm is Not Right

Faking an orgasm is not the right thing for a woman to do because it causes a woman to experience an unsatisfied sex life. The woman experiences an unsatisfied sex life because if she is busy faking an orgasm by moaning and writhing, she is actually missing out on the actual sexual pleasure that she could be feeling. The woman is setting herself up for a vicious cycle of having to fake an orgasm every time she has sex and not experiencing true sexual pleasure at its maximum. This will cause a woman to experience sexual frustration. This sexual frustration can damage a relationship, and result in the termination of the relationship between a man and a woman.

Every time the woman fakes an orgasm, the man thinks he has done something that felt good to the woman making her climax, when in reality he has not done anything that felt good to the woman to make her climax. By the woman faking an orgasm, she is not letting the man know how to make her climax during sex. Faking an orgasm deprives the man and the woman of the best things about sex, which are intimacy and honesty. However, since the man is not aware that the woman is faking the orgasm, faking an orgasm causes only the woman to feel emotional distress, even though it is depriving both the man and the woman of intimacy and honesty. Faking an orgasm is an effect, and not a cause. Faking an orgasm is a result of a sexual difficulty. The sexual difficulty is caused by poor communication and sexual unease. It is not right to let the effect continue without dealing with the cause.

The Solution to Faking an Orgasm

A man should not become angry if he thinks his woman is faking an orgasm. Becoming angry with the woman for faking an orgasm will not help. It will simply make matters worse. Anger will only drive both people apart. It will hinder the ability of the couple to overcome the sexual problem that is causing the woman to fake an orgasm. The man should know that no woman in the world wants to have to fake an orgasm, and this thought should be enough to keep the man calm and relaxed. The man should help the woman overcome her faking by being supportive, kind, and nice. The man should ask the woman to tell him, what makes her climax during sex. He should ask her where she likes to be stimulated during sex with his penis, and how she likes to be stimulated there. If necessary, the man should ask the woman to show him, by masturbating in front of him. When the woman masturbates, she should point out to the man where she likes to be stimulated and how she likes to be stimulated.

If the man never suspects that his woman is faking an orgasm, then it is up to the woman to let the man know that she has been faking an orgasm. She should not be worried about him becoming angry because he should be sympathetic towards her and supportive. Most men will be sympathetic and supportive. But if the woman is with a man that will become angry and will not be supportive of her, then the woman is better off being with someone else. Once the woman explains to the man that she has been faking orgasms, she should let him know where she likes to be stimulated during sex and how. If necessary, the woman should show the man through masturbation where she likes to be stimulated during sex and how.

In both situations, when the woman shows the man where she likes to be pleased sexually and how, then that should be enough to have the man satisfy the woman sexually so that her orgasms become genuine orgasms and not fake orgasms. In both situations, when the woman shows the man where she likes to be pleased sexually and how, then that should give the couple the best things about sex, which is intimacy and honesty. By having honesty in the relationship, the couple will have stability and understanding in the relationship. Intimacy, honesty, stability, and understanding in a relationship will all contribute to the man and the woman being relaxed during sex, which is an essential part to pleasurable sex.

Chapter 25

Safer Sex

It would be irresponsible to offer advice about sexual interaction without discussing the safety aspects of it. In this day and age, with the presence of numerous sexually transmitted diseases, some of which can be deadly, safety is important. Safety is important during sexual interaction because it takes only one sexual partner, and one sexual encounter to be at risk. Safety is important because a person can be infected with a STD, show no symptoms, not know it, and pass the STD on to his or her sexual partner. Safety is important because a person can be infected with a STD, show no symptoms, be dishonest with his or her partner about the STD, and pass the STD to his or her partner. Even if a person is very close to his or her partner, the partner may still be dishonest about his or her STD because he or she may be too embarrassed to tell the person. A second reason why the partner may still be dishonest about his or her STD is because the partner might be afraid to lose the person if the person finds out that he or she has a STD.

Sexual interaction involves a person's health, body, and future. It is up to the person to take control of his or her sexual safety. The person should never rely on the partner for sexual safety. A person's health is too important to risk, therefore sexual safety is imperative. Sexual safety shows that a person is considerate to the partner's health, comfort, and protection, as well as to his or her own health, comfort, and protection. Sexual safety is the foundation for great sex, since it lets both people feel protected, comfortable, and relaxed, thus allowing them to experience sexual pleasure and sexual intimacy to its maximum. A person should never be embarrassed to take safety measures during sex, because he or she is acting responsibly. If a person's partner does not want to deal with safety issues during sex, then the partner is not ready for sex, and is not the right person to have sex with.

Being safe and careful during sexual interaction should be a matter of self-respect to a person. Due to a person's self-respect, he or she should be honest about his or her health status with his or her partner, no matter how casual the sexual relationship might be. Due to a person's self-respect, he or she should make sure that he or she does not unknowingly pass a disease on to a lover. Without protection there is not an excuse for a person to participate in a sexual relationship with a partner, whose health he or she is not 100 percent sure about.

Safety Precautions During Sex

There is really only one way to be 100 percent sure that a person does not get a sexually transmitted disease and for the couple not to have an unwanted pregnancy. That way is to practice sexual abstinence. However, this is unrealistic for most people. The second safety precaution that a person could take is for the person and his or her partner not to have unprotected sex, or sex without a condom, unless both people are in a monogamous relationship, and neither of them is cheating on the other. Both people must have been in the monogamous relationship for at least six months and tested negative for all STDs after being in the monogamous relationship for six months before they can have unprotected sex. The six-month time period is crucial, since after being infected with HIV it can take up to six months for a person's immune system to show antibodies for the HIV and for the person to test HIV-positive. Every sexually active couple should have two sexually transmitted diseases tests: one at the beginning of the relationship and another after being in the monogamous relationship for six months. If both people test negative for all STDs at the first STDs test at the beginning of the relationship, then both people can have sex, but using condoms. After six months, if both people get tested for STDs and the STDs test results are negative, then both people can have unprotected sex with no condoms, provided that both of them remained monogamous during the six months and will do so until the relationship ends. If a person suspects that his or her partner will cheat on him or her in the relationship, then the couple should use condoms every time they have sex.

The third safety precaution that a person could take if he or she cannot be in a monogamous relationship is to reduce the number of sexual partners at the same time period and over a lifetime. A person can reduce the risk of contracting a STD by limiting the number of his or her sexual partners at the same time period and over a lifetime. The fourth safety precaution that a person could take if he or she is not in a monogamous relationship is to get to know his or her sexual partners. A person could do that by exchanging information about his or her health, number of sexual partners, and sexual habits including whether he or she practices safer sex, in exchange for the same information from his or her partner. A person should remember not to believe everything his or her partner tells him or her since people lie sometimes. Therefore, the fifth safety precaution that should be taken if a person is not in a monogamous relationship is for him or her to make sure that safer sex is always practiced during every sexual encounter. That means that latex condoms should be used every time there is vaginal sex, anal sex, or fellatio. Also, during cunnilingus the man should use a dental dam every time he performs oral sex on the woman. Correct usage of latex condoms each time a person has any form of sex that requires its use will reduce the risk of getting a sexually transmitted disease. Correct usage of dental dams each time a woman receives oral sex will reduce the risk of getting a sexually transmitted disease. Also, an STD can be spread by contact with sores on the skin of the genital or anal area. The STDs that may be spread that way include herpes, human papillomavirus, and syphilis. These STDs can infect another person during sex, despite the fact that a condom is used during sex. These STDs can infect either partner on places on the genital area and anal area not protected by a condom during sex. Therefore, as part of practicing safer sex, before sex a person should take the time to look at his or her partner's genital area for sores since this could be a sign of a sexually transmitted disease. If a person finds such a sore on his or her partner's genital area, then they should refrain from any form of sex.

The sixth safety precaution that a person should take during sex if he or she is not in a monogamous relationship is to make sure that the sex toys are clean before using them, if he or she uses any. If a person shares a sex toy with his or her partner, he or she should wash it before using it and after each use. A person should do so, so that he or she does not catch any sexually transmitted disease from the sex toy, and so that he or she does not transmit any sexually transmitted disease to his or her partner from the sex toy. If the sex toy is not washed well, bodily fluid could remain on the sex toy and transmit a sexually transmitted disease to the user.

Low risk behavior is behavior that does not involve penile penetration. It is sometimes known as outercourse. Outercourse or low risk behavior includes hugging, cuddling, massage, mutual masturbation, sharing fantasies, and one person masturbating in front of his or her partner. When in a relationship some people try not to have safer sex but engage only in outercourse to reduce the risk of getting a sexually transmitted disease. But these efforts are usually in vain, since most people eventually end up having sex. They do so because over time they are not satisfied sexually only by outercourse. Since outercourse is not usually effective, it is not included as a safety precaution.

Safer Sex Guidelines

Sexual intercourse can be mind-blowing, but it can also be dangerous if a person's sexual partner has a sexually transmitted infection. Safer sex is a way of having sex that will help reduce the risk of getting a sexually transmitted disease. It will also reduce the risk of a couple having an unwanted pregnancy. Safer sex means the correct usage of condoms every time a person engages in vaginal sex, anal sex, and fellatio. Safer sex means the correct usage of a dental dam every time a person engages in cunnilingus. Safer sex means the inspection of the partner's genital area before sex for sores because sores could be a sign of a sexually transmitted disease.

Sexually transmitted diseases are passed by body fluids during vaginal sex, anal sex, or oral sex. These fluids include semen, vaginal fluids, and blood. A latex condom acts as a barrier during vaginal sex, anal sex, and fellatio to prevent body fluids from being exchanged. A dental dam acts as a barrier during cunnilingus to prevent body fluids from being exchanged. A few STDs such as herpes, human papilloma virus, and syphilis can infect either partner on places on the genital area that are not protected by a condom during sex. These STDs are transmitted through contact with a sore during sex. Careful inspection of a partner's genital area before sex for sores, and abstaining from sex if any sores are found, should prevent a partner from being infected with a STD.

When a person is engaging in safer sex, he or she should make sure that the male condom used is a latex condom. Latex condoms should be used because they are effective in blocking the smallest organisms, including the HIV virus. They are effective against sexually transmitted diseases. They are more elastic than polyurethane condoms. However, condoms made of polyurethane have been shown to be effective against sexually transmitted diseases also, including HIV. Around ten percent of the population is allergic to latex. So if a person is allergic to latex and engaging in safer sex, polyurethane condoms should be used. Although lambskin condoms might feel more comfortable and might prevent pregnancy, they should not be used if a person is engaging in safer sex, because they are not effective against sexually transmitted diseases, including HIV.

Condoms should be kept in their packs, in a cool and dry place. A person should avoid storing condoms at hot temperatures. A person should also avoid exposing condoms to direct sunlight. Storing condoms at hot temperatures or exposing them to direct sunlight can cause them to become brittle or gummy, and not be of any good use. For example, storing condoms in a wallet or a car glove compartment is not advisable. It is important that the condoms are never past the expiration date because if they are then they are not any good.

If the packaging of the condom is damaged, a person should discard of the condom. When a person opens the condom wrapper, he or she should be careful not to damage the condom. He or she should not use his or her teeth, fingernails, scissors, jewelry, belt buckle, or any other sharp object to open the wrapper. A person should not use a sharp object to open a condom wrapper because this might tear the condom. A person should use his or her fingers to open the condom wrapper. When a person takes out the condom from the wrapper, he or she should inspect it to see if it looks damaged in any way. A person should look for tears or holes in the condom. A person should also see if the condom is not the same color all over, since this is a sign of a damaged condom. A person should see if the condom is stiff, dry, sticky, gummy, or brittle since these are signs of a damaged condom. If the condom is damaged, then it should be discarded. Unrolling the male condom completely while it is not on the erect penis to check it can damage the condom and should not be done. Filling the condom with air or water to check it can also damage the condom and should not be done.

When the person takes out the condom, if the condom is made of latex, he or she should make sure that the latex condom does not come in contact with any oil in any form, since oil causes latex condoms to deteriorate and not be effective. Forms of oil that the latex condom should not come in touch with include petroleum jelly, baby oil, mineral oil, vegetable oil, and baby powder. Baby powder contains oil, and should be avoided when using a latex condom. Mineral oil is found in lotions, creams, and baby care products. Therefore, lotions, creams, and baby care products that contain oil, should not come in contact with the latex condom.

The man or the woman should put the male condom on the man's penis as soon as it becomes erect. The male condom should be put on before foreplay and before the penis gets near any of the woman's body openings. This should be done to avoid the exchange of body fluids between the man and the woman, so that sexually transmitted diseases or sperms are not transferred in the body fluids. Remember fluids released from the penis during the early stages of the erection, can cause pregnancy or pass on a STD.

The condom should be handled gently and carefully, so that it does not get damaged. The man or the woman should hold the male condom, so that the rolled up ring is on the outside. He or she should leave half an inch of space at the tip of the male condom to hold the semen. He or she should squeeze the tip of the male condom gently so no air is trapped inside. Then the man or the woman should unroll the male condom a little bit while holding it in his or her hand. He or she should then place a few drops of water-based lubricant inside the tip to increase the sensitivity and pleasure to the man. He or she should insert the lubricant while continuing to squeeze the tip of the male condom gently, leaving half an inch of space at the tip of the condom. If the man has a foreskin on his penis, then he or the woman should pull the foreskin back before putting on the male condom. Then the man or the woman should hold the tip of the male condom, while he or she unrolls the male condom all the way down to the base of the penis or pubic hair. If the male condom does not unroll, it is on wrong. Then the man or the woman should throw it away, and start over with a new male condom. When the male condom is rolled all the way down to the base of the penis or pubic hair, the man or the woman should make sure it covers the entire penis and smooth it by squeezing out any air bubbles. The man or the woman should check the male condom on the erect penis for any damage.

Plenty of water-based lubricant should be put on the outside of the male condom because that decreases the chance that the condom will break. Not enough lubricant is one of the major reasons that condoms break. Plenty of lubricant on the outside of the male condom will make sex more pleasurable for both the man and the woman. Only a water-based lubricant should be used, because it does not damage the latex condom. Oil-based lubricants should not be used, because they can cause latex condoms to be damaged. It is important not to put spermicide when practicing safer sex because it can cause a vaginal irritation and tiny tears in the vaginal mucous membranes, which will increase the risk of a STD transmission.

As soon as the man ejaculates, his penis must be withdrawn. The man should withdraw the penis while it is still erect and while holding the base of the male condom, making sure it does not slip off. The man should not wait after ejaculation to withdraw his penis because his penis may become soft and the male condom can slip off, releasing the semen. Then the man should throw away the condom. After that the man should either wash off his penis or put on a new male condom before he and the woman continue to caress one another. It is advisable for the man to wash his hands after throwing the condom away because he might have some semen on his hands. If he has semen on his hands and puts his fingers inside the woman's vagina, there is a risk of pregnancy or STD transmission. There is a risk of pregnancy or STD transmission since sperm can live outside the body for up to 48 hours. It is important that the male condom is never reused and that a new condom is used for every new sexual act.

Sometimes a male condom slips off or breaks because it was not put on correctly. Other times a male condom slips off because it was not held during withdrawal. If the male condom slips off or breaks, the woman should urinate and insert spermicidal foam, cream, or jelly into her vagina. She should leave the spermicide in her vagina for at least an hour. She should do so to help destroy the sperm, viruses, and bacteria. A woman could also take the morning after pill the next morning if she is concerned about getting pregnant. The morning after pill is a birth control pill that prevents pregnancy if taken the next day.

The anus does not have much lubrication on its tissue inside the anal passage like the vagina does, and its tissue inside the anal passage is very fragile. Therefore, its tissue is more likely to tear during anal sex than the vaginal tissue during vaginal sex. Thus it is easier for STDs, including HIV, to enter the body during anal sex than during vaginal sex. In fact, anal sex is the riskiest form of sex for getting HIV. Therefore, using a male condom during anal sex is very important. Using a water-based lubricant during anal sex is important, because it will help reduce the risk of the male condom breaking. After anal sex, the man should never have vaginal sex unless he washes his penis with soap and water and puts on a new condom. This is important because the anus is filled with bacteria that cause serious infections if they get into the vagina.

The female condom is a pouch with flexible rings at each end. It looks like a giant male condom with flexible rings on each end. Before vaginal sex the ring inside the pouch is inserted deep into the vagina holding the condom in the vagina. The penis is inserted into the pouch through the ring at the open end. The ring at the open end and part of the female condom stay outside the vaginal opening during intercourse. Usually, about one inch of the female condom hangs outside the vagina during sex. The female condom is highly effective in protecting the woman from sexually transmitted diseases. In fact, the female condom is better than the male condom in preventing sexually transmitted diseases. This is because the female condom covers more skin than the male condom. The woman's vulva and the base of the man's penis are more protected during vaginal sex with a female condom than with a male condom. Also, since the female condom covers more skin than the male condom, it is more effective against sexually transmitted diseases that are transferred from skin to skin contact, like herpes and genital warts.

The female condom can be made of polyurethane, latex, or some other material. It may feel like a tampon. A woman can wear a female condom before she goes out on a date and can leave it in, so that safer sex is not an issue. The female condom should not be left in the vagina for more than eight hours.

Female condoms put the woman in a position of power, since the woman no longer has to rely on the man in order to practice safer sex. However, the woman should never allow the man to use the male condom if she is using the female condom. Using both the female and the male condom at the same time does not make it safer for the couple. On the contrary, friction between the condoms could cause tearing in both condoms. Through these tears, bodily fluids could leak through, rendering both condoms ineffective. Some men and women find sex with the female condom to be more stimulating than with the male condom.

Dental dams are rectangular sheets of latex used in dentistry. Sometimes they are made of other material. They are also used during cunnilingus as a safer sex barrier against sexually transmitted diseases. Many sexually transmitted diseases can be transmitted during cunnilingus including syphilis, gonorrhea, herpes, and genital warts (HPV). The dental dam should be placed over the vulva of the woman during cunnilingus. It must be held in place to prevent exposure to vaginal secretions, sores on the woman's genital area, or sores on the man's mouth. To increase the pleasure of the woman during cunnilingus, a water-based lubricant should be placed on the woman's genital area or on the side of the dental dam that is touching the woman's genital area.

Excuses People Give Not to Practice Safer Sex

Despite the risks involved in sex, some people do not like to practice safer sex. They give excuses why they do not practice safer sex and take the risk of getting a sexually transmitted disease. One common excuse is that they enjoy sex without a condom. They claim that they enjoy the feel of the nice warm skin of their partner compared to the feel of the latex or polyurethane of the condom. However, it is obvious that the risk of a serious infection or the loss of a person's life for a few minutes of naked pleasure is not worth it. Another excuse that some people give for not practicing safer sex is that they do not think that their partner has a sexually transmitted disease because he or she is too cute or successful to have it. This thinking is incorrect, since no one is immune from having a sexually transmitted disease. A person's age, race, or socio-economic status does not matter when it comes to having a sexually transmitted disease, since sexually transmitted diseases do not discriminate. A third excuse that some people give for not practicing safer sex is that they got caught up in the passion of the moment and forgot to practice safer sex. This is no excuse, since a person should never forget to take care of his or her health. A fourth excuse that some people give for not practicing safer sex, is the man's penis is too big for a condom. This excuse is totally ridiculous since a condom can stretch to fit any size penis.

A fifth excuse that some people give for not practicing safer sex is that condoms decrease the pleasure for both the man and the woman during sex. Condoms tend to desensitize the penis a little bit, but they do not prohibit the enjoyment of sex. Rather, they make sex more enjoyable to both the man and the woman. They make it more enjoyable to the man because he can last longer before climaxing as a result of his penis being desensitized a little bit. They make it more enjoyable to the woman because the man lasts longer before climaxing, giving the woman a greater probability to climax through sexual intercourse. Also, as a result of the man lasting longer the couple will feel more intimate. They will enjoy the sex more as a result of this intimacy. Furthermore, as a result of condoms both people can relax during sex and enjoy sex more because they are not worried about sexually transmitted diseases or pregnancy.

Ways to Make Safer Sex More Enjoyable

Safety during sex is essential, but it does not have to undermine the fun to be enjoyed during sex. Putting on a condom during vaginal sex or fellatio does not have to interrupt the momentum or excitement of the sexual experience. Instead, by the man sharing the procedure of putting on a condom with the woman, they can actually increase the play or erotic factor, thus increasing the pleasure during sex. One way for the male condom to be put on to increase pleasure is for the man and the woman both to put it on together, using both a man's hand and a woman's hand simultaneously to roll it down. Another way for the condom to be put on to increase the pleasure during sex is for the woman to put the condom on the man's penis using her mouth. She should hold the condom tip between her lips, and then put the condom on the man's penis with her lips. Then she should roll down the condom on the man's penis with her lips, making sure to smooth it out on the penis using her lips. A third way for the male condom to be put on to increase pleasure is for the man to touch and caress the woman's breasts and other parts of her body while she puts on the condom. A fourth way for the male condom to be put on to increase pleasure is for the man to put on the condom while the woman touches and caresses his buttocks and other parts of his body. Putting on the condom in any of these methods will ensure that the putting on of the condom is felt as part of the sexual encounter and does not take away from it any pleasure.

Another way to make sure that the sexual encounter with the male condom is pleasurable is to place a water-based lubricant the size of a jelly bean in the nipple end of the condom before it is put on. This will enhance the sensation for the man by reducing that stuck-on feeling. It will make the condom adhere better to the skin. Also, to make sure that a man's sensitivity is not reduced with the male condom, the man or the woman is to find condoms that fit the man well. Furthermore, using a lot of water-based lubricant on the outside of the male condom will make the sexual encounter more pleasurable.

Male condoms could also be used as sex toys, since they come in different sizes, shapes, colors, and features. The man and the woman could vary the size of the male condom from one sexual encounter to another, so that they vary the sensations produced to the man and the woman during sex, thus making the sex more pleasurable. The sensations will vary based on how tight or loose the male condom is as a result of its size. The couple could also vary the thinness of the male condom from one encounter to another to produce different sensations for the man and the woman during sex, making the sex more pleasurable for both. The couple could also vary the shape of the male condom to produce different sensations for the man and the woman during sex, making the sex more pleasurable for both. A ribbed condom has ridges in the latex of the condom, thus changing the shape of the condom. This difference in the shape of the male condom produces a different sensation for the man and the woman during sex.

There are glow in the dark condoms. A man could wear the glow in the dark condom during sex in a dark room, making the sex more exciting and pleasurable. The man should be sure to wear a reputable condom under the glow in the dark condom, so that he is protected to the fullest extent from sexually transmitted diseases and the risk of getting a woman pregnant. Male condoms also come in a variety of colors. The couple could change the color of the male condom during sexual encounters in a dark room, making the sex more pleasurable for both of them. There are also scented male condoms available on the market. The scents include orange, banana, strawberry, and mint. The couple could change the scent of the condom from one sexual encounter to another, making the sex more pleasurable and exciting.

Male condoms also come in different flavors. The couple could change the flavor of the male condom from one fellatio encounter to another, making the fellatio encounters more pleasurable and exciting. However, during fellatio no lubricated condom should be used. Rather, a flavored lubricant should be used on the outside of the condom, to make the fellatio more pleasurable to the man and the woman. There are a variety of flavored lubricants available. A person can change the lubricant's flavor from one encounter to another, making the fellatio encounter more pleasurable and exciting. The dental dams also, come in a variety of flavors and scents. The couple could change the flavor and scent of the dental dam from one cunnilingus encounter to another, making the encounter more pleasurable and exciting. A person can have fun with condoms and dental dams once he or she knows how to use them properly. The more a person gets used to using a condom and a dental dam during his or her sexual encounters, the more he or she won't mind using them.

Chapter 26

Sexually Transmitted Diseases

Sexually transmitted diseases are also known as STDs. STDs are any disease that is passed by body fluids, during vaginal, anal, or oral sex. These body fluids include semen, vaginal fluids, and blood. Some STDs can also be spread by contact inside of the mouth. Some STDs can be spread by contact with the skin of the genital or anal area if the infection is present. Some STDs have symptoms, while others do not. On the other hand, some STDs have symptoms that show and then disappear while the STD remains in the body. So a person cannot always rely on symptoms to know whether he or she is infected with a STD. Most STDs can be treated, while others can only be controlled. If a person is sexually active he or she is at risk of contracting a STD, regardless what his or her age, race, occupation, or sexual preference is. STDs, should not be taken lightly. They are not minor diseases. STDs, if untreated can become a major problem, sometimes causing sterility and even death.

The key to reduce the risk of contracting a STD is to be informed about all STDs. By a person being informed about STDs, he or she will know the necessity of taking control of his or her sexual health. A person will know how important it is for him or her to be safe and careful in order to prevent contracting a STD. By knowing more about STDs, a person can learn to recognize STD symptoms if he or she has them, and get early treatment. By doing so, a person can quickly and painlessly cure most STD infections that he or she has symptoms for. A person will also know the seriousness of having to get a general checkup for STDs from time to time, even if he or she is married, so that he or she finds out as soon as possible if he or she has a STD that has no symptoms. By doing so, a person can quickly and painlessly cure most STD infections that he or she has.

Preventing Sexually Transmitted Diseases

A person should take responsibility for his or her sexual health and make sure that he or she does not get any sexually transmitted diseases. A person taking care of his or her body against sexually transmitted diseases should be as normal as taking care of his or her teeth. Just as a person would not let a day go by without brushing his or her teeth, likewise a person should take care of his or her sexual health at all times. A person should make it a point, to take precautions to prevent the transmission of sexually transmitted diseases. The first precaution that a person should take is to reduce the number of sexual partners he or she has. The larger the number of sexual partners he or she has, the greater the risk is to contract a sexually transmitted disease. The second precaution that a person should take is to choose a sexual partner that seems or admits to limit his or her sexual partners. By a person choosing a sexual partner that limits his or her sexual partners, he or she is reducing the risk of contracting a STD.

A third precaution that a person should take is to get to know his or her partner. Honest communication is important when a person is about to have sex with a new sexual partner. The person should ask his or her partner if he or she has a STD. If the new partner does have a STD, then the person should not have sex with him or her. Rather, the person should wait until the new partner has treated his or her STD and is no longer infected with it. If the new partner says that he or she does not have a STD, then the person should inquire as to how recent the STD test results were. If they are not recent, then the person could decline to have sex with the new partner until the new partner has gotten tested for STDs, and made sure that he or she has none. A fourth precaution a person should take, is to make sure that his or her partner will not cheat on him or her. If the new partner does not agree to be sexually exclusive with the person, or if the person does not believe that the new partner will be sexually exclusive, then the person should practice safer sex. Practicing safer sex is the fifth precaution that a person should take. Read the chapter on Safer Sex for more information about it.

What Should a Person Do if He or She Suspects or Knows that He or She Has an STD?

No one should ever ignore suspicious symptoms. If a person suspects or knows that he or she has a STD, then he or she should take action quickly. A person should take action quickly because many STDs can be successfully treated if caught in the early stages. Delaying treatment can cause the infection to get worse. The first thing that a person should do is to go to a doctor or a clinic for professional diagnosis and treatment. If the doctor confirms that the person has a STD, then the person should follow the doctor's instructions in regards to the treatment and medications to take.

Second, the person should tell his or her sexual partner or partners that he or she has a STD immediately after he or she finds out. There is no doubt that breaking the news can be difficult and awkward, but the person's sexual partner or partners need to know for their own health. They need to know so that they get treated, so that they do not reinfect the person after he or she has healed from the STD, and so that they do not spread the STD to other people. Third, the person should avoid all sexual contact until he or she has completely healed from a STD, in order to prevent others from being infected. Fourth, a person should be more careful than usual to wash his or her hands every time he or she touches his or her genital area if he or she is suspicious that he or she has a STD. A person should do so in order to avoid transferring infections to others. If a person has herpes, he or she should wash his or her hands every time he or she touches his or her genital area to avoid transferring herpes to other parts of his or her body. Fifth, when a person heals from the STD, he or she should reduce the likelihood of acquiring a STD in the future by practicing safer sex.

List of Sexually Transmitted Diseases

The following is a list of the most common sexually transmitted diseases, along with a brief description of them. This list is for general information. It is not proper for a person to diagnose himself or herself when it comes to his or her personal health. This task should be left to a professional doctor.

Non-specific Urethritis (NSU)

Non-specific urethritis is on this list because it can be caused by chlamydia. NSU can be caused by chlamydia or it can have a non-sexual origin. Both men and women can be carriers of NSU. Some men and women that have NSU experience no symptoms at all, but others have symptoms like a whitish discharge, and burning or pain when urinating. NSU is sometimes associated with pink eye. If a person suspects that he or she is infected, then he or she should be treated for NSU, even when there are no obvious symptoms.

Chlamydia

Chlamydia is caused by a bacterium that is also a parasite, meaning it needs other cells to exist and survive. It is often called the silent STD because in women it may not cause any symptoms in 75% of the cases and can linger for months or years before being discovered. The symptoms that could occur in women include unusual vaginal bleeding or discharge, pain of the abdomen, painful sexual intercourse known as dyspareunia, fever, painful urination, or the urge to urinate more frequently than usual. In women it can cause a bacterial infection deep within the fallopian tubes, causing chronic pain, tubal pregnancies, or infertility. In men chlamydia causes inflammation of the urethra in about 50% of the cases. The symptoms that could occur in men include a painful or burning sensation when urinating, an unusual discharge from the penis, swollen or tender testicles, or fever. In men, if the chlamydia is left untreated, it is possible for it to spread to the testicles, causing epididymitis. Epididymitis in rare cases can cause sterility in men, if not treated within 6 to 8 weeks.

Chlamydia is spread through sexual intercourse, including oral sex. With oral transmission, chlamydia can give a person an upper respiratory infection. Chlamydia can also be passed from mother to child during birth, causing eye, ear, and lung infections in newborns. The good news is that chlamydia is easily cured with antibiotics, but it must be tested for specifically.

Trichomoniasis

Trichomoniasis is the most common curable sexually transmitted disease in the world. It is also one of the three most common vaginal infections in women. It is caused by a one-celled parasite called Trichomonas Vaginalis. It affects both men and women. The vagina is the most common location of trichomoniasis infections in women. The symptoms of trichomoniasis in women could include a yellowish green vaginal discharge, a fishy odor, pain during urination and sexual intercourse, and genital itching or irritation. On the other hand, the urethra is the most common location of trichomoniasis infection in men. Usually men do not show trichomoniasis symptoms, but some may experience discharge from the penis, burning during urination, or burning during ejaculation.

Pelvic Inflammatory Disease (PID)

The pelvic inflammatory disease is the inflammation of the female reproductive system, particularly the fallopian tubes, ovaries, and uterus. It is usually the result of an untreated STD, such as gonorrhea or chlamydia. The main symptoms of the pelvic inflammatory disease are pain in the lower abdomen, fever, backache, and an irregular period. The pelvic inflammatory disease can affect the woman's fertility by blocking and scarring the fallopian tubes.

Pubic Lice (Crabs)

Pubic lice, or crabs, are lice that live in the pubic hair of the man or the woman. They infest the area where the pubic hair is located by biting the skin, feeding on blood, and laying eggs. The public lice may not be immediately visible because they are tiny, but microscopic examinations can provide a definite diagnosis. The main symptoms of the pubic lice are that the person will notice an intense irritation and itching of the pubic region and possibly small flakes of dried blood in the pubic hair. A person can get pubic lice from his or her sexual partner.

Candidiasis

Candidiasis is an inflammation of the vagina and vulva caused by an overgrowth of yeasts that are found normally in the vagina. This may be triggered by antibiotics, stress, a high sugar diet, diabetes, too much bathing with highly scented bath products or soaps, or wearing very tight pantyhose or jeans. The symptoms of candidiasis are a thick white vaginal discharge, irritation of the vagina, and a burning sensation during intercourse. Although candidiasis is not a sexually transmitted disease, it is included in this section because a woman can pass it on to a man during sex. Once it is passed to a man, it can cause the man to experience it as an inflammation of the glans of the penis. When the man experiences it as an inflammation of the glans of the penis it is known as balanitis.

Cystitis

Cystitis is the inflammation of the urinary bladder. It causes frequent, painful urination. It more often affects women, but can affect men also. It affects all age groups, but it more frequently affects sexually active women ages 20 to 50. It can also occur in women and young girls that are not sexually active. Although it does occur in males, it is rare in males. Females are more prone to the development of cystitis than males because of their relatively shorter urethra. The shorter urethra in females allows the bacteria to travel a shorter distance than in the male's urethra to enter the bladder. A second reason why females are more prone to the development of cystitis than males is because there is a shorter distance between the opening of the urethra and the anus in females than in males. This makes it easier for bacteria from the anus to enter the urethra in women than in men.

Although cystitis is not a sexually transmitted disease, it is included in this section because sexual intercourse may increase the risk of cystitis. Sexual intercourse increases the risk of cystitis because bacteria can be introduced into the bladder through the urethra during sexual activity. Once bacteria enter the bladder, they are normally removed through urination. However, when bacteria multiply faster than they are removed by urination, a cystitis infection results. When bacteria causes the cystitis, it is known as bacterial cystitis. In sexually active women, the most common cause of bacterial cystitis is from the bacteria E. coli and staphylococcus saprophyticus. There is a second type of cystitis, traumatic cystitis. Traumatic cystitis is the most common form of cystitis in the female. It occurs after intercourse, because the urethra, which lies close to the vagina, gets bruised by the thrusting movement of the penis and the bladder gets bruised by sexual intercourse. Cystitis is called the honeymoon disease since traumatic cystitis often occurs after overenthusiastic intercourse in the early days of a relationship. In both types of cystitis, the urethra and bladder are irritated and inflamed.

Gonorrhea

Gonorrhea is a sexually transmitted disease that is caused by a bacterial infection. It is transmitted from one person to another through vaginal, oral, or anal sexual relations. It is highly contagious through any contact with the penis, mouth, anus, and vulva, even without penetration. In some people, both male and female, gonorrhea can be completely without any symptoms. However, in others gonorrhea has symptoms, and they develop within two to thirty days after infection. In a man, the symptoms for gonorrhea are a yellowish discharge from the penis and frequent, painful urination. In a man, the infection may move into the prostate, seminal vesicles, and epididymis, causing pain and fever. Untreated, gonorrhea can lead to sterility in the male.

Less than half the women with gonorrhea show any symptoms. If a woman shows symptoms for gonorrhea, the symptoms could include a vaginal discharge, difficulty urinating, off-cycle menstrual bleeding, vomiting, fever, and bleeding after sexual intercourse. Women who leave gonorrhea untreated will usually have the infection spread to the uterus, fallopian tubes, and ovaries, causing pelvic inflammatory disease. In women, if the gonorrhea is untreated, it can cause permanent damage including sterility, tubal pregnancies, and chronic pain. In both men and women, if gonorrhea is left untreated it may spread throughout the body, affecting joints and even heart valves. The good news is that if gonorrhea is detected early, it is easily curable with antibiotics.

Syphilis

Syphilis is a sexually transmitted disease that is transmitted through vaginal, oral, and anal sex. It can also be transmitted by contact with infected sores, rashes, and open wounds on the skin. It can also be transmitted through blood transfusions and by sharing infected needles. Syphilis develops in three distinct stages. In the first stage, a firm painless ulcer known as a chancre appears on the genital area. The ulcer, or chancre, heals in 6 to 10 weeks. In the first stage, local lymph glands in the groin may also become enlarged.

In the second stage, bacteria have spread to all parts of the body, causing diverse symptoms. The diverse symptoms can include skin rashes, headaches, mild fever, hair loss, swollen lymph glands, and wart-like growths on the genital area and around the anus. The third stage occurs any time between three and 25 years after initial infection. In the third stage, the body's internal tissues start to be destroyed. This sometimes causes permanent damage to the heart, brain, eyes, and joints. This can also, eventually cause damage to the cardiovascular or nervous system. Damage to the cardiovascular, or nervous system can lead to death. Many babies born to mothers with syphilis die during childbirth, or are born with abnormal features. The good news is, if syphilis is detected early then syphilis is curable with strong doses of antibiotics.

Herpes

There are two viruses that cause herpes. The first one is herpes simplex I which occurs orally, and is known as oral herpes. When there is an outbreak of herpes simplex I there are cold sores on, around, or inside the lips and mouth. The second virus that causes herpes is herpes simplex II, which occurs on the genital area. When there is an outbreak of herpes simplex II, there are itchy bumps or tiny blisters on the genital area. In men, the itchy bumps or tiny blisters typically appear on the shaft of the penis at the end of the foreskin or near the head of the penis. They could also appear near the anus. In women, the itchy bumps or tiny blisters typically appear near or inside the vagina. They also appear on the labia. They could also appear near the anus. In both men and women herpes lesions can appear in areas related to the genital area by nerve endings, but that are not actually part of the genital area. An example of that is herpes lesions appearing on the buttocks and thighs.

Herpes simplex I and II are easily transmitted by direct contact with a lesion or the body fluid of an infected individual. Herpes is highly contagious when physical contact is made during an outbreak, but it can also be contagious when the virus appears to lie dormant. This is because it can reactivate without symptoms in some people with herpes. If a person has a herpes outbreak, he or she should not have vaginal sex, oral sex, anal sex, nor kiss his or her partner. A person should not do so, so that he or she does not infect his or her partner because the chances are very high that he or she will infect him or her. If an infected person with herpes does not have an outbreak he or she can have vaginal sex, oral sex, anal sex, and kiss his or her uninfected partner without infecting his or her partner, although there is a chance that the uninfected partner could get infected. As a matter of fact, there are many married couples where one person is infected and the other is not, and during an outbreak they do not have vaginal sex, anal sex, oral sex, nor kiss. However, when there is not an outbreak they have vaginal sex, oral sex, anal sex, and kiss. The vast majority of these couples after a long duration of time (many years) had the uninfected person remain uninfected with herpes.

There is no cure for herpes. Once a person is infected with the virus, it remains in his or her body for life. The virus resides in the sensory nerves of the person as a latent virus. It does so for the duration of a person's life. However, a person infected with herpes will get an outbreak from time to time. Over time, the episodes of an outbreak decrease in frequency and in severity. As a matter of fact, after several years some people will become perpetually asymptomatic and will no longer experience outbreaks, though they may still be contagious to others. Although there is no cure for herpes, there are some medications available that reduce the symptoms of the herpes outbreaks and decrease the possibility of another outbreak.

The chances of a herpes outbreak occurring increases greatly because of stress and being in the sun. Herpes can be stressful, both physically and emotionally. Physically, herpes can be tiring. When the herpes outbreaks occur, they are uncomfortable to the person that experiences them. They are also embarrassing and awkward to the person that experiences them.

Although it might seem embarrassing and awkward to a person to tell his or her sexual partner that he or she has herpes, it is important for the infected person to be honest with his or her sexual partner and let him or her know that he or she is infected. Most people, when their partner tells them that he or she has herpes, appreciate his or her honesty and continue to pursue the relationship with him or her. They continue to pursue the relationship, but they refrain from sex during the times that the partner is having an outbreak. Most people who are uninfected with herpes continue to pursue a sexual relationship with a person infected with herpes. They do so because they know that the vast majority of people that do so do not become infected if they avoid any form of sex and kissing at times that their partner is having an outbreak.

There is a real danger of herpes to an unborn child. Herpes is usually transmitted during delivery and causes painful blisters and damage to the eyes, brain, and internal organs of a new born baby. Sometimes it can be fatal, to a newborn baby. The good news is that when a pregnant woman is infected with herpes, a cesarean delivery is done to prevent damage to the child. However, a cesarean section is done only if there is an active lesion present because the risk is very low for a baby to get herpes from his or her mother during delivery if no lesion exists. The risk of neonatal herpes, or a baby being born with herpes because the mother or father has it, is very unlikely.

Genital Warts (HPV)

Genital warts is a highly contagious sexually transmitted disease that is caused by some subtypes of the human papillomavirus or HPV. There are many strains of the human papillomavirus. Some strains cause some visible genital warts while others do not cause any warts at all. Genital warts in the man are growths that appear on the penis, scrotum, groin, or thighs. In women the warts could occur on the outside and inside of the vagina, on the cervix, or around the anus. Genital warts can develop in the mouth or throat of a person who has had oral sex with an infected partner, but this rarely happens. The genital warts could be flat or raised, single or multiple, and small or large. The genital warts are spread through direct skin to skin contact during oral, genital, or anal sex with an infected partner.

Once cells are invaded by HPV, a quiet or latent period of months to years may occur. HPV can last for several years, without a symptom. If a person has sex with a sexual partner whose HPV infection is latent and shows no outward symptoms, the person is vulnerable to becoming infected. Because the HPV can lie dormant for years, a person may suddenly have an outbreak after being monogamous for years. Warts are the most easily recognized symptom of the genital HPV infection. Not everyone infected with HPV develops warts. Some people do not develop warts and can still transmit the virus. Some strains of HPV cause genital warts, while other strains of HPV cause cervical cancer. Also, some strains of HPV cause anal cancer. The strains that cause genital warts are not the same strains associated with cervical cancer. There is no cure for HPV, but there are methods to treat the visible warts. Genital warts may disappear without treatment, but sometimes eventually develop into small, fleshy, and raised growths. There is no way to predict whether the genital warts will disappear on their own or become small, fleshy, and raised growths.

Hepatitis B

Hepatitis B is an infection caused by the hepatitis B virus. It is spread through infected semen, vaginal secretions, and saliva. A person can get hepatitis B from vaginal sex, oral sex, and anal sex. A person can get infected with the virus through direct contact with an infected person's open sores or cuts. This means that if someone in a person's house is infected, a person can get hepatitis B from using the same razor or toothbrush.

Sometimes hepatitis B might be entirely asymptomatic, and go unrecognized. Other times, a person may not know that he or she has hepatitis B in its mildest form. However, when symptoms of hepatitis B appear, they are very much like those of the stomach flu. The symptoms can include nausea, loss of appetite, vomiting, mild fever, unexplainable tiredness, dark urine, and the yellowing of the eyes and skin. The illness lasts for a few weeks, and then gradually improves in most affected people. However, a few people may have more severe liver disease, and may die as a result of it.

However, there is a possibility that a person will have a chronic infection with hepatitis B. If a person has a chronic infection with hepatitis B, he or she might be asymptomatic. But if the person shows symptoms for the chronic infection, then these symptoms include nausea, loss of appetite, vomiting, mild fever, unexplainable tiredness, dark urine, and the yellowing of the eyes and skin. Chronic infection with hepatitis B can lead to a chronic inflammation of the liver, leading to cirrhosis. Chronic hepatitis B may eventually cause liver cancer, a fatal disease. Chronic hepatitis B increases the possibility that a person will get liver cancer. Chronic carriers of hepatitis B are encouraged to avoid consuming alcohol, as it increases the risk of cirrhosis and liver cancer. Once hepatitis B is contracted, a person has a small chance of becoming a carrier for life. The good news is that there is a vaccination for hepatitis B.

Hepatitis B is easily passed from mother to unborn child. It can also be transmitted to babies and young children from one of the parents. However, it can be prevented from being transferred to babies and young children by vaccinating the infants at birth.

HIV/AIDS

HIV stands for human immunodeficiency virus. AIDS stands for acquired immune deficiency syndrome. HIV and AIDS are not the same thing. HIV is the predecessor of AIDS. AIDS comes from HIV. A person cannot get AIDS without having HIV. However, a person can have HIV, but not have AIDS. Most people with an HIV infection will progress to AIDS within 10 years of being infected. Some will progress much sooner, and some will take much longer.

HIV is a sexually transmitted disease spread through bodily fluids like blood, semen, vaginal fluids, and the mother's breast milk. HIV can be transmitted by any activity that involves the exchange of bodily fluids, including both heterosexual and homosexual sex. As a matter of fact, unprotected vaginal sex, anal sex, and oral sex are the most common routes of infection for HIV. Unprotected vaginal sex, anal sex, and oral sex expose a person to his or her partner's semen or vaginal fluids. The risk of HIV transmission by intercourse increases if a person has torn or ulcerated skin on or around his or her genital area. This is why sores and ulcers on the genital area caused by herpes or syphilis make HIV transmission more likely.

HIV can also be transmitted through infected blood. Drug users who share needles and are exposed to each other's blood can get infected with HIV from sharing the same needles. If blood transfusions are not screened for the HIV virus, they can be a source of HIV infection. Infected pregnant women can pass HIV to their babies during pregnancy or delivery. Infected mothers can infect their babies with HIV through breast milk.

HIV is not an airborne virus and cannot be spread by casual contact. Touching, food, coughing, mosquitoes, toilet seats, swimming in pools, and donating blood do not spread HIV. It is possible to find HIV in the saliva, tears, and urine of an infected person, but the risk of being infected through them is negligible. The risk of a person being infected with HIV from French kissing is negligible. However, in a few remote cases HIV has been transmitted from an infected person to an uninfected person through French kissing, from the open bleeding gums or mouth sores of the infected person. However, usually a person can French kiss as much as he or she likes without worrying about being infected with HIV because the risk of getting HIV from French kissing is negligible.

When a person tests positive for HIV, his or her immune system has been exposed to it and is presenting an immune response to it. There are usually no symptoms accompanying HIV. People can get the virus and feel terrific for many years. A small percentage of people will develop an acute mononucleosis-like illness at the beginning of the HIV infection. Left untreated, the HIV virus almost always leads to AIDS. Because when a person has AIDS the immune system fails, the symptoms for AIDS can look like anything from a cold to cancer. Although there is no cure for AIDS, there are treatments that slow down the effect that HIV has on the immune system.

There are several clades, or types of the HIV virus. The several types are A, B, C, D, E, F, M, and O. Within each clade, there are different strains. Some strains appear to be more virulent than others. So even if a man or a woman is already HIV positive, he or she can still become infected by another form of the HIV virus. This may happen because he or she is more susceptible to infection, given the already weakened state of the immune system. A person can get infected with another strain that is more virulent than the one that he or she already has.

After being infected with HIV, it can take up to six months for a person's body to show that it is infected when the person is tested. Every sexually active man and woman should have two HIV tests, one after risky behavior and another after waiting six months. The six month waiting period, will ensure a clean bill of health. The person's clean bill of health is important, before having unprotected sex with any new partner. However, how soon after initial infection the person's body shows that it is infected when tested, depends upon the virulence of the strain. Some strains, could almost immediately show a HIV diagnosis when the person is tested. Since there is no cure for AIDS, the only way for a person to protect himself or herself against it is to practice safer sex.

Chapter 27

Premature Ejaculation

Premature ejaculation is the most common sexual problem for men. It occurs when the man does not have control of his ejaculation. Some men that experience premature ejaculation will ejaculate before their penis enters the woman's vagina or upon anticipation of entry. Some other men that experience premature ejaculation will ejaculate as soon as their female partner touches them, even though they have not inserted their penis inside the woman's vagina yet. Others will ejaculate once entry is attempted, or within a few seconds after entry is made. The most common pattern of premature ejaculation is when the man ejaculates after four or fewer penile thrusts inside the woman's vagina. Most men have ejaculated prematurely once in a while when they were very excited or anxious. It is not considered premature ejaculation if a man ejaculates prematurely once in a while. It is considered premature ejaculation when a man ejaculates prematurely in more than half of his sexual experiences with a woman.

Some people extend the definition of premature ejaculation even further. They say that if a man ejaculates before he or his female partner wants the ejaculation to occur, then this is premature ejaculation. They view premature ejaculation as the man's inability to delay ejaculation long enough for his sexual pleasure and for the woman's sexual pleasure. Also, it is interesting to note that women are more likely than men to view a situation as being a premature ejaculation situation.

Men who experience premature ejaculation are not sloppy lovers. They are genuinely unable to prevent themselves from ejaculating prematurely. They are unable to prevent themselves because they do not have the skill to overcome premature ejaculation. Some of these men are too lazy to learn how to prevent premature ejaculation from happening. Overcoming premature ejaculation is a skill which could be acquired by most men, if they put in the effort. Premature ejaculation is something that a man should fix as soon as he experiences it so that he enjoys his sex life to the maximum. A man should not live with premature ejaculation because it becomes an involuntary habit. Fortunately, premature ejaculation is one of the easiest sex problems to overcome with the proper training.

Causes of Premature Ejaculation

Many men who suffer premature ejaculation actually learned to ejaculate quickly from an early age. From the time they were pre-teens or teens, they may have gotten used to masturbating to ejaculation quickly because of the fear of being discovered. This pattern of ejaculating prematurely became an involuntary habit. Also some men that suffer premature ejaculation as adolescents and as young adults they learned to have sex in a rush, and bring themselves to ejaculation very quickly. They did so because they had sex with their female partner in a setting where the couple did not feel safe from intrusion on their privacy. For example, they might have had sex in the parent's living room, or in their own bedroom. Then it became an involuntary habit for them to have a premature ejaculation. Some men that suffer premature ejaculation might have needed to get sex over quickly several times. They might have needed to do so because of circumstances. Then they find themselves trapped in a pattern of premature ejaculation. In all three instances, the men rush to ejaculation without focusing on the good feelings produced. They unconsciously trained themselves to experience sex in a rush.

Some men that experience premature ejaculation do so because they believe the concept that reaching the goal quickly is good. So when they apply this concept to sex, and they want to ejaculate as soon as possible, they experience premature ejaculation. In sex, however, success is when the man takes longer to achieve an ejaculation. A man will provide himself and his female partner with the greatest pleasure during sex when he is able to slow down, take his time, and control the experience. Other men that experience premature ejaculation do so because of anxiety. They are anxious if they will have a premature ejaculation. Once or twice they might have ejaculated prematurely because they were excited, but as a result of this they might be anxious that they will have a premature ejaculation again. This causes them to concentrate mentally on trying to control their ejaculation. This concentration causes them to have a premature ejaculation. It gets in their way of maintaining their erection and hinders their freedom to enjoy themselves during sex.

Premature ejaculation is generally a young man's problem. However, some men that are not young experience it. Most males that are not young do not experience premature ejaculation because they can last longer and they became better lovers as they grew older. Young males experience premature ejaculation because they are inexperienced.

They come quickly because the sex feels so good that they do not know how to hold off from ejaculating. They are not aware of how rapidly they are coming to a climax.

Effects of Premature Ejaculation on the Man and the Woman

When the man and the woman come to have sex for the first time together, they expect that their sexual encounters will be satisfying and delightful. They have great passion and desire for the sexual encounters. There is no thought that the sexual encounters that they will have together will not be satisfying to the both of them. They assume that the sexual response is a natural one and that as long as they do what comes naturally everything will be just fine. For some couples, this expectation is not fulfilled. They have the problem of premature ejaculation getting in the way of their sexual enjoyment. During the first several sexual encounters the man and the woman might notice that the man ejaculates prematurely but they might not be concerned about it. They believe that this problem will go away on its own and that it is not something important. However, after a while the couple sees that the problem is not going away and that it is affecting them negatively.

The woman, as a result of premature ejaculation, starts to feel used and unfulfilled. She begins to resent the fact that she is not being fulfilled sexually from the sexual encounters with the man. She resents that she cannot climax during the sexual encounters because they are too short as a result of the man's premature ejaculation. The woman may think that if the man just tried, he would be able to control his ejaculation. She fails to realize that premature ejaculation is involuntary, and that he cannot stop it at will. She might feel that the man does not really care about her, and that is why he is ejaculating prematurely during sex with her. She may think that the reason why the man is experiencing premature ejaculation is because of her. She might imagine that she is not attractive enough for him, or that her sexual techniques and abilities are not good enough for him. She may begin to lose confidence in herself and feel anger towards him.

The man might feel frustrated regarding his premature ejaculation and might resent how it affects the woman. It may cause the man personal distress that he and his woman are not getting sexual satisfaction from the sexual encounters because they are too short due to his premature ejaculation. The man might try to stop the premature ejaculation by willing it, but his attempts will be unsuccessful. He will find out that he will ejaculate prematurely, regardless how hard he tries not to. The man may try to distract himself during sex by thinking of something else, like counting from 100 to zero backwards. However, his attempts will be unsuccessful in stopping premature ejaculation. His preoccupation with trying to postpone ejaculation will hinder his ability to fully enjoy the sexual experience. The man might know that he has a problem, but will not know how to deal with it. Lack of control of his body's functioning leaves him feeling unsure of himself. He could begin to doubt his masculinity and feel inadequate. He could lose his self-esteem and feel embarrassed as a result of premature ejaculation. He might also begin to dread the sexual encounters with the woman because he is anxious about whether he will have a premature ejaculation. He may begin to suspect that the woman might be causing his premature ejaculation because of her sexual techniques.

As a consequence of premature ejaculation, the couple's relationship will suffer. Both the man and the woman will begin to withdraw from each other sexually, not wanting to enter an experience that is going to end up frustrating to both of them. There is likely to be hostility in the relationship as a result of premature ejaculation. The man might seek to prove that he is adequate sexually by cheating on his current woman and becoming involved with another woman The woman might cheat on her current man with another man to get the sexual fulfillment that she craves. As a result of premature ejaculation, sometimes the relationship between the man and the woman ends. Therefore, it is important that the man overcomes his premature ejaculation as soon as possible.

Most men feel like the man described previously as a result of premature ejaculation. However, there are a small number of men that are insensitive. They do not care that their premature ejaculation is causing the woman not to get what she needs and deserves in terms of sexual pleasure. They might not care because they view intercourse as the male's prize for seduction. They may not be concerned because they believe that only the man should get pleasure from the sexual experience, and not the woman. They might not care because they are selfish. Also, they may not be concerned because they are negligent. They might continue to have sex without worrying about their premature ejaculation and the effects that it is having on the woman. In these cases, after a while the woman either leaves the relationship because she is not fulfilled sexually, or she might let the man know that she expects him to do something about his problem because she is not being satisfied sexually. If the man does not listen to her and do anything about his premature ejaculation problem, then the woman most often will leave the relationship or begin cheating on him to get the sexual fulfillment that she needs.

Incorrect Methods of Dealing With Premature Ejaculation

Some men might try to deal with their premature ejaculation by using incorrect methods. One incorrect method that men use to try to stop premature ejaculation from happening is by using some form of mental distraction during sex. For example, they might count from one hundred to zero backwards, or imagine themselves in a nonsexual situation during sex. They might also try to distract themselves with thoughts of baseball, taxes, or the stock market during sex. They might also try to distract themselves by thinking of something repulsive during sex. These attempts are not successful and might lead to anxiety. A second incorrect method that men use to try to stop premature ejaculation from happening is by using willpower. They try to force themselves using their willpower not to have a premature ejaculation. This is usually not successful, since the more a man tries not to have a premature ejaculation, the more likely he is going to have a premature ejaculation.

How to Make Sex with Premature Ejaculation Enjoyable

When the man ejaculates prematurely, the woman is disappointed because she will not get a chance to orgasm during sex. Therefore, when the woman comes to have sex with the man, she is worried that he will ejaculate prematurely. However, premature ejaculation does not have to be a negative experience for the woman. The man can still have the woman climax with his penis inside her, even though his penis is limp. The man can do that by doing the following. He can lie flat on his back with his legs straight, and the woman can sit on top of him, either facing him or facing away from him. Her legs should be in a kneeling position, straddling the man's pelvis. The man inserts his limp penis in the woman's vagina. Then the woman can simply rub her clitoris and the areas surrounding it with her hand until she climaxes. She will feel fulfilled sexually when she climaxes with a limp penis inside of her. The man will also feel satisfied and happy that the woman climaxed with his penis inside of her. The man could do the rubbing until the woman climaxes as an alternative, instead of the woman rubbing her clitoris. This alternative contributes to the couple's pleasure, because it offers another way to climax the woman.

Even though the man climaxed prematurely, there is a second way he can use his limp penis to satisfy the woman sexually so that she is not disappointed. He can do that by having the woman lie on her back with her legs straight. Then he lies on top of her, with his legs straight. His limp penis should be lying on the clitoris of the woman. Then the man should make thrusting movements with his hips, causing the limp penis to rub the woman's clitoris. The man should continue to do these thrusting movements, until the woman climaxes. This is very sexually fulfilling to the woman because there is a lot of concentration on the clitoral area from the limp penis.

Thrusting for Premature Ejaculation

If a man suffers from premature ejaculation, he should consider how the thrusting of the penis into the vagina during intercourse is occurring. The way to enhance the man's ejaculatory control and satisfy the woman during intercourse, is to thrust using the grinding technique. During the grinding technique the penis remains deep inside the woman's vagina at the same depth while the man or the woman thrusts in a circular motion. The one doing the thrusting is the one in control in that particular sex position.

This technique causes the penis to rub against the woman's vaginal walls during thrusting and it causes the man's pelvis to rub against the woman's clitoris stimulating it. The stimulation of the woman's clitoris by the man's pelvis usually causes the woman to orgasm the same time as the man. The thrusting in this technique is not the traditional in and out thrusting. This technique stimulates more areas of the penis and vagina than the traditional in and out thrusting. It also makes the man's erection last longer during sex and makes it more likely that the woman will orgasm during sex. This technique is extremely pleasurable for both the man and the woman. This technique is very pleasurable to the woman because it stimulates her clitoris in a circular motion the same motion she rubs her clitoris during masturbation. This technique is very pleasurable to the man if he is prone to quick ejaculation since it makes him last longer before ejaculating. Although this thrusting technique makes it easier for the man to last longer before ejaculating during sex, this does not mean that the man suffering from premature ejaculation cannot use the traditional technique of thrusting in and out of the vagina during sex.

The Most Favorable Positions for Premature Ejaculation

The woman on top position seems to be the most effective sex position for the man to have intercourse in if he suffers from premature ejaculation. In this position the man lies flat on his back with his legs straight and the woman sits on top of him, kneeling on her knees. Her knees should be straddling the man's pelvis. Her face should be facing his face. Even though the woman is controlling the thrusting in this position, the man has more ejaculatory control in this position. The man has more ejaculatory control in this position because he does not have to support his weight and can just relax, enjoying the sex. Even though the woman is controlling the thrusting, the man can decrease his sexual arousal and delay ejaculation by asking the woman to hold off and slow down when he needs her to.

Another position that is effective for the man to have intercourse in if he suffers from premature ejaculation is the modified missionary position. It gives the man more ejaculatory control. In this position the woman lies on her back, with a small pillow under her back for comfort. Her legs are raised in the air and her knees bent. The man is on his knees between her legs facing her. The man then should insert his penis inside her vagina and thrust his penis in and out of the vagina. The woman should not rest her legs on the man's shoulders during sex in this position if she can, so that she decreases the muscle tension in the man's body. But if she has to rest her legs on his shoulders due to exhaustion then that is okay, the position is still effective for premature ejaculation. Since the man in this position is using his knees instead of his arms to support most of his weight, the man minimizes muscle tension throughout his body so that he has more ejaculatory control.

Another position that is effective for the man to have intercourse in, if he suffers from premature ejaculation, is the side-by-side position. In this position the man lies on his side and the woman lies on her side facing him. Both the man and the woman have their legs straight. The man then inserts his penis inside the woman's vagina and he thrusts his penis in and out of the vagina. This position allows a man more ejaculatory control and allows him to last longer during intercourse before climaxing. In this position the man can also thrust using the grinding technique. The man can also have sex in the side-by-side position with the woman facing away from him. In this position, the man lies on his side and the woman lies on her side. But the man is facing the back of the woman's head. Both the man and the woman should have their legs straight. Then the man should insert his penis inside the woman's vagina from behind. This position also allows a man more ejaculatory control, and allows him to last longer during intercourse before climaxing. In this position the man can also use the grinding technique to thrust.

Overcoming Premature Ejaculation

Premature ejaculation can be corrected. It is not only the man's problem; it is a problem for the couple. Both the man and the woman are affected by it. As with any sexual problem, it requires the active involvement of both the man and the woman. The solution to premature ejaculation when the couple is willing to deal with it is very simple. Since premature ejaculation is very troubling to some men the woman should be sympathetic and kind to her man if he suffers from it.

The first step to overcome premature ejaculation is for the man and the woman to have the proper attitudes. First, the man must desire to overcome premature ejaculation and must believe it can occur. Second, the man must be willing to allow his female partner to participate with him in the process. This means that he should be willing to relax, and enjoy receiving pleasure from her. Third, the woman should believe that the man can overcome premature ejaculation, and she should be willing to work towards it. She must understand that her participation in it is important. Fourth, the woman should feel comfortable with the man's genital area. If she is not comfortable, then the woman should spend some time touching and feeling the man's genital area until she is comfortable with it.

Once the couple has the proper attitudes, the next step for them to overcome premature ejaculation is to have open communication with each other about the problem. The couple might have never talked about the problem with each other. They might have been in denial or embarrassed to talk about it. It is important that they talk about it openly, without leaving any details out of the conversation. In the communication the man should let the woman understand what he feels as a result of premature ejaculation, including describing any feelings of inadequacy. The man should let the woman know how he feels about her. The woman needs to let the man know how she feels about him. She needs to explain to him how she feels about his premature ejaculation. She should let him know that he should not feel inadequate because of his problem. She should make it clear to him, that she will be fully involved in helping him overcome his premature ejaculation.

Once the couple has the proper attitudes and has communicated with each other, the next step for the couple is to try a simple method to overcome premature ejaculation. The simplest and easiest way to overcome premature ejaculation is for the man to slow everything down during sex. Women tend to approach their climax more gradually than men. A man's quick penile thrusting will have less effect on the woman than slow penile thrusting that causes the woman a gradual buildup towards climax. If a man does eighteen penile thrusts within 2 minutes it will have less of an effect on the woman than if the man does eighteen penile thrusts within 4 minutes. A man will provide himself and his woman with the greatest pleasure when he is able to slow down, take his time, and control the experience. The man should overcome his natural inclination to rush through the experience. Rather, he should enjoy the process and make it longer by going slower. He should enjoy the good feelings that he experiences during sex and focus on them instead of rushing to release. This might work for some men in overcoming premature ejaculation, but for many it might not work. If this works for the man the man should continue doing it until he feels that having sex without premature ejaculation is a habit. Once it becomes a habit the man can have sex any way he wants and not worry about premature ejaculation. For it to become a habit it usually takes two to three weeks.

If slowing down does not work for the man, then the man should try showering or bathing with the woman in a relaxed way. This allows both of them to enjoy touching each other and get used to each other's body in a relaxed atmosphere without the pressure of climaxing. This could contribute to the couple becoming relaxed before sex. The man could also have the woman massage his body from head to toe. She could massage both the front side of his body and the back side of his body. The man should be in a relaxed position lying down, with his legs straight. While massaging the front side of the man's body, the woman should focus on his genital area. She should gently caress the penis and scrotum, so that he gets used to having her touch them while remaining relaxed. This also causes her to get familiar with his genital area and get used to touching it. The massage should cause the man to become very relaxed. After showering and having a massage, the man should try to have sex slowly as before. Some men that were not able to prevent their premature ejaculation before might be able to now. They are able to now because they are more relaxed as a result of the massage and showering with the woman. If this works for the man, the man should continue doing it until he feels that having sex without premature ejaculation is a habit. Once it becomes a habit, the man can have sex any way he wants and not worry about premature ejaculation.

If the relaxation techniques and the slowing down during sex don't help the man overcome premature ejaculation, then the man should try masturbating an hour or two before having intercourse. The man should masturbate an hour or two before intercourse, and then shower with the woman before sex. After that, the woman should massage the man's body. After the massage the man and woman should have sex, with the man slowing down his movements. This should help a number of men to overcome their premature ejaculation if they were not able to do so previously. If this works for the man, the man should continue doing it until he feels that having sex without premature ejaculation is a habit. Once it becomes a habit the man can have sex any way he wants and not worry about premature ejaculation.

If the masturbation technique does not work for the man in overcoming premature ejaculation, then the man should squeeze his PC (pubococcygeal) muscle anytime he feels he is becoming highly aroused and approaching ejaculation during sex. Such an action will help the man reduce the urge to ejaculate, and will help delay or prevent ejaculation. This will allow the man to overcome premature ejaculation. A strong PC muscle works like a good set of brakes in a car. Just as brakes in a car are used to control the car's speed, the PC muscle is used to control a man's arousal and sexual excitement. Squeezing the PC muscle slows down the man's sexual excitement and sexual arousal, which delays the man's ejaculation. Some men prefer one big hard squeeze of the PC muscle that lasts at least for ten seconds, while others use a series of short light squeezes. Whichever method the man chooses, he should take a deep breath after each squeeze. A man can squeeze his PC muscle at several instances during each lovemaking session. If a man squeezes his PC muscle during sex, he will have more control during penile penetration of the vagina and during penile thrusting into the vagina. This technique might work for a number of men, but for others it might not work. If this works for the man, the man should continue doing it until he feels that having sex without premature ejaculation is a habit. Once it becomes a habit the man can have sex any way he wants and not worry about premature ejaculation.

If squeezing the PC (pubococcygeal) muscle does not work for the man in controlling his premature ejaculation, then the man should try keeping his penis inside the woman's vagina still, as soon he feels he is becoming highly aroused and approaching ejaculation. When the man's penis is still in the woman's vagina, the man can ask the woman to stop moving for a while until he resumes thrusting. The man should keep the penis still in the woman's vagina until he feels his sexual arousal has decreased and his urge to ejaculate has vanished. Then the man could resume thrusting his penis inside the woman's vagina. The man's arousal decreases far more quickly than the woman's arousal. Therefore, when the man and woman resume intercourse, the woman will have kept much more of her original level of arousal than the man. This allows the woman to be able to maintain her gradual buildup towards a climax. Also, as a result of the man keeping his penis still in the woman's vagina for a while, the man is able to prolong the sexual encounter until the woman climaxes. He is able to prolong the sexual encounter since he cools off quite a bit when he stops thrusting, while keeping his penis still in the vagina. The man can stop thrusting, while keeping his penis inside the vagina, several times throughout the sexual encounter. This technique might work for some men, but for others it might not work. If this works for the man, the man should continue doing it until he feels that having sex without premature ejaculation is a habit. Once it becomes a habit the man can have sex any way he wants and not worry about premature ejaculation.

If the man's action of keeping his penis inside the woman's vagina still as soon he feels he is becoming highly aroused does not work then the man should try another method. The other method that the man should try is to withdraw his penis from the vagina so that only the head of the penis remains inside the woman's vagina. The man should remain motionless for 10 to 30 seconds and should ask the woman to do likewise. The man will begin to lose his erection as a result of this. If the man waits until the urge to ejaculate begins to subside before entering the vagina again, he will begin to learn ejaculatory control. The man will also be able to prolong the sexual experience until the woman climaxes as a result of this method. The man can do this method several times during a sexual intercourse session. After several sexual encounters using this method, the man will begin to need to withdraw his penis less often. Although this technique might work for some men, for others it might not work. If this works for the man, the man should continue doing it until he feels that having sex without premature ejaculation is a habit. Once it becomes a habit the man can have sex any way he wants and not worry about premature ejaculation.

Then the man needs to undergo some training in order to overcome his premature ejaculation if the method of withdrawing the penis from the vagina so that only the head of the penis remains inside does not work. Premature ejaculation can be cured with the proper training. The training allows the man to be more in tune with his body, and with his sexual arousal during sex. It allows the man to recognize the sensations that precede ejaculation, so that he knows when he is about to ejaculate. The man's ability to recognize when he is about to ejaculate is important in order for him to learn how to control or delay the process. If the man can recognize when he is about to ejaculate, he can relax just enough so that he does not reach the point of ejaculation until he is ready. The man can stay at a level of excitement during sex without getting to the point of ejaculation until he is ready because he can tell when he is getting close to the point of ejaculation.

The training works by weakening a reflex response that has become a habit that is causing premature ejaculation. It allows the man to establish a new reflex response that becomes a habit that does not cause premature ejaculation. The training allows the man to bring the ejaculation process under greater voluntary control, by frequently approaching the threshold of ejaculation without actually reaching it. This raises the threshold of ejaculation with time and practice. In other words, with time and practice the time needed for the man to reach ejaculation becomes longer, as a result of approaching the point of ejaculation but not actually reaching it during training.

The training not only improves the man's sexual ability, it also improves his relationship with his woman. The training builds intimacy and trust between the couple. It draws the couple closer to each other and increases the pleasure of their times together during sex. Since the training gives the couple a common goal, it improves communication between them. It lets the couple act as a team to solve a frustrating, sometimes finger pointing problem. By the couple acting as a team, they share the problem and take joint responsibility for the solution.

The training is made up of two exercises. One exercise is a masturbation exercise, and the second exercise is a sexual intercourse exercise. During these two exercises a man can use one of four methods to stop his sexual arousal, and cause his urge to ejaculate to go away. The four methods are the squeeze technique, the stop-start technique, the testicle pull down technique, and the pull technique. The man can choose any one of the four techniques that he feels more comfortable with to cause his urge to ejaculate to subside. In the squeeze technique, when the man is getting close to the point of ejaculation, he or his woman place the thumb on the underside of the penis on the frenulum, and then places the next two fingers on the top of the penis on either side of the coronal ridge. Then these fingers squeeze the head of the man's penis firmly, until his urge to ejaculate subsides. The squeeze is done so that the intensity of the man's sexual arousal is lessened, and so that ejaculation is delayed from happening. The squeeze of the tip of the penis might cause the man to lose his erection partially, but he will regain it once stimulation of the penis is resumed. The frenulum is the piece of skin on the underside of the penis below the head.

The second method is the stop-start method. In this method, when the man is getting close to the point of ejaculation, stimulation of the penis stops until the urge to ejaculate subsides. Then stimulation of the penis resumes. The third technique is the testicle pull down technique. In this technique when the man is close to the point of ejaculation, he pulls down his testicles either by holding them between his legs or by gently tugging them down with one hand until the urge to ejaculate subsides. As an alternative, the woman could also pull down the man's testicles by tugging them down with one of her hands. If the man's testicles are pulled down, then he won't ejaculate, because if the testicles do not undergo at least a partial elevation during sex then ejaculation won't happen. The fourth method is the pull technique. In the pull technique, when the man feels close to ejaculation, either the man or woman, using the thumb, gently squeezes and pulls down on the top of the man's scrotum. The top of the man's scrotum is where the scrotum and the penis meet, not the testicles. The squeeze should be held until the urge to ejaculate passes, which usually takes 10 to 30 seconds.

The first exercise in the training is a masturbation exercise. The man can learn to control his ejaculation by masturbating in a specific way. He can try to masturbate with a dry hand at first, or have the woman masturbate him with a dry hand. When the penis is masturbated the frenulum should be stimulated, because it is one of the most pleasurable areas in the penis. Also, the ridge around the head of the penis known as the coronal ridge should be stimulated because it too is one of the most pleasurable areas in the penis. The shaft of the penis should also be stimulated because it is a pleasurable area to stimulate. The man should try to last for a full 15 minutes before ejaculating. He can last for so long by doing the following: He can have his penis stimulated until he feels he is close to ejaculation. Once he feels close to ejaculation, he should cause the ejaculation to subside using one of the four methods. Once the ejaculation subsides, then masturbation of the penis should resume until the urge to ejaculate arises. Once that happens, then the man should cause the urge to ejaculate to subside, using one of the four methods. Then stimulation of the penis should resume. This process should go on until fifteen minutes have elapsed. Once fifteen minutes have elapsed, the man should allow masturbation of his penis to continue until he ejaculates.

During this exercise the man should completely be relaxed and focus on the sensations in his body. He must learn to let himself experience pleasure rather than feel he has to do something for his woman. After a while, this training exercise should allow a man to last longer than before, in regards to ejaculation. The man should be able to last longer than before without resorting to any of the methods to stop the ejaculation. Once a man can last easily up to 15 minutes using any of the four methods to control ejaculation when his penis is masturbated with a dry hand, then he should do the same process but this time his penis should be masturbated with a wet hand. Once the man can last up to 15 minutes easily using any of the four methods to control ejaculation when his penis is masturbated with a wet hand, then he should consider if he is ready to try the second exercise.

In the second exercise, the man and woman should kiss and touch each other as they see fit until they are both aroused. The woman needs to be aroused, so that she is fully lubricated. It might be a good idea to use a lubricant, so that the woman is fully lubricated. Then the man should lie flat on his back with his legs straight, and the woman should kneel on both knees next to him. Then she should massage his upper body, from the face to the stomach. Once she feels the man has had enough, then she should massage his lower body, from his toes to the upper legs. She should not touch his genital area. Once she feels that she has massaged his lower body enough, then she should sit on top of him in a kneeling position, facing him as he lies flat with his legs straight. Her knees should be straddling his pelvis. Then she should guide the man's penis into her vagina. After the woman has inserted the penis, she should sit quietly without making any movement. The man should do likewise. They should do that for two or three minutes. This step is very important, because it helps the man learn to be quiet inside the vagina. This may be very difficult for him because he usually ejaculates quickly, and hence moves rapidly the moment entry has taken place. The woman might find it hard not to move with the penis inside her. Both the man and the woman might find that this period of having the penis inside the vagina without moving as going against what their bodies naturally want to do.

After the woman sits still with the man's penis inside her for two or three minutes, then she should begin to gently move her pelvis in a mildly thrusting manner. When the man feels he is close to ejaculating, he should let the woman know and the woman should quickly move off the man. Then she should immediately apply one of the four methods, to cause his ejaculation to subside. Once the man's ejaculation has subsided, usually within thirty seconds, the man should let the woman know. Then the woman should return to her original kneeling position, straddling the man's pelvis with his penis inside her. Then she should thrust gently, until he is close to ejaculation. She should continue this process, until fifteen minutes have elapsed. Once fifteen minutes have elapsed, then the woman should continue thrusting with her pelvis until the man ejaculates in her vagina. It is important that the woman thrusts gently during this exercise, so that she and the man experience the sexual pleasure to the greatest extent. During this exercise, the man should be completely relaxed, and focus on the sensations in his body. He should let himself experience sexual pleasure instead of feeling he has to do something for his woman. The couple should continue to do this exercise until the man can easily do this exercise. The man should easily remain fifteen minutes without ejaculating using any of the four methods.

This exercise should make the man's confidence in his sexual ability grow. As a result of this exercise, the man should be able to last longer than before, before ejaculating during sex. He should be able to do so without using any of the four methods. Once the man feels that he is ready, he could have sex in any position that he likes without using any of the four methods to subside his ejaculation. When he does so, he should find out that he has overcome his premature ejaculation. However, from time to time the man might need to resort to one of the four methods to stop him from ejaculating prematurely, which is normal. Also the man can use one of the four methods during sex even though he is not going to ejaculate prematurely, to make the sex longer. The training exercises are the most effective way to help a man overcome premature ejaculation.

When doing these two training exercises, several problems arise. The first problem is that some men feel uncomfortable at being the total focus of the pleasuring. They find it hard to just lie back and enjoy. They feel they must be doing something for their woman or she will become upset. The man should not have such feelings since the woman wants him to overcome premature ejaculation and does not expect him to do anything for her during these exercises. The man should not feel uncomfortable at being the total focus of the pleasuring. He should not feel uncomfortable just lying back and enjoying the experience, since that is what needs to be done for him to overcome premature ejaculation. The second problem is that some men sometimes during the exercises are unaware of when they are about to ejaculate, so they find that the ejaculation happens suddenly without any warning. The man should not be discouraged by this but should proceed more slowly during the exercises, so that he gives himself the time to become aware of when he is about to ejaculate. He should learn to be aware of his level of arousal. If the man ejaculates suddenly during any of the exercises, the couple should not be upset, but should continue to enjoy the experience. The man should then proceed to satisfy his woman sexually, using manual or oral stimulation. A third problem that some men experience during these exercises is that sometimes they ejaculate despite using one of the four methods to control ejaculation. This happens because they wait too long after they are close to ejaculating before they use one of the four methods to control the ejaculation.

Seeking Professional Help

Premature ejaculation is one of the easiest sex difficulties to overcome. Despite the fact that there are self-help methods for a man to overcome premature ejaculation, a tiny percentage of men find their premature ejaculation so severe that they cannot overcome it on their own. The pattern of premature ejaculation might be so deeply ingrained, that a man might need the help of a competent sex therapist to overcome his problem. If the man after reading and trying the techniques outlined in this chapter, finds that he still cannot overcome premature ejaculation, then he should seek the help of a trained certified sex therapist. Since this is a very common problem, a man should not be embarrassed to get help.

Chapter 28

Sex during Menstruation, PMS, and Menopause

Menstruation is the periodic discharge of blood and tissue from the lining of the uterus, occurring approximately monthly from puberty to menopause in non-pregnant women. It also called the menses, menstrual period, or period. It occurs because once a month the lining of the uterus thickens, preparing to house the fertilized egg if the woman were to get pregnant that month. However, because most months the woman does not get pregnant, her body has to shed this pumped up uterine lining. It sheds the uterine lining monthly, during the period. The menstrual fluid flows from the uterus, through the small opening in the cervix, and through the vagina, passing out of the body. Most periods can last from 1 to 8 days, with the average being 4 to 5 days. The length of the period can vary from time to time. Also, the length of the period can vary from woman to woman. The flow of menses, is usually a sign that a woman has not become pregnant. When a woman is having her period, she may have physical symptoms also. The physical symptoms that she might experience include bloating, abdominal cramps, constipation, swelling or tenderness in the breasts, cramps or tension in the vulva, and joint or muscle pain.

Menstruation is part of the menstrual cycle. The menstrual cycle is a cycle of physiological changes that occurs in fertile females. It helps a woman's body prepare for the possibility of pregnancy each month. A menstrual cycle begins on the first day of bleeding, and continues up to but not including the first day of the next period. A menstrual cycle can range from 21 days to 35 days or more.

However, the average menstrual cycle is around 28 days long. The length of a woman's cycle can change a little from month to month. Also, the length of the menstrual cycle varies from woman to woman. Both the length of the period and the menstrual cycle are affected by the woman's diet, stress, exercise, travel, or if she is taking any medication.

Premenstrual Syndrome (PMS)

The premenstrual syndrome, or PMS, is a collection of physical and emotional symptoms related to a woman's menstrual cycle that result from the hormonal changes that the woman experiences before menstrual flow begins. These symptoms usually occur regularly, during the ten days prior to menses. They usually vanish either shortly before or after the start of menstrual flow. The three most prominent emotional symptoms associated with PMS are irritability, tension, and dysphoria (unhappiness). Other emotional symptoms associated with PMS include stress, anxiety, mood swings, increased emotional sensitivity, and changes in libido. The physical symptoms associated with PMS include bloating, abdominal cramps, insomnia, headache, fatigue, constipation, swelling or tenderness in the breasts, cramps or tension in the vulva, and joint or muscle pain. The physical symptoms associated with PMS are the same that are associated with the menstrual cycle, but the presence of the physical symptoms alone during the menstrual cycle, without the presence of the emotional symptoms, is not considered PMS.

Most women with PMS experience only a few of the physical and emotional symptoms described earlier. The PMS symptoms and their intensity vary from woman to woman, and even from cycle to cycle. A majority of women experience PMS during their lifetime, but not all. Many women do not develop PMS until their 30s and 40s. PMS tends to worsen as the woman ages.

Reducing Menstruation and PMS Symptoms

There is no cure for PMS nor for the menstruation symptoms, but a healthy lifestyle can reduce the PMS and the menstruation symptoms. A healthy lifestyle could include exercise, getting enough sleep, reducing stress, not smoking, and a healthy diet. Sex during menstruation could help reduce the physical symptoms that the woman experiences. Sex during PMS could help reduce the physical and non-physical symptoms that the woman experiences. In addition to sex, a woman could masturbate. Sex, masturbation, and exercise will reduce the stress that a woman is experiencing, thus reducing the symptoms that a woman experiences during menstruation and PMS. Also, masturbation and sex both relieve the woman's cramps and tensions in the vulva by sending blood into that area. In addition, if a woman gets enough rest during PMS and menstruation, that should reduce the menstruation and PMS symptoms that she is experiencing.

Horniness and Period

From an evolutionary standpoint, a person would think that both men and women would be like the lower mammals (squirrels and rabbits) and non-human primates (apes and monkeys), having almost all sexual activity take place when the female is ovulating (producing eggs), and the rest of the time neither party would be interested in sexual activity. However, with the human female there is no consistent pattern when she feels horniest. Some women say they feel horniest towards the end of their menstruation, while others feel horniest at the beginning of their menstruation. Still others feel horniest at the middle of their menstruation, while other women never see a change in their horniness level during the menstrual cycle. It is important to note that a considerable number of women feel horniest at the beginning, and in the middle of their menstruation. The woman's subjective experience of the sexual response and her physiological response during the sexual response are the same throughout the menstrual cycle. They do not vary at all. This is true in all women's cases. As for the man's sexual interest it does not vary during the month.

Sex During PMS and Period

Some men are under the wrong impression that women cannot have sex during their PMS. This is far from the truth. As a matter of fact, sex and orgasm during PMS decrease the emotional and physical symptoms of PMS. They make PMS less unpleasant.

Some men are under the wrong impression that women have no sexual desire during their period. In fact, as mentioned earlier, a large number of women report an increase in their sexual desire before or during menstruation. There is no reason why a woman who craves sex during her period should deny herself sexual gratification. Plenty of people have sex when the woman has her period. As a matter of fact, sex and orgasm have been shown to be instant cures for menstrual cramps and menstrual migraines. Although sex during a woman's period seems totally natural to some people, it feels gross to others. It feels gross to some people because it seems messy to them. Also, some people object to sex during menstruation for religious reasons.

However, the only reason not to have sex during the woman's period is HIV. Unprotected vaginal intercourse during menstruation increases the risk of female-to-male transmission of HIV. This is because although HIV is present in vaginal secretions, it is present in much higher concentrations in blood, and sex during a woman's period brings the man into direct contact with her blood. Also, unprotected vaginal intercourse during menstruation can be hazardous to the woman's health if it is the man who is infected with HIV. It is dangerous to the woman's health because the woman is more vulnerable to HIV during menstruation. The woman is more vulnerable during menstruation because the menstrual blood flushes away some of the mucus that partly plugs the cervix, making it easier for the HIV virus to penetrate the deeper regions of her reproductive system. Also, the vagina is fairly acidic, which helps kill invading microorganisms. But during the woman's period, the menstrual blood decreases the acidity of the woman's vagina, making her more susceptible to HIV infection.

But the couple could practice safer sex and still have sex during the woman's period. The use of a condom during sex during a woman's period not only ensures that it is safer for the couple to have sex, it also makes it cleaner for the man to have sex. A woman could also use a diaphragm or cervical cap to decrease the amount of blood that escapes during sex, thus making sex during a woman's period less messy. Placing a towel under the woman's bottom during sex during her period, will protect the sheets from being stained with blood. During a woman's period, her vagina dries out a little. Therefore, it is a good idea for the woman to use lubrication when having sex during her period. Also, a woman should use some form of birth control if she has sex during her period. A woman should do so because it is possible that she gets pregnant during her period.

In conclusion, a man and a woman can have unprotected sex during the woman's menstruation, provided that both parties are not infected with the HIV virus. If the HIV status of the man or the woman is uncertain, then the couple could have sex during the woman's menstruation, provided that they practice safer sex. The woman's menstrual blood during sex is just a minor aesthetic problem that should not interfere with the man and the woman's enjoyment of sex. Finally, oral sex is okay during the woman's period. Some men like the taste of menstrual blood during oral sex.

Best Time for the Woman to Get Pregnant

In order to get a woman pregnant, it is not just a matter of having unprotected sex. The couple needs to have sex when the woman is ovulating. The woman usually ovulates around the middle of her cycle. In order to get the woman pregnant, it is a good idea for the couple to have sex anytime during the time period that starts two days before the middle of the menstrual cycle and ends two days after the middle of the menstrual cycle. It is important to remember, that each woman has a different menstrual cycle length.

The following is an example if the woman had an average cycle, which is a 28-day cycle. If the woman's cycle is an average 28 day cycle, the woman ovulates on day 14. Sperm can live for up to 5 days and the egg can survive for about one day or even up to two days after it is released. Therefore, on a 28-day cycle the best time to have sex to get the woman pregnant would be from day 12 through day 16. Day 12 and day 13 are good days since the sperm can survive up to 5 days, fertilizing the egg when it is released on day 14. Day 15 and day 16 are good days, since the egg can survive up to two days if it is released on day 14.

Sex During Menopause

Menopause is the end of fertility in the female, which is indicated by the permanent stopping of the monthly menstruation. Menopause does not happen suddenly, but it is a gradual transition that takes two to seven years. The menopausal transition begins with variation in the menstrual cycle length and ends after a woman has experienced 12 months without menstrual bleeding. It is important to note that menopause is not complete until the woman has not experienced menstrual bleeding for 12 months. The usual age range for menopause is between 40 to 60, but the average age is 51. The symptoms of menopause are insomnia, irritability, and stress incontinence. Stress incontinence is when the woman loses urine when she laughs, sneezes, or during sex. Menopause also causes the opening to the woman's vagina to gradually grow smaller, especially if the woman is not sexually active. The depth and width of the woman's vagina gradually shrinks, making it less elastic. The vagina becomes drier as a result of menopause. Its ability to produce lubrication during arousal is reduced as result of menopause. It takes the woman longer to lubricate her vagina due to menopause.

The most common myth surrounding menopause is that in addition to the loss of the reproductive function, menopause marks the end of the woman's sexuality. This myth came to exist because many women, as a result of menopause, have their sexual desire decrease. But even though their sexual desire decreases, women retain their interest in sexual activity and are fully capable of good sexual functioning. Menopause is not the end of the woman's sex life and should not be the end of the woman's sex life. Some women even experience a sort of sexual rebirth after menopause, freshly rediscovering their husband or boyfriend, paying more attention to their own appearance, and suddenly becoming interested in daytime trysts. For them, the occurrence of menopause is liberating. It is liberating because there is the freedom from the fear of pregnancy and the inconvenience of menstruation. However, for some women menopause is a long-awaited excuse to abandon sexual activity because they never enjoyed it anyway. However, all women after menopause are fully capable of sexual functioning, and should continue to have an active sex life to keep their body healthy. They should continue to have sex, too, to keep their relationship with their husband or boyfriend well.

After menopause, there are several things that a couple could do to ensure that the sex remains a pleasant and satisfying experience to both the man and the woman. First, the vagina is thinner and more delicate as a result of menopause. Therefore, during sex the man should be gentle with his penile thrusts. Second, a man should not be too fast or too rough during sex, and the woman should make sure that her vagina is well-lubricated. They should do so because if they do not, a mild burning sensation during sex will result, and this sensation lasts sometimes for hours or even days. Third, as a result of menopause, a woman needs more foreplay than usual before sex to get her in the mood for sex. Fourth, after menopause, the woman can keep her body healthy and keep the changes that occur to it to a minimum by having sex regularly, thus ensuring a satisfying sex life. Fifth, the woman should communicate her feelings openly with her partner, and her partner should respond positively and reassuringly. This will ensure that sex remains a pleasant and satisfying experience to the woman. Sixth, after menopause, it is important that the man be gentle and reassuring during sex, to ensure that the sexual experience is pleasant and satisfying.

Chapter 29

Sex and Pregnancy

The most ideal sex position for conception is the missionary position. In this position, the woman lies on her back with her legs straight up towards the sky and spread wide, or she can draw her legs up to her chest while keeping them spread wide. The man lies on top of the woman with his legs straight. This way when the man ejaculates, the sperm is at the correct angle to swim toward the ovum. After sex, the woman can remain on her back with her legs either straight up towards the sky and spread wide or drawn at her chest and spread wide. The woman can remain like this for 10 to 30 minutes, encouraging the sperm to swim upward.

Sex During Pregnancy

Almost every newly pregnant couple worries whether they can continue to have sex when the woman is pregnant. It is usually perfectly safe for the couple to continue to have sex when the woman is pregnant. It won't hurt the baby. Having an orgasm won't throw a woman into labor or trigger a miscarriage. The man's penis won't harm the baby and sperm inside the woman won't cause an infection or harm the baby. A pregnant woman might feel increased movement of the fetus after orgasm, but that is normal, a result of small harmless contractions of the uterus. As a matter of fact, satisfying sex is good for pregnancy. Although usually it is perfectly safe for the pregnant woman to have sex, in some cases it is not advisable. It is not advisable if a woman is considered high risk or has any condition that would make sex during pregnancy dangerous. Some of the conditions that would make the woman high risk and would make sex during pregnancy dangerous include if a woman has a history of miscarriages, has a dilation of the cervix, has had premature labor in the past, or is pregnant with twins or more. A woman should talk to her doctor to make sure that it is okay for her to have sex during pregnancy. It is important to point out that unless the doctor has indicated a concern, there are no physical reasons why a healthy pregnant woman should not have sex.

The pregnancy is divided into three trimesters. In the first trimester, many women report feeling nauseous, vomiting, and being very tired. They also have painful, swollen breasts. This makes sex a very low priority for most women during the first trimester. It also decreases the sex drive of most women during the first trimester. However, not all women suffer from these symptoms during the first trimester, and a few women are lucky to enjoy a normal or even a heightened sex drive during the first trimester.

In the second trimester, many women have their bodies adapted to the new hormone levels and are feeling much more normal. Their nausea often subsides, their breast tenderness abates, and their fatigue diminishes. They are feeling normal and able to enjoy sex. They have their energy levels high, their appearance healthy, and their sex drive increased. Most women during the second trimester are feeling sexy and have an active sex life. In the second trimester, most women's bodies retain more fluid than usual, which means that their bodies will be permanently partially aroused and responsive. Also during the second trimester, there is an increase in blood flow in the woman's genital area and the pelvis. This makes it easier for most women to achieve an orgasm, and the orgasm is more intense than usual. Some women even have their first orgasm during the second trimester, while some other women have their first multiple orgasms during the second trimester. If a woman still has a low sex drive during the second trimester, then she should not worry because that is normal, too.

In the third trimester, the woman is likely to feel very large, tired, and immobile. She will most likely have a very low sexual desire. Also, she will have a heavy vaginal discharge, and will have colostrum leaking from her breasts. Colostrum is a liquid that will nourish the newborn for several days before the true breast milk comes in. Just about every pregnant woman feels tired, if not exhausted, during the final trimester. In addition, sleep is usually difficult for the woman during the third trimester, because it is increasingly hard to find a comfortable position. The vaginal discharge, fatigue, and leaking breasts will deter a woman from frequent intercourse. Therefore, some women choose to have other forms of gratification instead, that do not involve penetration. The other forms of gratification that some women enjoy are oral sex, masturbation, massage, hugging, cuddling, and mutual masturbation. During the third trimester, the baby's head drops, creating pressure and discomfort during intercourse. It becomes more difficult for a woman to have an orgasm during the third trimester. If a woman has an orgasm during the third trimester, her contractions last for several minutes and can be frightening, but not harmful. Having sex during the third trimester won't harm the baby. In the third trimester, pressure in the pelvic area intensifies the need for an orgasm. If the woman finds intercourse difficult, she should try masturbating instead in order to relieve the need for an orgasm.

Sex during pregnancy is natural. It is important that sex is not interrupted during pregnancy, but rather continue even though a woman might have a low sex drive. It should be continued during pregnancy because if it is not the feelings of love that the couple has for each other will decrease. Another reason why it should be continued during pregnancy is so that the feelings of love that the couple has for each other continue. Furthermore, it is important that sex continues during pregnancy so that the man does not feel deprived. As a matter of fact, sex during pregnancy is better than usual. It is better than usual because during pregnancy the blood flow increases to all parts of the body, including the genital area. As a result of the increase in blood flow, the vulva may feel engorged and sensitive. This can lead to more intense orgasms than usual, or even to multiple orgasms. The engorged vagina also hugs the penis more tightly during intercourse if the woman is pregnant, making the feelings of pleasure during sex more intense to both the man and the woman. The freedom of not having to worry about birth control during sex when the woman is pregnant makes the sex more pleasurable to both the man and the woman. Sex during pregnancy allows the couple to strengthen the emotional bond that they have together, increasing their intimacy.

Sometimes a woman does not feel like having sex during pregnancy, and that is normal. The couple should not be concerned that the woman does not want to have sex sometimes. The couple could gratify themselves and demonstrate their love and caring to each other in other ways besides intercourse when the woman does not feel like having sex, or if the doctor has notified her not to have sex during pregnancy. The other ways include oral sex, masturbation, mutual masturbation, hugging, cuddling, massage, and caressing one another. The other ways include also showering together and kissing. Kissing does not have to be a precursor to sex. The couple could find kissing to be all the stimulation needed to bring them pleasure and demonstrate their love and care to one another. Fellatio and cunnilingus are both safe during pregnancy, as long as the man does not blow air into the vagina during cunnilingus. Masturbation, mutual masturbation, and cunnilingus are good methods to provide the woman with sexual relief if she does not feel like having intercourse.

Sexual Positions and Methods During Pregnancy

Mother Nature never intended for a woman to stop having sex when she became pregnant. Some women report their best sex ever is during their pregnancies. They enjoy the sex while being pregnant because they could climax more easily. The couple should experiment when the woman is pregnant to see which sex positions will work for the pregnant woman. As a general rule, the couple should choose positions that do not let the man rest his body weight on the woman's abdomen or her sore breasts during sex. Therefore, the couple should avoid the missionary position, since the man's body puts too much pressure on the woman's abdomen in that position.

There are several sex positions that are pleasurable for a pregnant woman. The first position that is pleasurable for a pregnant woman is the woman on top position. In this position, the man lies on his back with his legs straight and the woman sits on top of him, either facing him or facing away from him, with her legs straddling his hips. The woman on top position is the most comfortable for a pregnant woman, because she controls the movement during sex, ensuring no movement that makes her uncomfortable is done. This position takes pressure off the woman's abdomen, which makes it very pleasurable. The second sex position that is pleasurable for a pregnant woman is the side-by-side position with the man from behind. In this position, the woman lies on her side and the man lies on his side behind her. This position is one of the most comfortable positions for a pregnant woman in the late stages of pregnancy, since all the pressure is taken off the woman's abdomen and back during sex. In this position, the man still has access to the woman's clitoris with his fingers. In this position the woman is able to move freely, while the man can stimulate her breasts.

The third sex position that is pleasurable for a pregnant woman is the doggy style position. In this position, the woman is on her hands and knees like a dog. The palms of her hands are resting on the floor with her hands straight, while she is kneeling on both knees. Her back is kept straight in a horizontal position. The man penetrates her from behind while in a kneeling position. In this position, the man's hands are free and he can use them to grasp her legs and pelvis as he thrusts. This position is very comfortable for the couple because the woman's pregnant belly does not get in the way. This position also allows the man to give the woman clitoral stimulation very easily. Underneath the woman's stomach, a man can place pillows so that her stomach rests on them. This is not necessary, but the couple could do it if they find that the woman feels better with the pillows underneath. The fourth sex position that is pleasurable for a pregnant woman is the sitting position facing the man. In this position, the man sits on the chair with the woman sitting on top of him, facing him. This position is good for women in the late stages of pregnancy since it allows the woman to control the movement during sex, ensuring that she does not cause herself any pain.

There are several things that could be done to make sex during pregnancy more pleasurable. First, women whose breasts are sore during pregnancy might find it a good idea to wear a bra during sex, so that the breasts ache less. They will ache less because they are not moving during sex as a result of the bra. Second, pregnant women can use pillows during sex to transform an awkward sex position into a pleasurable one. Third, the man could be very gentle and careful with the woman during sex, making sure that he does not cause her any discomfort.

Things to Avoid During Pregnancy

There are two things that a pregnant woman should avoid. The first thing that should be avoided is the man blowing air into the vagina during cunnilingus, because it could have the serious but rare result of causing an embolism. The embolism could harm the woman and the baby. An embolism is an air bubble that could pass into the woman's blood stream, which can be fatal to both her and the baby. In some rare cases, pregnant women died as a result of the man blowing air into the vagina during cunnilingus. During pregnancy, an embolism is more likely to occur because the veins of the uterus are dilated in order to get more blood to the baby. The second thing that should be avoided is the pregnant woman having sex with a man carrying a sexually transmitted disease. Under no circumstance should a pregnant woman have sex with a man carrying a sexually transmitted disease, because a newly born infant can contract potentially fatal infections during delivery, if the mother's birth canal has been contaminated by sexually transmitted diseases.

Sex and Condoms During Pregnancy

During pregnancy, if a woman is in a stable monogamous relationship with a male partner and both are disease-free, then there is no need for a condom to be used during sex. However, safer sex is even more important during pregnancy if the woman is not in a monogamous relationship. Also, safer sex is even more important during pregnancy if the woman has a new partner whose health status she is not certain of. Safer sex is more important during pregnancy to protect the woman and the baby from sexually transmitted infections if the risk is present.

Sex After Pregnancy

It is standard medical advice for the woman to wait six weeks after she gives birth before resuming sex. The woman should do so because after delivery everything is very raw inside her, and the tissues need time to heal. Another reason why the woman should do so is because there is a big danger that bacteria may attach to sperm cells, swim up into the uterus, and cause an infection. However, sometimes if a woman has an episiotomy she cannot resume sex within six weeks like she is supposed to. Rather, she might have to wait up to four months after delivery before resuming sex. This is so because the episiotomy does not heal within three weeks like it is supposed to, but rather it might be painful for as much as four months after delivery. An episiotomy is a small incision made in the perineum to enlarge the woman's vaginal opening during delivery, which is later closed with stitches called the husband's stitch. Any woman who has had an episiotomy is unlikely to feel relaxed about sex until the wound has healed, because sex before the episiotomy wound has healed is only painful. Furthermore, women who receive a cesarean section usually recover in six weeks, and can have sex in six weeks. However, sometimes recovery might take longer, and the woman should avoid sex longer than six weeks, until the cesarean wound has healed. A cesarean section is a surgical incision in the walls of a woman's abdomen and uterus that allows for delivery of the baby.

A woman usually receives a six-week postnatal checkup by her doctor after delivering the baby. During this checkup, it is an excellent time for the woman to discuss with the doctor whether it is advisable to resume sex at this stage. When the woman does get the okay from the doctor to resume sex, most women find that their sexual desire is low. The woman's sexual desire might be low because she might be fearful of another pregnancy or anxious about being in pain or discomfort during sex. Her sexual desire might also be low because she might find that the sex has become painful. The sex might be painful for several months after giving birth. A third reason why the woman's sexual desire may be low is because the hormone that helps the woman's body produce milk, prolactin, decreases the woman's sexual drive. Prolactin also can decrease the sensations during sex, making it more difficult to achieve an orgasm. A fourth reason why a woman's sexual desire may be low, is because her breasts leak after childbirth, especially during sex, making sex uncomfortable for her and her partner. A fifth reason why a woman's sexual desire may be low is because the woman usually suffers vaginal dryness after giving birth, making the sex uncomfortable and painful. A sixth reason why a woman's sexual desire may be low is because after delivering the baby some women do not find the sex enjoyable because of slack vaginal muscles. A seventh reason why a woman's sexual desire may be low is because shortly after delivery most women suffer through a mild mysterious depression called the baby blues. The baby blues is also known as postpartum depression. Postpartum is the transition period following delivery, beginning immediately after the birth of a child, and extending for about six weeks.

The woman should not pressure herself to return to an active sex life right away. The couple's sexual activities, usually, gradually return to previous levels. For some couples, it takes more than a year to return to pre-pregnancy levels of sexual relations. However, the woman should try her best to have sex with her male partner as much as she can if she wants the relationship to last. At times when the woman cannot have sex, the couple should use other means to gratify themselves. The other means include oral sex, masturbation, mutual masturbation, hugging, cuddling, massage, kissing, showering together, and caressing one another. Also, the couple should use oral sex, masturbation, and mutual masturbation to relieve the sexual feelings of the man and the woman when the woman does not feel like having sex. It is important that the sexual feelings of the man are relieved regularly, either by sex or by other means, so that the man does not feel deprived and the relationship does not turn sour.

Sexual Positions & Methods to Have Sex after Pregnancy

Pregnancy does not have to hurt a woman's sex life after giving birth. Every couple has their own pace to return to normal levels of sexual relations after giving birth. When the woman is ready to have sex for the first time since having the baby, the man and the woman should make sure that they slowly work up to intercourse. They should spend a lot of time on foreplay, stroking, massaging, and kissing each other to give the woman's vagina time to lubricate and expand. The couple should use lubricants the first couple of times to decrease the friction of the penis across the vaginal opening, making the sex more pleasurable. The couple should do so since after giving birth and during breast feeding estrogen levels are low, which may cause vaginal dryness and painful intercourse. The woman should not be surprised if the sensations in the vagina are not as intense as they were prior to the pregnancy, because it might take a few months for the nerves in the pelvis to recover. Orgasms also come back slowly for most women after giving birth, sometimes taking as much as several months.

During the first few sexual encounters after giving birth, emotionally, the woman's self-esteem might be low because she might feel that she is unattractive. She might feel that she is unattractive because of stubborn pregnancy pounds that she did not lose as yet. The woman's low self-esteem will lower her enjoyment of sex and the male partner will sense that, decreasing his pleasure during sex as well. The woman should not let her self-esteem become low and feel unattractive because she did not lose some pregnancy pounds. Rather, the woman should have a high self-esteem by changing her attitude towards herself and thinking positively about herself, seeing herself as attractive.

During the first several sexual encounters after giving birth, the woman's breasts will leak. This may be uncomfortable for the woman and the man. One way to deal with this situation is for the woman to feed the baby before she has sex, so that her breasts are not as full, decreasing the possibility that her breasts will leak. Another way to deal with this situation is for the woman to wear a bra with pads during sex. This will hide the fact that the breasts leak during sex. It is important for the couple to remember that breast feeding is not a sure contraceptive. The couple should use some kind of birth control while the woman is breast feeding to ensure that the woman does not get pregnant again.

During the first several sexual encounters after giving birth, the vagina may feel different. The woman may worry that labor and delivery have changed the size of the vagina greatly, to the extent that she and her male partner will no longer enjoy sex. The woman should not worry because the vagina will return to normal size in time. A woman could do Kegel exercises to help return the vagina to its normal size. The Kegel exercises will strengthen the muscles that surround the vagina, making the vagina tighter. The Kegel exercises will also increase blood flow to the pelvic floor muscles, making the sex more pleasurable. Also, during sex a woman can contract the pelvic muscles, increasing stimulation for the man and the woman during sex. Such an act will compensate for the large vagina size.

Most women suffer depression the first six weeks after giving birth. That is normal and the woman should not worry about it. This should not affect the woman's sex life since the woman won't be having sex the first six weeks after giving birth. After six weeks the depression should go away, and it should have no effect on the woman's sex life. However, if the depression persists beyond six weeks after giving birth, the woman should seek the advice of a doctor.

After giving birth, the woman's breasts most likely will feel tender for a while, whether she breast feeds or not. Therefore, when having sex the woman may ask the man to avoid touching her breasts or to touch them very gently. If the woman has undergone a cesarean section, then during sex she should avoid positions that put weight or pressure on her abdomen, since that can be very uncomfortable or painful. She should do so until the cesarean wound heals.

To accommodate the woman's tender tissues and healing scars after childbirth, the couple should choose a sex position that allows the female to control the angle and depth of the penetration. The best sex position that does that is the woman on top position. In that position, the man lies on his back with his legs straight and the woman sits on top of him, either facing him or away from him, with her legs straddling his hips. This position gives a couple the maximum pleasure from sex since it is the least painful for a woman recovering from childbirth. Another thing that a couple could do is to have the woman try positions in which she keeps her legs straight and closed, so that the tension within the vaginal walls increases. One such position has the woman lying on her side and the man lies on his side from behind her. A second such position has the woman lying on her side and the man lies on his side facing her. These two positions compensate for the larger than usual vaginal opening that a woman has after childbirth by increasing the tension within the vaginal walls.

Motherhood and Sex

Some women and some men stop enjoying sex after the woman gets pregnant and after she gives birth. They do so because they incorrectly feel that being a mother and making love cannot go together. They feel it is not right for a mother to enjoy sex. Having a baby is a life changing event, but it does not change a woman from a sexual to a non-sexual being. A woman is a sexual being when pregnant and when she is a mother. Even though a woman has become a mother, she has all the same parts, hormones, and sexual abilities that she had before she gave birth. Her capacity to enjoy sex after giving birth is the same as before she gave birth. Therefore, these men and women should change their incorrect attitudes and accept the fact that being a mother and having sex go together. They should also accept the fact that it is right for a mother to enjoy sex. This change in attitudes will let these women and men resume enjoying sex, during pregnancy and after pregnancy.

Exercise and Pregnancy

During pregnancy and after pregnancy, exercise should be a way of life to a woman. Exercise will help a pregnant woman maintain a healthy pregnant weight without gaining too much weight. It will also help reduce a pregnant woman's depression if she has any. It will also improve a pregnant woman's sexual desire and increase her stamina during sex. Exercise after a woman gives birth will help get her body back into shape. It will also be good for her mind, reducing depression if she has any. It will also make the woman more capable of enjoying sex, because of her increased stamina and increased sexual desire.

Chapter 30

Naturally Enlarging the Penis

Unfortunately, most people are misinformed about the penis. Most people incorrectly think that a man cannot do anything about his penis size or sexual pleasure. The penis can be worked on to become larger in size and for the sexual pleasure to increase. The penis has the potential to gain 1-3 inches in length and thickness naturally. This chapter shows how a man can increase his penis size and sexual performance naturally, without resorting to surgery or pumps.

Natural Penis Enlargement: How it Works

The basic principle behind natural penis enlargement is to increase the blood flow of the penile chambers. By doing so, the penis gains an average of 1-3 inches in length and thickness over the course of a few months. This result is permanent.

The penis has three chambers that run along its length. The smallest chamber is known as the Corpus Spongiosum and is located on the bottom of the penis. It is used for urinating and ejaculating. This chamber is not responsible for the erection size of the penis. The other two chambers, known as the Corpora Cavernosa, are responsible for the penis size. These two chambers are the largest in the penis and are located above the smaller Corpus Spongiosum chamber. When a man gets sexually aroused, the Corpora Cavernosa swell up to several times the usual size with blood, causing an erection. The extent to which these chambers can expand and the amount of blood they can hold during an erection determines the erection size. Since the size of the Corpora Cavernosa determine the size of the penis, these chambers are important in naturally enlarging the penis size. Therefore, the principle behind natural penis enlargement is to enhance the potential of the Corpora Cavernosa chambers so that they are able to hold greater volumes of blood and expand further. The ability of the Corpora Cavernosa chambers to hold greater volumes of blood increases steadily, causing a steady increase in penis size over a short period of time. The chambers permanently hold a greater amount of blood, therefore the increase in penis size is permanent.

The increase in blood flow in the penis not only increases the penis size permanently, but it leads to more blood flowing to the pubococcygeus muscle or PC muscle. The increase in blood flow to the PC muscle causes a stronger PC muscle. There are various natural penis enlargement methods which work to promote blood flow in the penis. Three of these methods are jelqing, supplements, and topical oils.

Jelqing

Jelqing is an ancient penis enlargement technique that originated in the Middle East. It is very effective in making the penis thicker and longer naturally. It is also known as milking. The purpose of the jelq exercise is to force more blood into the flaccid penis, which will essentially stretch the tissues of the penis, thus allowing more blood to enter the penis. As a matter of fact, the jelq exercise forces more blood into the Corpora Cavernosa which is the spongy tissue that makes up the penis. This expands and stretches the cell walls of the Corpora Cavernosa to allow larger quantities of blood to enter the penis. Thus, the capacity of the Corpora Cavernosa to hold more blood is increased as a result of the jelq exercise. The jelq exercise will increase the size of both the flaccid and erect penis, but most noticeably in the erect penis.

To start the jelq exercise the man needs to do a warm up. The warm up is usually around five minutes long and involves putting a wash cloth in warm water, then holding it around the penis until it cools. Once the wet wash cloth cools, the man should take it and put it in warm water again. Then he should hold it around the penis again until it cools. He should continue to do that until five minutes have elapsed and the penis is in a partial erection. If the penis is not in a partial erection after five minutes, then the man can massage it so that it becomes in a partial erection. The cloth should not be too hot, but it should be as warm as possible without inflicting pain on the penis. The heat from the cloth will draw more blood into the penis, allowing the jelq exercise to be more effective. This warm up is necessary because it makes the penis and testicles very relaxed, and gets the penis in a semi-erect state. This gets the man ready for the jelq exercise because the man cannot do a jelq exercise unless the penis is in a semi-erect state.

Once the man has finished the warm up he should put sufficient lubricant on both his hands and his penis. The lubricant should be fairly long lasting and should be reapplied when necessary. It is better to use a water-based lubricant than an oil-based lubricant. A man should not use soap during jelqing because soap dries and irritates the skin. Soap also causes high levels of urethral irritation.

The level of the erection during jelqing is important. The penis should be around 50% erect. It is important that the erection level is around 50% for the jelqing exercise to be most effective. If the erection is around 50%, the man can effectively push blood throughout the penis. If the erection is around 50%, the fibers and tissues in the penis are limber enough to stretch and contract as blood is forced through the shaft. If the erection level is too low or too high, then the jelqing exercise won't be effective. Jelqing should never be performed on a fully erect penis because that may damage the penis. Jelqing should never be performed if the penis is fully erect because the fibers and tissues in the penis are not limber enough to stretch and contract as blood is forced through the shaft. In general, if the erection is a little over 50%, like 60%, then the jelqing exercise will have more of an effect on girth. Likewise, if the erection is a little below 50%, like 40%, then the jelqing exercise will have more of an effect on length. That explains why some people gain length as a result of jelqing easily while others only gain girth easily.

To start the jelq exercise the man should make sure the erection is around 50%. If it is below that he should stimulate the penis with his hands until it is around 50%. If it is more than that then he should wait and let the erection decrease to around 50%. Once the erection reaches 50% then he should start the jelq exercise.

To start the jelq exercise, the man with the thumb and forefinger of one hand should make an okay sign or circle around the base of the penis and grip it firmly. The man should have the thumb and forefinger meet when making the okay sign in a way that it traps blood effectively. The man should place the grip as close to the pubic bone as possible. He should move his hand slowly towards the head of the penis. The man should stop his hand before it reaches the glans. This will force blood from the base of the penis through the shaft to the head. When the hand stops before it reaches the head of the penis, the man should form an okay sign around the base of the penis with the free hand. When the hand that is close to the glans releases the penis, the second hand at the base of the penis should start moving towards the glans of the penis. This process should be repeated in a continuous motion. The man should not stimulate the head of the penis during jelqing.

To ensure that the entire penis is worked out thoroughly the grip should be varied during the course of a jelq session. The ideal jelqing pressure as a result of the grip is one that does not hurt but effectively forces blood up the penis. If the man feels the need to ejaculate during the jelq exercise, he should take a break and let the feeling go away. Jelqing while standing increases the initial pressure of the blood in the penis, thus the effectiveness of the exercise. Also, jelqing in a sitting position with the legs raised above the level of the penis is effective. This posture encourages a slumped back which allows easier access to the base of the penis and increases the downward angle when jelqing. If the man does the jelq exercise only 15 minutes every day that should be enough time for him to achieve his goal of a larger penis. However, it is not uncommon for some men to do this exercise for a half hour.

As an extra, sometimes when the man does the jelq exercise he could tighten his PC muscle every time his hand is getting very close to the head of the penis. He could keep the PC muscle tightened until the hand close to the head of the penis releases the penis. By the man tightening the PC muscle during the jelq exercise more blood is pushed into the penis during the jelq exercise, making the exercise more effective.

After the jelq exercise is completed the man needs to do a warm down. The warm down is usually around five minutes long and involves putting a wash cloth in warm water, then holding it around the penis until it cools. Once the wet wash cloth cools the man should take it and put it in warm water again. Then he should hold it around the penis again until it cools. He should continue to do that until five minutes have elapsed. The cloth should not be too hot, but it should be as warm as possible without inflicting pain on the penis. The heat from the cloth will draw more blood into the penis during the warm down. This will relax the tissues, minimize the chances of injury, and will allow the jelq exercise to be more effective.

Sometimes as a result of the jelq exercise red pin prick spots will appear on the penis as a result of burst capillaries. They should disappear within a day or two even though a person is continuing his jelq exercise daily. Sometimes larger red or purple spots appear on the penis as a result of the jelq exercise. These spots indicate a more substantial damage in capillary or vein walls. Taking a couple of days off from jelqing is a good idea if these spots appear on the penis. Black pin prick spots that sometimes appear on the shaft of the penis as a result of the jelq exercise indicate that there was insufficient lubrication during the exercise. They should heal quickly even though the man is continuing his jelq exercise daily provided that he uses sufficient lubrication from the time they appear. Bruise-like discoloration located toward the end of the shaft and often more noticeable on the bottom is common among jelqers. These are caused by blood being pushed through the membranes under pressure and having no route to return. Even though a person is continuing his jelq exercise daily, the bruise-like discoloration should go away provided the man starts warming up and down thoroughly and when he moves his hand during the jelq exercise he does it less intensely than before.

Sometimes as a result of the jelq exercise a small hard lump or coagulated blood occurs. In this situation continued jelqing can aggravate the problem dramatically. A break of at least 3 days is essential. With intense or long jelq exercise sessions, fluid is pushed towards the end of the shaft where it collects. In circumcised men this can result in a large swelling around the circumference of the penis near the glans and in minor pain. The swelling is temporary and will subside within a few hours.

For uncircumcised men the equivalent is swelling of the foreskin which will subside within a few hours also.

Sometimes the discoloration on the penis that resulted from the jelq exercises will fade very slowly. Sometimes even after halting the jelq exercises for a period of months the discoloration on the penis will remain. Sometimes even after halting the jelq exercises for a period of years the discoloration on the penis will remain. This is normal, and a man should not worry about it.

The jelq exercise can add up to 3 inches in length and girth to the man's penis. The fact that the jelq exercise forces more blood into the penis chambers not only enlarges the penis but will give the man rock hard erections during sex. The jelq exercise will also make the penis stronger and the man's sensations during sex more heightened. It will also lengthen the duration of the orgasms during sex and will make them more explosive. It will also improve the man's stamina during sex, making the erections last longer. These changes, as a result of the jelq exercise, are permanent.

The jelq exercise is like a regular exercise: it needs to be carried out on a daily basis. It also needs to be done for a period of time. It is common to achieve noticeable changes in the first month as a result of the jelq exercise. More pronounced results can be seen after several months. The jelq exercise is usually done for a time period of several months to a year. The man will usually cease to do the jelq exercise once he has attained the results he wants or once a year of continuous jelq exercising has elapsed, whichever comes first.

Supplements

Many natural male enhancement supplements are available to men. Men should look for a male enhancement supplement that has L-Arginine in it. The reason is because L-Arginine is the only scientifically tested ingredient that stimulates genital blood flow. L-Arginine is a natural amino acid which stimulates extra blood flow to the penis. It works naturally to increase blood flow to the penile chambers.

Results are much faster with a supplement that has L-Arginine in it than with jelq exercises. The reason is the pills work on the inside to stimulate blood flow, while jelq exercises stimulate blood flow from the outside of the penis, which takes longer. With a natural male enhancement supplement results appear within weeks. As a matter of fact, over the course of the first three months men notice a change in the penis size and sexual performance. The average increase in penis size that a man experiences as a result of the supplement is 1-3 inches in length and thickness. The man's erection becomes much stronger as a result of the supplement. These changes, as a result of the supplement, are permanent. They are permanent because over time the penis stretches as a result of more blood flow circulating through it.

Oils

Erection oils are applied to the penis to increase blood flow through the penis, thus providing a quick erection that is firmer and longer than usual. They are meant to be used prior to sex, and they offer immediate results that last as long as one hour before another application of oil is needed. Once another application of the oil is done to the penis, it provides a quick erection boost. Erection oils work because they usually contain ingredients which stimulate blood flow instantly. The most popular ingredient used in a large number of erection oils to stimulate blood flow through the penis is L-Arginine. The difference between erection oils and supplements is that the results of the oils are instantaneous but wear off within an hour, while the results of the supplements are over a couple of weeks but they are permanent.

Chapter 31

Multiple Orgasms for Men

Most people incorrectly believe that a man can only have a single orgasm, simultaneously with an ejaculation. They do not know that a man can have multiple orgasms. They are not aware that a man can have an orgasm without an ejaculation. Most important of all, they do not realize that a man can learn how to have multiple orgasms. They do not understand that a man can learn how to have an orgasm without an ejaculation.

Male multiple orgasms are when the male has more than one orgasm with the same erection and with no refractory period. In other words, the man experiences more than one orgasm without him losing his erection or getting soft. The multi-orgasmic male is a man who can have two or more orgasms in a row without resting. If a man has two or more orgasms in the same night, with a period of rest or breaks in between, that is not multiple orgasms. He is not multi-orgasmic. A multi-orgasmic man maintains his erection, even though he has the first orgasm, and continues making love from orgasm to orgasm. He can continue to a second, third, or even fourth orgasm without resting. A multi-orgasmic male, is usually capable of experiencing a non-ejaculatory orgasm. A non-ejaculatory orgasm is an orgasm without an ejaculation. As a matter of fact, in order for a man to experience multiple orgasms, he should be able to have a non-ejaculatory orgasm. A non-ejaculatory orgasm feels as good, if not better than a conventional orgasm.

History of Male Multiple Orgasms

Male multiple orgasms are nothing new. Eastern cultures have been aware of male multiple orgasms and non-ejaculatory orgasms for many years. Male multiple orgasms and non-ejaculatory orgasms were originally introduced in Chinese Taoist philosophy during the Chou Dynasty (770-222 B.C.). Those teachings were incorporated into Tantra, an Eastern sexual practice. It is not difficult to find references to multiple orgasms and non-ejaculatory orgasms in Tantric literature and Eastern historical literature.

In 1948, Alfred Kinsey's book, *Sexual Behavior in the Human Male*, was published. In the book, Kinsey clearly reported that several of the normal men he studied experienced the sensation of orgasm without ejaculation. He also noted that several of the normal men he studied experienced more than one climax with the same erection. Today, male multiple orgasms and non-ejaculatory orgasms are well-documented in professional publications. They are documented in numerous books and journal articles, available at most college libraries in the U.S.

The idea that a man can learn to have multiple orgasms or learn to have non-ejaculatory orgasms is not new. Teaching a man to have multiple orgasms or non-ejaculatory orgasms was originally introduced in Chinese Taoist philosophy during 770-222 B.C. These teachings were incorporated into Tantra. However, in the West most people thought that men were either born multi-orgasmic or were born not multi-orgasmic. It was not until the 1970s that experts came to the conclusion that male multiple orgasms and non-ejaculatory orgasms could actually be learned. This was good news to many people because that meant a man does not have to be lucky to be multi-orgasmic. It was good news that a man can acquire the ability to be multi-orgasmic, regardless of his age, experience, or talents.

Ejaculation Versus Orgasm

Many people incorrectly assume that orgasm and ejaculation must occur at the same time in the male body. Ejaculation and orgasm are two distinct functions. Ejaculation is the emission of semen out of the penis. Orgasm consists of involuntary contractions along the seminal duct system and the penis. Ejaculation produces the sensation of semen coming out of the penis, while orgasm produces an intense feeling of pleasure. A man can have an orgasm without ejaculating. Also, a man can ejaculate without having an orgasm. A man can experience many orgasms with the same erection, but as for ejaculation, a man usually can only ejaculate once with the same erection. Since orgasm and ejaculation are two distinct functions, a man's capacity to repeatedly reach orgasm is not limited by his capacity to ejaculate. This is one of the sexual secrets of the multi-orgasmic man.

The Ejaculation Process

It is important that a man has a full understanding of the ejaculation process in order for him to become multi-orgasmic. Ejaculation actually occurs in two phases. The first phase is called the emission phase and the second phase is called the expulsion phase. During the emission phase, the sperm move through the vas deferens as the prostate gland contracts at intervals of eight-tenths of a second. The semen then collects near the base of the penis, ready for expulsion. During the expulsion phase, the PC muscle (pubococcygeal muscle) starts to contract, forcing the semen up through the urethra and out of the penis. In other words, during the emission phase the penis is loaded, and during the expulsion phase the penis is fired. The entire ejaculation process takes about two seconds.

Why Men Usually Do Not Have Multiple Orgasms

A man usually only has one orgasm, and then his penis goes limp. Then he needs a resting period to get hard again and to experience a second orgasm. The reason the penis goes limp after the man has one orgasm is because the man's orgasm is accompanied with an ejaculation. When the ejaculation happens and the semen spurts out of the penis, the excess blood in the penis returns to the rest of the body. This excess blood is what makes the penis hard. If the man does not ejaculate, but has a non-ejaculatory orgasm, then the excess blood will remain in the penis and the penis will remain erect. Then the man could experience more than one orgasm with the same erection.

How a Man Can Have Multiple Orgasms

Remember in the Male Sexual Response Cycle chapter, I said that it is very rare that a man experiences more than one orgasm. The reason it is rare is because most people do not know it could be done. Also, most people if they know that it could be done do not know how to do it. I am going to tell you in this section how a man can train himself to have multiple orgasms. The first step for a man to have multiple orgasms is for him to know that multiple orgasms do not mean having repeated ejaculation. The man should know that orgasm and ejaculation do not have to happen at the same time. A man can have an orgasm without ejaculating. It is possible, but not easy, for a man to have contractions along the seminal duct system and the penis without ejaculation occurring. Disconnecting the orgasm reflex and the ejaculation reflex is the basis of male multiple orgasms. A man should be able to disconnect both reflexes, so that he experiences an orgasm without ejaculation happening. This type of orgasm is a non-ejaculatory orgasm. By the man experiencing a non-ejaculatory orgasm he is delaying ejaculation.

A man's capacity to experience an orgasm is usually not limited. However, his ability to experience ejaculation is limited. Usually a man can experience ejaculation once before it becomes necessary for him to rest. This resting period is known as the refractory period. During this period, a man cannot continue having intercourse. He has to wait until after this period is over with for him to continue having intercourse. Since the capacity to ejaculate is limited, if the man does not separate both reflexes, then the man's capacity to orgasm will be limited by his ability to ejaculate. However, if the man separates ejaculation and orgasm, a man's capacity to orgasm is not limited and he can experience multiple orgasms. He could delay ejaculation until the last orgasm.

Orgasm without ejaculation can be the result of a retrograde ejaculation. A retrograde ejaculation occurs when the valve between the bladder and urethra does not close, and the ejaculation is forced back toward the bladder rather than out of the urethra. A retrograde ejaculation is neither painful nor harmful, and it does not affect the pleasure of an orgasm. As a matter of fact, when a retrograde ejaculation happens, the orgasm might even be more pleasurable.

A retrograde ejaculation and a non-ejaculatory orgasm are the result of a strong PC (pubococcygeal) muscle. For most men, the contraction of the PC (pubococcygeal) muscle during sex is an involuntary process. It usually happens during the expulsion phase of the ejaculatory process. During the expulsion phase, the PC (pubococcygeal) muscle contracts, forcing the semen up through the urethra and out of the penis. However, if the man takes control of the PC (pubococcygeal) muscle, he can voluntarily delay or prevent ejaculation. A person can take control of the PC (pubococcygeal) muscle by squeezing his PC (pubococcygeal) muscle as hard as he can for ten seconds when he feels that ejaculation is going to happen. Usually, the man feels ejaculation is going to happen at the point of no return, which is also known as the point of ejaculatory inevitability. Therefore, at the point of no return, a man should squeeze his PC (pubococcygeal) muscle. Remember in the Male Sexual Response Cycle chapter, I said that at the point of ejaculatory inevitability the man has to ejaculate no matter what happens. Well, there is one exception to that fact, which is if the man squeezes his PC (pubococcygeal) muscle he does not have to experience ejaculation at this point. Instead, he will experience a non-ejaculatory orgasm.

During sex, when the man is about to ejaculate because he has reached the point of no return, he should squeeze the PC (pubococcygeal) muscle. The man should squeeze the PC (pubococcygeal) muscle as hard as he can for ten seconds. At the point of no return, the man feels that his ejaculation is inevitable, but in reality, he has plenty of time to stop it if he wants to. When the man squeezes his PC (pubococcygeal) muscle, he and the woman should stop stimulating the penis so that it is easier for him to contain himself. If they are having intercourse both people should remain still, but the penis should remain inside the vagina. A man and woman can agree on a signal, which the man gives to the woman so that she stops stimulating his penis because he is clenching his PC muscle. When the man squeezes the PC (pubococcygeal) muscle, he should experience a full orgasm including rapid heart rate, muscle contractions, and the incredible sensation of release without an ejaculation. The PC (pubococcygeal) muscle has stopped the ejaculation, while still allowing the body to go into orgasm. Then the man should feel the urge to ejaculate subside. The penis should remain erect.

After feeling the orgasm and feeling the urge to ejaculate subside, stimulation of the penis should resume. However, it should resume extremely slowly, accompanied by slow breathing from the man. Once the man is in control of his breathing again, then the speed of the stimulation of the penis can increase, but still remain slow. If the man is having intercourse, the speed of thrusting can increase but still remain slow. A person repeats this process several times, so that he experiences multiple orgasms. Clenching the PC (pubococcygeal) muscle allows the man to maintain his erection and experience multiple orgasms with the same erection and with no refractory period. When the man wants to stop making love, he has a final orgasm, but this time without squeezing the PC (pubococcygeal) muscle and he ejaculates.

A multi-orgasmic man can delay his ejaculation until he and his partner are ready to stop having sex. If they want to have intercourse for a long time, then he simply delays his ejaculation for a long time. If they want to have intercourse for a short time, then he simply delays his ejaculation for a short time. The important thing is that the length of the sexual encounter is their decision. It is not imposed upon them by circumstances. Usually, a multi-orgasmic man can delay his ejaculation until the woman climaxes, so that they both climax simultaneously.

Squeezing the PC (pubococcygeal) muscle at the point of no return is easier said than done. Some men are naturals and can prevent themselves from ejaculating by squeezing the PC muscle at the point of no return without any ejaculatory control training. However, many men try to prevent themselves from ejaculating by squeezing the PC (pubococcygeal) muscle at the point of no return, but their timing is off and they end up ejaculating. They need to learn ejaculatory control in order to prevent themselves from ejaculating using the PC muscle. In order for a man to learn ejaculatory control, there are three techniques that he could use. He can use either one of the three, or all three.

The first technique is called the squeeze technique. In the squeeze technique, the man simply masturbates to the point he is about to ejaculate and then stops. He squeezes the tip of the penis tightly just before ejaculation, with the thumb underneath and the next two fingers on top. He usually squeezes the tip of the penis, for a short time. Usually, the time period is 10 to 30 seconds. He squeezes the tip of the penis, until the urge to ejaculate subsides. While squeezing the tip of the penis, he should begin to have the experience of reaching orgasm without ejaculating. Then, after the urge to ejaculate subsides, the man should start to masturbate again. He should bring himself to the brink of ejaculation and stop the ejaculation using the squeeze technique three or four times before letting go and experiencing an ejaculation. A man can do this technique with the woman by having her stimulate his penis until he is about to ejaculate. Then she could squeeze the tip of the penis tightly, just before ejaculation, with the thumb underneath and the next two fingers on top. This technique is effective, because it helps the man's body learn to gain control over the ejaculation process. It enables the man to control, whether he ejaculates or not.

A second ejaculatory control technique that is effective is called the stop-start technique. This technique also helps the man's body learn to gain control over the ejaculation process. In the stop-start technique, the man masturbates to the point he is about to ejaculate and then stops masturbating. He waits until the urge to ejaculate subsides, then he resumes masturbating. He does that three or four times, before letting go and experiencing an ejaculation.

A third ejaculatory control technique that is effective is called the testicle pull down technique. This technique also enables the man's body to learn to control the ejaculation process. Before ejaculation, the man's testicles usually rise up very close to the body. If the testes do not undergo at least a partial elevation, the human male will not ejaculate. So a man can pull down his testicles either by holding them between his legs or by gently tugging them down with one hand, just when he feels he is about to ejaculate in order to prevent an ejaculation. In the testicle pull down technique, the man masturbates to the point he is about to ejaculate and then he stops masturbating. Then he pulls down his testicles by gently tugging them down with one hand. He keeps them pulled down until the urge to ejaculate subsides. If the man pulls down his testicles then he won't ejaculate, but will delay the ejaculation. After the urge to ejaculate subsides, he could continue masturbating. Then when the urge to ejaculate comes again, he stops masturbating and pulls down his testicles until the urge goes away. He does that three or four times before letting go and experiencing an ejaculation. Doing this will enable the man to learn to control the ejaculation process. A man could have a woman involved in this exercise by having her gently tug his testicles down with one hand instead of him using his hand to pull down his testicles.

If a man does any of these ejaculatory control techniques, it is a good idea that he does them regularly, three to five times a week, for several weeks. If he finds that he needs longer than several weeks, then he should go longer than several weeks. Most people find the squeeze technique to be the most effective ejaculatory control technique, while some do not. When a man is using any of the ejaculatory control techniques to train to become multi-orgasmic, the man may experience a number of new and unusual feelings before he has the first set of multiple orgasms. The man might feel he missed an orgasm. He might feel that he had a partial orgasm. He might feel that he had a partial ejaculation with the orgasm. He might feel that he had a partial ejaculation without an orgasm. All these feelings are normal. The man should not worry about any of them. In fact, these physiological experiences are clear signs that the man is on his way to have the first set of multiple orgasms. These are good signs and not bad signs.

Some men will become multi-orgasmic quickly within several weeks, while others will take a long time to become multi-orgasmic. The key to improvement is practice. Although most men can learn to become multi-orgasmic, it is important to note that some men will never become multi-orgasmic, no matter how hard they try. Those that become multi-orgasmic will retain that ability for the rest of their lives. Those that learn to become multi-orgasmic can get tremendous pleasure for themselves and their female partners. Their sexual experience will be much more intense, and it will be more intense for their female partner. Those that do not become multi-orgasmic, even after trying, the worst that can happen to them is nothing. Nothing happens to them, since there are not any harmful effects from trying to be multi-orgasmic.

Benefits of Male Multiple Orgasms

If a man can have multiple orgasms, it will be very beneficial to him and his woman. First, if the man is capable of climaxing more than once, it tends to make the woman less anxious during sex. The woman is less anxious during sex because she knows the man is going to keep climaxing until she has an orgasm, too. She is not worried that the man will climax and stop the sex before she has climaxed. The fact that the woman is less anxious during sex makes the sex more pleasurable. Second, if the man is capable of having multiple orgasms, he will enjoy the sexual act more because he is not under stress worried whether he will make the woman climax. He is not worried since he knows he can keeping going until the woman climaxes. Third, it is thrilling to the woman to know that the man that she is with can climax and still keep going. The woman is so excited by that fact that she actually reaches her climax much sooner than she and the man anticipated. Fourth, the fact that the man can have multiple orgasms means that the couple can experience a climax simultaneously. A simultaneous climax is very much desired by the couple. It is also extremely pleasurable to the couple.

Furthermore, touching is pleasant and oral sex is nice, but some women need more intercourse to feel satisfied. They desire long sessions of lovemaking. They desire their man to stay erect longer than he usually does, so that they climax from intercourse and not another way. Some women in their daydreams, when they think of the perfect sexual experience, imagine the man going on for hours thrusting. The fact that the man can experience multiple orgasms makes long sessions of lovemaking a reality and not just a dream. The fact that the man can have multiple orgasms means that the man's orgasm is not the end of the couple's lovemaking. Also, the fact that a man can experience multiple orgasms makes it possible for the man to orgasm without disturbing the couple's erotic connection. Male multiple orgasms allow the man to satisfy the woman's sexual needs. It results in a more relaxed atmosphere for both the man and the woman.

Male Multiple Orgasms Should Not Be a Demand

Some men will attempt to train themselves to orgasm without ejaculating. It is important to keep in mind that although for some men it will be easy and quick to become multi-orgasmic, for others it might take a long time. Some might never be able to become multi-orgasmic. Some might not be able to experience non-ejaculatory orgasms, but will experience a partial ejaculation with the orgasms. Every man's body is unique and will respond in a unique way when the man tries to train himself to have multiple orgasms. A man and his woman should accept whatever the man's ability in regards to multiple orgasms is. The woman should be helpful, never judge nor criticize the man in regards to his multi-orgasmic ability. The man's drive to become multi-orgasmic should not be a result of his woman's demand. Rather, it should come from within himself. Many women are satisfied if the man has only one orgasm. Most women are satisfied if the man has one orgasm and uses manual stimulation or oral stimulation to bring them to climax. Therefore, a man should not make it a demand on himself to become multi-orgasmic because most women are satisfied if the man is not multi-orgasmic. Also, both the man and the woman should keep in mind that orgasm should not be the goal of sex. Rather, a couple should enjoy the sexual pleasure during intercourse, whether the man or the woman orgasms. If the man or woman focuses only on orgasm, he or she will run the risk of rushing past the pleasure to be enjoyed along the way to orgasm. Also, the man or woman will run the risk of denying oneself the pleasure to be enjoyed along the way to orgasm if he or she focuses only on orgasm.

Chapter 32

Conclusion

When a man is deeply in love with a woman at the beginning of a relationship, both people usually do not talk much about their sexual knowledge or sexual experience. Rather, they hope and expect that the excitement and joy that they have with each other will carry over into their sexual relationship, making the sex very satisfying. However, without the proper sexual knowledge many couples find they have difficulty transferring their passion towards each other into their sexual encounters. This makes their sexual encounters not very pleasurable. This might even lead to the end of their relationship.

Many couples might not think there is anything to sex other than the man putting his penis inside the vagina and thrusting. They might think that sex is a mechanical act. They also might think that sex is from the time the man starts thrusting until the time the man orgasms, regardless whether the woman orgasms or not.

However, this should not be the case with the reader of this book. Whether the reader is a man or a woman, he or she should have all the proper knowledge to make his or her sexual encounters more pleasurable as a result of reading this book. After reading this book the reader should be aware of several things. He or she should be aware how to enjoy his or her body and his or her partner's body during sex. He or she should also be aware of the natural bodily responses during sex and not view them as abnormal. His or her expectations for the sexual encounters should be realistic and not unrealistic. He or she should realize that the man and the woman's genital size do not matter for wonderful sex. He or she should know how to keep the sex life exciting and alive in the relationship no matter how long the relationship lasts, by having variety in his or her sexual encounters. He or she should know about safer sex, and sexually transmitted diseases in order to protect himself or herself, and in order to give himself or herself peace of mind. This peace of mind will allow him or her to enjoy the sexual encounter.

After reading this book the reader should know that sex is not just a mechanical act. He or she should know that although, physically, the sexual response is the same in all men and the same in all women, what might be pleasing to a person during sex might be different from one person to another, from one sexual encounter to another, and from one minute to another.

After reading this book the reader should know how a man can get the woman to orgasm at the same time that he orgasms during sex. However, the reader of the book should most importantly know that a person having a nubile body and doing acrobatics during sex is not the secret to great sex. He or she should also know that orgasming during sex is not the secret to great sex. He or she should know the secret to great sex is sharing love, affection, and romance with his or her partner. The intimacy, emotional closeness, caring, and love that the couple shares during sex are fulfilling in their own right. As a matter of fact, they are more fulfilling than an orgasm.

Sexual fulfillment is a person's right. A person should never be embarrassed or ashamed by the fact that he or she is a sexual being. A person should understand his or her sexuality. If a person has an amazing sex life, this can lead to a more committed happy relationship and can make both people feel compatible. The man or woman's capability as a lover depends on the sexual knowledge he or she knows and puts to use. This book has provided the reader with more than enough sexual knowledge for him or her to put to use to make himself or herself a great lover.

Everyone creates his or her own individual sexuality. Everyone is unique sexually, and sex is only his or her own unique sexual expression. Although there is an abundance of techniques for a person to use after reading this book, a person will usually pick some techniques, and others he or she will not care for. However, the more sex techniques and variations he or she knows, practices, and masters during sex, the more fantastic his or her sex life will be. As a person becomes a better lover he or she will develop greater self-confidence in bed. Sex is a person's physical expression of love to his or her partner, and this book provides the reader with the proper knowledge to physically express his or her love towards his or her partner in an exciting and pleasurable way.

Bibliography

This book was based on the research work of Shere Hite, Alfred Kinsey, Masters and Johnson, and other sources. Some of the sources used are listed in this section.

Angier, Natalie. *Women: An Intimate Geography.* New York: Anchor Books, 2000.

Barbach, L. *For Yourself: The Fulfillment of Female Sexuality.* New York: Anchor Books, 2000.

Berman, Jennifer. *For Women Only: A Revolutionary Guide to Overcoming Sexual Dysfunction and Reclaiming Your Sex Life.* New York: Henry Holt and Co., 2001.

Block, Joel. *The Secrets of Better Sex.* New York: Parker Publishing Co., 1996.

Brauer, A. *ESO (extended sexual orgasm).* New York: Warner Books, 1983.

Cane, William. *The Art of Kissing.* New York: St. Martin's Press, 1995.

Chalker, Rebecca. *The Clitoral Truth.* New York: Seven Stories Press, 2000.

Chichester, Brian. *Sex Secrets.* Pennsylvania: Rodale Press, 1996.

Crenshaw, Theresa. *The Alchemy of Love and Lust: How Our Sex Hormones Influence Our Relationships.* New York: Simon & Schuster, 1997.

Fisher, S. *The Female Orgasm*. New York: Basic Books, 1973.

Friday, Nancy. *Women On Top: How Real Life has Changed Women's Sexual Fantasies*. New York: Pocket Books, 1991.

Hart, Archibald. *The Sexual Man*. Texas: Word Publishing, 1995.

Hartman, W. *Any Man Can*. New York: St. Martin's Press, 1984.

Heiman, J. *Becoming Orgasmic: A Sexual Growth Program for Women*. New Jersey: Prentice-Hall, 1976.

Hite, Shere. *The Hite Report on Female Sexuality*. New York: Macmillan, 1976.

Hite, Shere. *The Hite Report on Male Sexuality*. New York: Ballantine Books, 1981.

Inkeles, Gordon. *The New Sensual Massage*. California: Arcata Arts, 1992.

Kennedy, A. *Touching For Pleasure - A Guide to Sensual Enhancement*. CA: Chatsworth Press, 1986.

King, Bruce. *Human Sexuality Today*. New Jersey: Prentice-Hall, 1999.

Kinsey, Alfred. *Sexual Behavior in the Human Female*. Philadelphia: Saunders, 1953.

Kinsey Institute. *The Kinsey Institute New Report on Sex*. New York: St. Martin's Press, 1990.

Lavinthal, Andrea. *The Hookup Handbook: A Single Girl's Guide to Living it Up*. New York: Simon Spotlight Entertainment, 2005.

Leiblum, Sandra. *Principles and Practice of Sex Therapy*. New York: Guilford Press, 2000.

Love, Brenda. *Encyclopedia of Unusual Sex Practices*. New York: Barricade Books, 1992.

Maines, Rachel. *The Technology of Orgasm: "Hysteria," the Vibrator, and Women's Sexual Satisfaction*. Baltimore: The John Hopkins University Press, 1999.

Massey, Doreen. *The Lover's Guide Encyclopedia*. New York: Thunder's Mouth Press, 1996.

Masters, William. *Human Sexual Response*. Boston: Little, Brown & Company, 1966.

Montagu, A. *Touching: The Human Significance of the Skin*. New York: Harper &Row, 1986.

Mumford, Susan. *Healing Massage*. New York: Plume, 1998.

Sherman, Alexa. *The Happy Hook-Up: A Single Girl's Guide to Casual Sex*. California: Ten Speed Press, 2004.

Stanway, Andrew. *The Joy of Sexual Fantasy*. New York: Carroll and Graf, 1991.

Taylor, Emma. *The Big Bang: Nerve's Guide to the New Sexual Universe*. New York: Plume, 2003.

Tiger, L. *The Pursuit of Pleasure*. Boston: Little, Brown & Company, 1992.

White, James. *The Best Sex of Your Life*. New York: Barricade Books, 1996.

Zilbergeld, Bernie. *The New Male Sexuality*. New York: Bantam Books, 1999.

Index

69 position 98, 99, 299

abstinence 352

affection 8, 114, 127

after sex play 187, 209–214

AIDS (see also "HIV") 92, 99, 108, 370, 371

alcohol 114, 132, 156, 297, 298, 334, 369

anal sex 2, 103–111, 299, 353–356, 366–370

anus 13, 37, 49, 50–52, 65, 72, 78, 87, 91, 97, 103–111, 151, 224, 259, 279, 281, 295, 296, 356, 365–368

arousal 6, 12, 16, 24–26, 29, 30–32, 38, 40, 52, 54, 60, 63, 66, 72, 78, 97, 117, 127, 130, 136, 137, 151, 158, 200, 210, 211, 220, 222, 223, 225–227, 232, 233, 242, 243, 247–250, 252, 254, 255, 261, 264, 265, 267, 288, 289, 294, 296, 299, 309, 317, 319–322, 378, 381–383, 386, 391

bathroom sex 270

beach sex 270, 271

Ben Wa balls 296

blindfold 154, 225, 291, 292

blue balls 27, 260, 261

breaks during sex 82, 217, 252, 254–256, 278, 281–283, 292, 295, 409

breasts 146, 147, 156, 348, 370, 394

breathing during sex 25, 33, 60, 66, 72, 78, 88, 90, 241, 242, 258, 316

butt plug 296

car sex 270, 271

casual sex 330

cervix 14, 17–19, 30, 31, 43, 46, 64, 65, 76–78, 137, 168, 169, 192, 252, 253, 312, 368, 387, 390, 394

chlamydia 363, 364

clitoris 14–17, 30, 32–34, 43, 45, 54, 56, 61–65, 67, 73–75, 77–79, 82, 84, 93–97, 109, 110, 152, 166, 168, 170–177, 179, 180, 182–186, 188–195, 198–204, 223, 225,

228, 246, 248, 254, 258–264, 279, 283, 286, 288, 294–297, 299, 300, 303–317, 319, 323, 337, 341–343, 377, 378, 396
cock ring 295
communication 98, 108, 158, 237, 307, 336, 337, 349, 362, 379, 383
condom 50, 51, 100, 101, 105, 108, 109, 219, 296, 300, 352–360, 390, 397
confidence 1, 3, 6, 121, 216, 229 298, 337, 375, 385, 418
Cowper's gland 9, 11, 14
crabs 364
cunnilingus 84, 93, 95, 97–100, 353, 354, 357, 360, 395, 397

dental dam 100, 111, 353, 354, 357, 360
desire 7, 30, 40, 84, 113, 116, 136–138, 140, 156, 159, 201, 220, 221, 228, 237, 244, 267, 269, 275, 319, 328, 329, 332–334, 375, 379, 389, 391, 394, 398, 401, 415
dildo 295, 296
dirty talk 237
doggy style (see also "rear entry sex") 192, 259, 315, 344, 396
dressing for sex 121, 122
duration of sex (see also "lasting longer during sex") 216–217

edibles 101, 277, 278, 296
ejaculation 1, 11, 12, 24–26, 38, 40–44, 47–49, 56, 61, 72, 92, 164–166, 188, 200, 201, 210, 211, 244–246, 260, 261, 289, 318, 347, 356, 364, 373–386, 409, 410–414, 416
enlarging the penis 403–408
enthusiasm 226, 229

epididymis 9, 10, 13, 366
erection 12, 13, 16, 24–27, 43, 49, 52, 82, 84, 88, 92, 136–138, 158, 200, 203, 210–212, 217, 219, 225–228, 242, 244, 246, 249, 259, 260, 262, 264–266, 287, 290, 294, 295, 297, 298, 303, 317, 321, 331, 332, 334, 335, 343, 347, 348, 355, 374, 378, 382, 383, 403–405, 407–411, 413
erogenous zone 49, 63, 142, 144, 145, 149, 153, 154, 279, 282, 313

faking an orgasm 306, 347–350
falling asleep after sex 7, 8, 210, 212, 306
fallopian tubes 14, 19, 20, 363, 364, 366
feathers 154, 280, 292
fellatio 84, 86–93, 99, 100, 101, 353, 354, 358, 359, 395
female condom 356, 357
female superior position (see also "woman on top position") 197, 198, 201, 205
fetishes 121, 275, 276
finger sucking 149, 283
food during sex 100, 101, 155, 156, 212, 278
foreplay 2, 24, 25, 31, 81, 82, 83, 85, 107, 113–117, 127, 128, 131, 134, 135–159, 163, 210, 211, 216, 217, 222, 227, 274, 321, 322, 355, 391, 399
foreskin 12, 355, 367, 407
fragrances 125, 273
French kissing 129, 130, 131, 239, 284, 370
frenulum 12, 59, 60, 71, 88, 89, 153, 223, 245, 383, 384

INDEX

frequency of sex 216, 274
full body orgasm 52, 65, 78, 170, 175, 193, 194, 204, 257, 258, 259, 260
furs 154, 280

genital warts 357, 368, 369
glans 12, 13, 16, 24, 25, 30, 88, 96, 110, 152, 223, 365, 405, 406
gonorrhea 357, 364, 366
G-spot 2, 43, 44–49, 54, 64, 65, 76–78, 96, 98, 103, 105, 110, 166–168, 170, 171, 175, 183, 188, 190, 192, 195, 198, 203, 207, 243, 246, 253, 258–260, 294, 298, 304, 312–315

healthy food 156
hepatitis 111, 133, 369
herpes 99, 100, 101, 133, 353, 354, 357, 363, 367, 368, 370
HIV (see also "AIDS") 92, 99, 100, 101, 108, 352, 354, 356, 370, 371, 370, 371, 389, 390
home 218
hotel 157, 270, 271
human papillomavirus (HPV) 353, 357, 368, 369

initiating sex 136, 142, 220, 221
intimacy 5, 6, 93, 116, 130, 134, 136, 137, 139, 155, 159, 162, 164, 171, 182, 183, 192, 195, 199, 200, 206, 212–214, 216, 230, 234–236, 266, 267, 269, 278, 329, 330, 335, 338, 339, 349, 350, 351, 358, 383, 395, 418

Kegel exercise 38–42, 48, 399
kissing 2, 86, 87, 95, 127–134, 136, 137, 146, 154, 155, 164, 211, 217, 220, 222–224, 230, 235, 238, 239, 242, 247, 249–252, 255, 267, 282–284, 287, 322, 329, 335, 343, 368, 370, 395, 398, 399, 419

labia majora 14, 15, 16, 30–32, 61–63, 73, 76, 95, 166, 224, 228, 254, 279
labia minora 14–16, 30, 31, 32, 61–63, 73, 75, 76, 95, 166, 224, 228, 254, 279, 281, 304
lasting longer during sex 56, 164, 200, 201, 240, 242–247, 358, 374, 378, 379, 384, 385, 407
length of penis 16, 341, 342, 344, 345, 403, 405, 407
letting go during sex 231, 320
lingerie 121, 122, 219, 275
locations for sex 157, 269–272
love 5, 6, 31, 37, 42, 57, 81, 84, 103, 114, 116, 124, 127, 130, 132–134, 139–142, 146, 148, 155–157, 162–164, 169, 174, 187, 192, 195, 198, 210, 212, 216, 219, 221, 224, 225, 228–230, 235, 236, 238, 250, 252, 266, 269, 270, 271, 273, 278, 280, 282, 288, 289, 307, 309, 322, 323, 325, 327–333, 336, 395, 400, 409, 413, 417, 418–420
lubricant 18, 59, 61, 67, 70, 73, 79, 88, 89, 100, 107, 109, 138, 271, 297, 299, 308, 316, 355–357, 359, 384, 404, 405

making circumstances right for sex 217
man on top position (see also "missionary position") 163
manual stimulation 2, 52, 69, 70–80, 180, 188, 263, 295, 298, 299, 305, 308–311, 314, 316, 318, 416

marriage 3, 6
married 6, 8, 57, 58, 122, 141, 361, 367
massage 41, 50, 51, 63, 75, 76, 89, 91, 98, 107, 109, 110, 141, 142, 144, 147, 150, 152, 153, 155, 183, 188, 190, 197, 206, 224, 225, 262, 276, 277, 281, 289, 353, 380, 381, 384, 394, 395, 398, 404, 420, 421
massage oil (see also "oils") 153, 276, 277
masturbation 1, 2, 8, 16, 55–67, 69, 80, 147, 280, 305–307, 309, 310, 350, 353, 378, 381, 383, 384, 388, 394, 395, 398
menstruation 19–21, 387–391
mirror 273
missionary position (see also "man on top position") 163, 165–168, 170, 171, 178, 200, 201, 243, 259, 284, 285, 293, 294, 311, 315, 344, 345, 378, 393, 396
monogamy 330, 339
mons veneris 14
multiple orgasms 2, 27, 33, 34, 38, 41, 42, 66, 198, 200, 263, 288, 294, 295, 298, 315–317, 347, 394, 395, 409–416
music 139, 140, 272, 273
mutual masturbation 80, 353, 394, 395, 398

nipple(s) 24, 31, 65, 78, 86, 91, 124, 131, 141, 146–148, 179, 198, 223, 224, 279, 280, 281, 283, 296, 348, 359
oils 14, 273, 355, 404, 408
oral sex 2, 52, 81–101, 209, 217, 255, 264, 295, 298, 299, 316, 318, 353, 354, 361, 364, 367–370, 390, 394, 395, 398, 415
orgasm 1, 2, 6, 7, 8, 12, 16, 19, 20, 23, 25–27, 29, 31–35, 37, 38, 40–44, 47, 49, 51–57, 60–66, 72, 74, 76, 78–82, 84, 88, 90–98, 110, 135–139, 142, 146, 148, 150–153, 158, 161, 163, 164, 166, 167, 170–172, 174, 175, 183, 187, 188, 192–194, 197–204, 207, 209–213, 217, 222–224, 227–234, 236–266, 281, 283–290, 293–300, 303–310, 312–323, 331–335, 342, 343, 347–350, 377, 378, 389, 393–395, 398, 409–416, 418–420
outdoor sex 271
ovaries 14, 20, 21, 54, 137, 364, 366
ovulation 19, 21, 169

passion 114, 115, 117, 130, 131, 134, 155, 159, 171, 174, 198, 216, 222, 234, 266, 267, 269, 329, 331, 334, 358, 375, 417
penis 2, 9, 11–13, 16–18, 23–26, 30, 31, 37–43, 49–52, 54, 55, 57, 59, 60, 70–72, 82, 84, 86–93, 95, 96, 103–111, 137, 138, 152, 153, 156, 163, 165, 166–176, 178, 180, 182, 183, 185, 186, 188–190, 192, 194, 195, 197–208, 210–212, 215, 217–219, 222, 223, 225, 227, 228, 235, 236, 240, 241, 243–246, 249–254, 256–262, 264, 266, 271, 278, 279, 281, 283, 285–291, 293–300, 303–306, 308, 311–315, 317–319, 322, 323, 328, 341–345, 349, 355–358, 364–368, 373, 377–385, 393, 395, 399, 403, 404–408, 410–413, 417
penis extension 296
penis length 344
perineum 15, 41, 49–52, 59, 70, 87, 91, 95, 151, 224, 258–260, 279, 281, 288, 397

plateau 23–25, 29–32
positions 2, 86, 93, 94, 98, 106, 161–164, 172, 173, 178, 180, 187, 188, 190–192, 197, 201, 234, 240, 241, 248, 250, 259, 260, 268, 284, 285, 291, 313, 314, 395, 396, 399, 400
positive body image 326, 327
pregnancy 19, 21, 66, 67, 79, 80, 82, 103, 111, 147, 164, 338, 352–356, 358, 370, 387, 391, 393–399, 401
premature ejaculation 40, 164, 188, 201, 373–382, 385, 386
premenstrual syndrome (PMS) 387–389
prostate 2, 9–11, 13, 14, 25, 40, 42, 43, 48–54, 257–260, 279, 294, 298, 366, 411
P-spot 49, 50, 52, 53, 54
pubococcygeal (PC) muscles 37–42, 44, 60, 66, 72, 78, 193, 197, 245, 288–290, 342, 381, 404, 406, 411–413

quickie 174, 178, 274

rear entry sex (see also "doggy style") 106, 161, 183, 192, 193, 195, 196, 315
rectum 17, 20, 49, 50, 51, 103, 104, 105, 107–111, 151, 259, 260, 294, 296
refractory period 2, 27, 33, 40, 210, 217, 247, 260, 263, 264, 298, 303, 315–317, 409, 411, 413
rejecting sex 219
relationship 2, 3, 5, 6, 8, 57, 58, 85, 113, 116, 119, 127, 128, 132, 133, 143, 220, 221, 228, 234, 236, 237, 239, 249, 266–269, 271, 290, 291, 306, 325–333, 335–339, 349, 350, 352, 353, 365, 368, 376, 383, 391, 397, 398, 417, 418
resolution 23, 26, 29, 34, 35, 210
rhythm 51, 60, 63, 66, 71, 72, 76, 78, 89, 91, 107, 139, 140, 144, 165, 180, 246, 249, 252, 255, 259, 272, 281, 307, 309, 313, 322
ribbed condom 359
romance 116, 117, 137, 140, 235, 236, 257, 328, 329, 418

sadomasochism 293
safer sex 2, 99, 351–360, 362, 363, 371, 390, 397, 418
scrotum 9, 10, 13, 24, 25, 50, 51, 52, 59, 70, 87, 91, 151, 199, 206, 258, 261, 279, 295, 368, 380, 383
semen 1, 9, 11–14, 18, 19, 26, 40, 44, 49, 84, 92, 93, 100, 101, 108, 164, 354–356, 361, 369, 370, 410–412
seminal vesicles 9, 11, 13, 14, 40, 366
serial monogamy 339
setting the mood 113–117, 136, 139, 148, 151, 221, 234, 264, 272, 392
sex toys 294, 353, 359
sexual response cycle 23–26, 29–32, 34, 210, 411, 412
sexual revolution 1
sexually transmitted diseases (STDs) 351, 352, 353, 354, 355, 356, 361, 362, 363, 364
showering with partner 224, 380, 395, 398
side-by-side position 110, 187–189, 259, 260, 314, 379, 396
simultaneous orgasm 249, 320
sitting position 176, 178, 180, 182, 183, 185, 197, 204–208, 396, 405

spanking 292
speed during sex 247, 286–288
sperm 9–14, 18–21, 25, 31, 40, 44, 49, 92, 300, 356, 390, 393, 397, 411
squeeze technique 383, 413, 414
standing position 173–175, 196
stimulating the whole body 240
stop-start technique 383, 414
stress 7, 8, 48, 56, 97, 140, 142, 143, 150, 219, 220, 231, 241, 264, 319, 332, 333, 365, 368, 388, 391, 415
stripping 140, 141
syphilis 353, 354, 357, 366, 370

talking dirty 116, 224, 237
talking seductively 224
testicles 10, 13, 24–26, 49, 54, 59, 70, 87, 152, 199, 206, 223, 225, 252, 261, 279, 281, 283, 318, 364, 383, 404, 414
thrusting 30, 59, 71, 91, 105, 110, 164–166, 169–172, 175, 180–183, 185, 192, 193, 197, 198, 200, 201, 203, 206, 217, 218, 235, 236, 238, 240, 241, 243–247, 249–254, 256, 264, 267, 268, 281, 285–287, 289, 291, 293, 294, 298, 303–305, 309, 311–315, 317, 318, 322, 328, 345, 365, 377, 378, 380–382, 385, 413, 415, 417
toe sucking 224, 283–284
tongue 81, 82, 84, 87–90, 94–98, 111, 128–131, 145, 146, 148, 154, 222, 223, 239, 240, 279, 281, 283, 308
touching 43, 45, 59, 63, 64, 70, 73, 75–77, 80, 100, 106, 111, 114, 115, 127, 129, 135–137, 142–147, 149–154, 164, 174, 179, 182, 190, 204, 205, 217, 220–224, 230, 232, 234, 235, 238, 247, 249–256, 267, 269, 277–280, 282, 285, 287, 308–310, 314, 317, 322, 323, 329, 330, 335, 357, 370, 379, 380, 400, 415, 420, 421

underwear 121, 123, 140, 141, 162, 275, 343
urethra 9–13, 15–17, 26, 37, 44, 54, 56, 65, 77, 212, 363–365, 411, 412
uterus 14, 17–21, 30–32, 34, 41, 54, 99, 137, 192, 257, 364, 366, 387, 393, 397, 398

vacation sex 271, 272
vagina 7, 12, 14–20, 25, 30–32, 37–39, 41–46, 49, 54, 56, 59, 62–67, 71, 74–79, 84, 92–97, 99, 103–105, 107–110, 137, 138, 147, 156, 164–170, 172–178, 180, 182, 183, 185, 186, 189, 190, 192–194, 197, 198, 200, 202–208, 215, 217–219, 222, 223, 225, 227, 228, 235, 236, 240, 241, 243–246, 248–254, 256–260, 262, 266, 278, 279, 283, 285, 286, 288–291, 293–300, 303–305, 308, 309, 311–315, 317, 318, 322, 323, 328, 341–345, 356, 357, 364, 365, 367, 368, 373, 377–379, 381, 382, 384, 385, 387, 390, 391, 395, 397, 399, 400, 412, 417
vaginal lubrication 30, 41, 138, 158, 227
vas deferens 9, 10, 11, 13, 40, 411
vibrator(s) 65–67, 78, 79, 209, 294, 295, 308
vulva 14–16, 30, 34, 67, 84, 100, 151, 166, 225, 262, 300, 357, 365, 366, 387, 388, 395

woman on top position (see also "female superior position") 178, 188, 197–206, 243, 260, 262, 285, 293, 294, 310, 311, 314, 344, 345, 378, 396, 400

www.ingramcontent.com/pod-product-compliance
Lightning Source LLC
Chambersburg PA
CBHW030238170426
43202CB00007B/38